ALZHEIMER'S DISEASE
AMYLOID PRECURSOR PROTEINS, SIGNAL TRANSDUCTION, AND NEURONAL TRANSPLANTATION

ALZHEIMER'S DISEASE
AMYLOID PRECURSOR PROTEINS, SIGNAL TRANSDUCTION, AND NEURONAL TRANSPLANTATION

Edited by Roger M. Nitsch, John H. Growdon, Suzanne Corkin, and Richard J. Wurtman

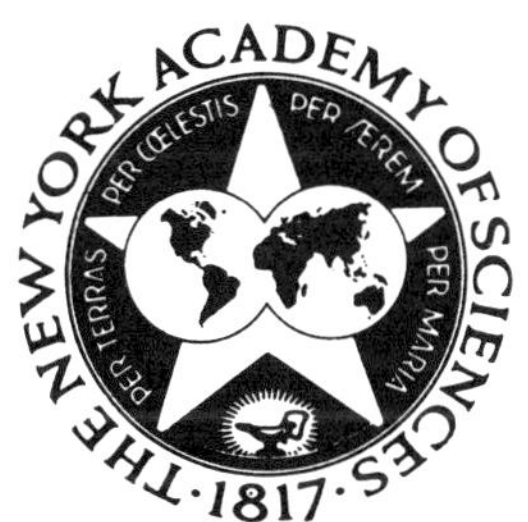

The New York Academy of Sciences
New York, New York
1993

Library of Congress Cataloging-in-Publication Data

Alzheimer's disease : amyloid precursor proteins, signal transduction, and neuronal transplantation / edited by Roger M. Nitsch . . . [et al.].
p.   cm. — (Annals of the New York Academy of Sciences, ISSN 0077-8923 ; v. 695)
Papers presented at the Seventh Meeting of the International Study Group on the Pharmacology of Memory Disorders Associated with Aging, held in Zurich, Switzerland on Feb. 12–14, 1993; organized by the Center for Brain Sciences and Metabolism Charitable Trust.
Includes bibliographical references and index.
ISBN 0-89766-853-7 (cloth : alk. paper). — ISBN 0-89766-854-5 (pbk. : alk. paper)
1. Alzheimer's disease—Pathogenesis—Congresses.   2. Alzheimer's disease—Pathophysiology—Congresses.   3. Alzheimer's disease—Molecular aspects—Congresses.   4. Amyloid beta-protein precursor—Metabolism—Congresses.   5. Alzheimer's disease—Treatment—Congresses.   I. Nitsch, Roger M.   II. International Study Group on the Pharmacology of Memory Disorders Associated with Aging. Meeting (7th : 1993 : Zurich, Switzerland)   III. Center for Brain Sciences and Metabolism Charitable Trust.   IV. Series.
[DNLM: 1. Alzheimer's Disease—metabolism—congresses. 2. Alzheimer's Disease—therapy—congresses.   3. Neural Transmission—in old age—congresses.   4. Signal Transduction—in old age—congresses.   5. Amyloid beta-Protein Precursor—physiology—congresses.   6. Nerve Tissue—transplantation—congresses.   W1 AN626YL v. 695 1993 / WM 220 A477816 1993]
Q11.N5 vol. 695
[RC523]
500 s—dc20
[616.8′31]
DNLM/DLC
for Library of Congress   93-26827
                                                                                          CIP

MC/PCP
Printed in the United States of America
ISBN 0-89766-853-7 (cloth)
ISBN 0-89766-854-5 (paper)
ISSN 0077-8923

Volume 695
September 24, 1993

ALZHEIMER'S DISEASE
AMYLOID PRECURSOR PROTEINS, SIGNAL TRANSDUCTION, AND NEURONAL TRANSPLANTATION[a]

Editors and Conference Organizers
ROGER M. NITSCH, JOHN H. GROWDON, SUZANNE CORKIN,
AND RICHARD J. WURTMAN

CONTENTS

[a] This volume comprises the proceedings of the seventh meeting of the International Study Group on the Pharmacology of Memory Disorders Associated with Aging, organized by the Center for Brain Sciences and Metabolism Charitable Trust, Cambridge Massachusetts. The meeting, entitled **Alzheimer's Disease: Amyloid Precursor Proteins, Signal Transduction, and Neuronal Transplantation,** was held on February 12–14, 1993 in Zürich, Switzerland.

Part III. Animal Models

*Financial aid was received from the following charitable institutions and
companies:*

- Alzheimer's Association
- The Helen Bader Foundation, Inc.
- The French Foundation
- The John D. and Catherine T. MacArthur Foundation

- Batelle Europe
- Boehringer-Mannheim
- California Clinical Trials Medical Group
- Central Soya Company, Inc.
- The Coca Cola Company
- Ferrer International

Preface

This volume contains the papers and poster abstracts compiled for the seventh meeting of the International Study Group on the Pharmacology of Memory Disorders Associated with Aging (ISG), that took place in Zürich, Switzerland, on February 12–14, 1993. The ISG was founded 14 years ago in the belief that the development of effective treatments for Alzheimer's disease (AD) and other dementias would be accelerated by periodic meetings of scientists and physicians from around the world who are actively working on issues related to dementia. There have been six previous "Zürich Meetings"—in 1979, 1981, 1984, 1987, 1989, and 1991. The proceedings of the second ISB meeting were published by Raven Press in 1982 (*Alzheimer's Disease: A Report of Progress in Research;* Corkin, Davis, Growdon, Usdin, and Wurtman, editors); the proceedings of the fourth ISG meeting were published by Springer-Verlag in 1988 as Supplement 24 of the *Journal of Neural Transmission* (*Topics in the Basic and Clinical Science of Dementia;* Wurtman, Corkin, and Growdon, editors); the proceedings of the fifth ISB meeting were published by Raven Press in 1990 (*Alzheimer's Disease, Advances in Neurology,* Volume 51; Wurtman, Corkin, Growdon, and Ritter-Walker, editors); and the proceedings of the sixth ISG meeting were published by the New York Academy of Sciences in 1992 (*Aging and Alzheimer's Disease,* Volume 640; Growdon, Corkin, Ritter-Walker, and Wurtman, editors).

The overall goal of the ISG meetings is to highlight discoveries that shed light on the potential causes of AD, its pathogenesis, and the biological mechanisms that might underlie its cure. This seventh meeting of the ISG considered three major topics:

> Principles of neural transmission in aging and dementia
> The amyloid precursor proteins
> Transplantation of neural tissues

The first session reviewed principles of first messengers and signal transduction pathways in synaptic transmission. Speakers in this section described changes in these mechanisms that occur with aging and AD. The second session concerned amyloid and its precursors. Here, speakers addressed the metabolism and function of precursor proteins (APP and others) in experimental systems and in AD. The role of tau was also discussed. The third session examined recent progress in attempting to use transplantation of neural tissue and various cell types to treat neurodegenerative diseases. Speakers discussed the range of cell types employed in transplantation experiments. Presentations on animal models and approaches to the pharmacology of Alzheimer's disease were also discussed.

The ISG fosters interactions among academic scientists, scientists in industry, clinical investigators, and administrators in public and private agencies concerned with dementia. The seventh ISG meeting continued in the tradition of its predecessors by stimulating research in dementia and by speeding the transfer of information from the basic sciences to physicians caring for persons with dementia and to the pharmaceutical industry.

The organizing Committee wishes to thank Ms. Kit Emory and Ms. Emily Rossie for excellent editorial and administrative assistance in the preparation of this volume.

ROGER M. NITSCH
SUZANNE CORKIN
JOHN H. GROWDON
RICHARD J. WURTMAN

Principles of Synaptic Transmission[a]

ROBERT Y. MOORE[b]

*Departments of Psychiatry, Neurology and Behavioral Neuroscience,
Center for Neuroscience and Alzheimer's Disease Research Center,
University of Pittsburgh, Pittsburgh, Pennsylvania 15261, USA*

ABSTRACT: Neurons in the central nervous system communicate almost exclusively by the production and release at synapses of a series of molecules that are designated transmitters. Three such molecules make up the major transmitters, GABA, glutamate, and acetylcholine. GABA neurons are the principal inhibitory neurons and, as such, are the major local circuit neurons of the brain. They also are projection neurons in a number of systems. Glutamate neurons are excitatory projection neurons, particularly of the cerebral cortex, thalamus and retina. Acetylcholine neurons are excitatory neurons in ascending brainstem and basal forebrain systems and in cranial and spinal motor neurons and neurons of the sympathetic and parasympathetic systems. The catecholamines, dopamine and norepinephrine, are transmitters in several systems in brain. Dopamine is present in midbrain neurons projecting to the neostriatum, basal forebrain and cerebral cortex. It is also produced by hypothalamic neurons projecting to the median eminence and pituitary. These systems are highly topographically organized in contrast to the norepinephrine systems. The locus coeruleus norepinephrine system projects principally to thalamus, cerebral cortex and cerebellar cortex whereas the lateral tegmental system projects primarily to basal forebrain, hypothalamus, brainstem and spinal cord. The serotonin neurons of the brainstem raphe also project widely over the neuraxis, midbrain raphe neurons primarily to diencephalon and telencephalon and pontine medullary neurons to brainstem and spinal cord. There are smaller neuronal groups that produce glycine or histamine.

At the present time, it appears that most, if not all, CNS neurons produce one of these small molecule transmitters. In many instances, these molecules are colocalized with one or more peptides that appear to modify the postsynaptic action of the small molecule transmitter.

A BRIEF HISTORY OF SYNAPTIC TRANSMISSION

Synaptic transmission has been studied for nearly a century (TABLE 1). It began with the establishment of the neuron doctrine as the fundamental unifying concept of neurobiology by Cajal and Sherrington's introduction of

[a] Some of the work reported in this review was supported by NIH Grant NS-16304.
[b] *Send correspondence to:* Robert Y. Moore, Center for Neuroscience, BST W1656, University of Pittsburgh, Pittsburgh, PA 15261, USA; TEL: (412) 648–8322; FAX: (412) 648–8376.

1

TABLE 1. History of Synaptic Transmission

1890–1910	Establishment of the neuron doctrine
	Identification of putative neurotransmitters
1919–1950	Acetylcholine and norepinephrine identified as PNS transmitters
	Pharmacology develops
1950–1975	Catecholamines, serotonin, acetylcholine and GABA Identified as CNS transmitters
	Mechanisms of transmitter release and disposition identified
	Beginnings of chemical neuroanatomy
	Development of single unit electrophysiology
	Second messengers identified
1975–1990	Amino acids and peptides become prominent
	Immunocytochemistry brings the flowering of chemical neuroanatomy
	Receptors identified
	Second messengers proliferate
	Patch clamping analyzes channels
	Tropic factors proliferate
1990–	Molecular biology invades the nervous system—receptor families, multiple channel types, trophic factor families, immediate early genes

the term "synapse" to designate the sites of functional interaction between neurons and between neurons and effectors. This era also witnessed the identification of the first putative neurotransmitters, the catecholamines. It was followed by a very long period in which acetylcholine and norepinephrine were demonstrated to be peripheral neurotransmitters and a fundamental pharmacology was developed.

Between 1950 and 1975, the catecholamines, serotonin, acetylcholine and GABA were identified in the CNS with a nonuniform distribution and shown to be transmitters. Pharmacology developed substantially and the fundamental mechanisms for transmitter disposition and degradation were discovered. A rudimentary chemical neuroanatomy arose with the development of acetylcholinesterase histochemistry and the Falck-Hillarp method for cellular localization of monoamines. A particularly important example of the power of the new methods and concepts for the study of neurotransmission was the discovery that the primary pathology in Parkinson's disease involved the loss of a major dopaminergic projection. And this led very rapidly to the development of a rational and effective therapy. This period also witnessed the development of single unit electrophysiology, the useful ancillary technique of microiontophoresis, and the discovery of second messenger molecules.

The period of approximately 1975 to 1990 witnessed a very rapid increase in our knowledge of synaptic transmission. Peptides, already known to be produced by hypothalamic neurons, were found to be colocalized with small molecule transmitters.[2] Amino acids were shown to be transmitters in a number of systems. GABA was recognized as the principal inhibitory transmitter.

Immunohistochemistry was refined and formed the basis for the demonstration of a new, and elegant, chemical neuroanatomy that has substantially enhanced our understanding of the functional organization of neuronal systems. Receptors were characterized by ligand binding studies, both with "bind and grind" techniques and receptor autoradiography. Second messengers proliferated and patch clamping added a new dimension to the study of channels. Trophic factors came of age.

The final era, from approximately 1990 and extending through this "Decade of the Brain" is to be dominated by molecular biology. Progress is now so rapid as to be nearly incomprehensible. Receptor families have been identified and are rapidly being characterized. New receptors are cloned, seemingly daily, and the array of such receptors, particularly those coupled to G proteins is bewildering. Multiple types of ion channels are being identified and their relationships to receptors characterized. Families of trophic factors are being identified and the multiple roles of trophic factors in neuronal function analyzed. A new type of intraneuronal messenger, the immediate early genes, is under intensive investigation. The outcome of this massive proliferation of information is the recognition that neuronal communication is vastly more complex than we had imagined, even a few years ago.

NEURONAL LOCALIZATION OF NEUROACTIVE SUBSTANCES

The evolution of the nervous system has provided a highly differentiated structure that serves to integrate the adaptation of an organism to its environment. The highly specialized organization of the nervous system can be analyzed from two perspectives, its anatomical organization and its chemical organization. Over the last four decades we have accumulated a wealth of information about the anatomical organization of the CNS but this has only recently been supplemented by similar insight into its chemical organization. This can be viewed at two levels, a neuronal level and a systems level.

The Neuron

Nearly all CNS neurons communicate by means of chemical transmitters. These can be divided into two broad categories: small molecule transmitters and peptides. There are at least eight small molecules that have fulfilled the criteria for identifying chemical transmitters (localization in the neuron, release on stimulation, and identity of action). These are listed in order of their occurrence in the mammalian CNS: GABA (approximately 50% of all CNS neurons), glutamate ($\sim$35%), acetylcholine ($\sim$5%), serotonin ($\sim$2%), dopamine ($\sim$1%), norepinephrine ($<$1%), histamine ($<$1%), glycine ($<$1%).

TABLE 2. Colocalization of Peptides with Classical Transmitters

Transmitter	Peptide	Location
GABA	Somotostatin, Neuropeptide Y	Cortex, Hippocampus
	Vasopressin, Vasoactive intestinal peptide	Hypothalamus
		Striatum
	Enkephalin, Substance P	
Glutamate	Substance P	Retina
	Enkephalin	Hippocampus
Acetylcholine	Vasoactive intestinal peptide	Parasympathetic neurons
	Galanin, CGRP	Nucleus basalis, motor neurons
Serotonin	Substance P, TRH	Raphe nuclei
Dopamine	Cholecystokinin, Neurotensin	Ventral midbrain
Norepinephrine	Neuropeptide Y, Galanin	Locus coeruleus
		Reticular formation

CGRP: calcitonin gene-related peptide; TRH: thyrotropin releasing hormone.

There is some evidence that sets of CNS neurons have the metabolic apparatus to produce DOPA or epinephrine but it is not established that they are released.

Over the last 20 years, it has become evident that neurons outside the classical hypothalamic neurosecretory systems produce peptides and that these peptides are usually colocalized with small molecule transmitters.[2] The list of peptides that are localized to specific neuronal systems is large, exceeding 40, but we have relatively little information on the function of neuronal peptides. This probably reflects two problems. First, the function of a colocalized peptide appears to be to modify the action of the small molecule transmitter. This is extremely difficult to analyze as the peptide may do this in several different ways. For example, it may alter or prolong the effect of the small molecule transmitter. Alternatively, it may have actions that are very prolonged and similar to that of trophic agents. Some examples of peptide colocalization with small molecule transmitters are listed in TABLE 2.

Synaptic Transmission

Synaptic transmission has presynaptic and postsynaptic components. On the presynaptic side, transmitters and other neuroactive substances are synthesized and distributed in the neuron in a manner that will result in appropriate release on stimulation. For small molecule transmitters, for example, enzyme(s) are produced in the cell body and transported to the axon terminal. Transmitter is synthesized and packaged in vesicles. Peptides must be synthesized in the cell body, packaged in vesicles, and transported to the axon terminal. On stimulation, transmitter and peptide are released into the synaptic cleft. They then interact with appropriate receptors which are coupled to second messenger systems with specific postsynaptic functions. Transmitter and peptide action is terminated in one of two ways. First, small molecule transmitters may be taken up into the terminal population from which they were released by specific transporters. Second, the transmitters and peptides are degraded by appropriate enzymes located either in neurons or in glial processes that envelop the synaptic field. Thus, synaptic transmission at the neuronal level has a number of determinants: 1) factors regulating the production of small molecule transmitters and peptides and their distribution to the presynaptic element; 2) neuronal input to the presynaptic neuron that determines firing pattern and, hence, release; 3) presence of autoreceptors or other local presynaptic events that will regulate release; 4) the availability of receptors, their specific subtypes and the second message and/or immediate early gene systems to which they are coupled; 5) the mechanisms of transmitter-peptide inactivation; and 6) the long-term effects of prior synaptic interaction. This is a complex interaction of multiple factors that clearly has the capacity for a precise regulation of synaptic events.

NEUROANATOMY—FUNCTIONAL SYSTEMS

GABA

GABA is the transmitter most commonly produced by CNS neurons, and is the major inhibitory transmitter. GABA neurons are found at all levels of the neuraxis from the olfactory bulb to the spinal cord. Although GABA is the predominant transmitter for local circuit, short axon neurons, it is also utilized by projection neurons. It is the transmitter of cortical granule cells where it may be colocalized with NPY, VIP or somatostatin. It is the transmitter of local circuit neurons in the thalamus, hypothalamus and brainstem but also is present in a series of projection neurons including those in the striatum, the thalamic reticular nucleus, the central nucleus of the inferior colliculus, brainstem reticular formation and cerebellar Purkinje cells. The distribution of GABA neurons in the CNS has been reviewed extensively by Mugnaini and Oertel.[7]

Glutamate

Although simple amino acids such as glutamate and aspartate have been suspected to be transmitters for 25 years, this has been difficult to establish.[2] The molecules are part of the general metabolic pool and, hence, are present in all neurons. Further, it is difficult to generate antisera against amino acids and a cellular localization of glutamate like that of the catecholamines (see below) has been hard to establish. There has been a recent massive interest in amino acid neurotransmission deriving from the demonstration of glutamate receptors and a putative role of glutamate in such things as the establishment of connections in development and in ischemic cell death. Glutamate appears to be an excitatory transmitter produced by pyramidal neurons of the cerebral and hippocampal cortices, thalamic projection neurons, retinal ganglion cells and a number of brainstem projection neurons. On this basis, glutamate can be viewed to be a major transmitter in the CNS, particularly of long-axon, projection neurons. Glutamate has been shown in some instances to be colocalized with peptides (TABLE 2).

Acetylcholine

Acetylcholine is the prototypical excitatory transmitter. It is present in a series of neuronal populations in the CNS that have been well-characterized.[8] These fall into two major groups, motor neurons and ascending projection neurons, but there are small populations that do not belong to these such as the striatal cholinergic interneurons and habenular neurons projecting to the interpeduncular nucleus. All alpha motor neurons are cholinergic as are the central autonomic motor neurons of the sympathetic and parasympathetic systems. Virtually all cranial motor neurons contain either galanin or CGRP and there is some evidence that the colocalized peptide regulates acetylcholine receptor number.[6] There are two major divisions of the ascending cholinergic projections. The cholinergic nuclei of the rostral pons, the dorsal tegmental nucleus and the pedunculopontine nucleus, project caudally into the deep cerebellar nuclei, the vestibular and other cranial sensory nuclei, the reticular formation and the pontine nuclei. They project rostrally into the tectum, substantia nigra, thalamus, hypothalamus and basal forebrain. The largest single population of cholinergic neurons is located in the basal forebrain in a series of nuclei including the nucleus of the diagonal band-medial septal complex and the preoptic magnocellular-substantia innominata-nucleus basalis complex. These neuronal groups project predominantly on the remaining telencephalon, particularly the hippocampal formation and cerebral cortex.

Serotonin

Serotonin-producing neurons are located predominantly in the brainstem raphe nuclei and have widespread projections over the entire neuraxis.[3] The largest group of serotonin neurons is in the nucleus raphe dorsalis. These neurons, and those in the nucleus centralis superior, project predominantly rostrally into the forebrain. There are very widespread projections to the thalamus, subthalamus, hypothalamus, basal forebrain (amygdala, septum, olfactory nuclei, ventral striatum), striatum and the entire cerebral cortex. The pattern of innervation is unusual in that serotonergic axons appear to make relatively few synaptic contacts. This is carried to its extreme in a widespread innervation of the inner ventricular wall of the lateral and third ventricles, the subependymal plexus, whose axons can only release serotonin into the CSF. The caudal brainstem raphe nuclei have many fewer serotonin neurons than those in the midbrain and project primarily to brainstem and spinal cord. Although there is a minor topography to serotonin neuron projections, the overall pattern is that individual neurons project widely over large areas of neuraxis. This is consistent with a view that an important function of serotonin neurons is behavioral state regulation.

Dopamine

Dopamine neurons are found in a number of locations in the brain, olfactory bulb, retina, hypothalamus and midbrain.[1] The majority are projection neurons but those in the olfactory bulb (juxtaglomerular cells) and retina (interplexiform cells) are local circuit neurons. The major groups of dopamine neurons are in the substantia nigra–ventral tegmental area complex and in the hypothalamus. The hypothalamic neurons include a posterior group that projects to the spinal cord and a large periventicular-arcuate group that projects in a highly topographically organized fashion on the median eminence and posterior pituitary. The substantia nigra–ventral tegmental area dopamine neurons are also topographically organized with respect to projections which are to forebrain. There is a massive nigrostriatal projection to the neostriatum. Neurons of the ventral tegmental area project to basal forebrain (olfactory tubercle, septum, nucleus accumbens and amygdala) and widely to both allocortex (piriform cortex, hippocampus) and to the entire neocortex.

Norepinephrine

Norepinephrine neurons are found in two groups along the brainstem reticular formation.[5] The most distinctive of these is the locus coeruleus. The locus is located predominantly in the central gray of the isthmic region. The principal projections to arise from the locus: 1) a large rostral projection to the thalamus and cerebral cortex, including the hippocampus; 2) a projection to the cerebellar cortex; and 3) a projection to spinal cord gray. The axons of locus neurons are highly collateralized and it is clear that a single neuron may project to cerebellum, thalamus and cerebral cortex. Locus neurons colocalize neuropeptide Y and galanin but appear to transport little, if any, to their terminal fields.[4] The highly collateralized projections of locus neurons and their very limited topography of projection renders them ideal candidates for participation in behavioral state regulation, attention and other non-specific functions. The other norepinephrine neurons, the lateral tegmental system, are located in loose groups along the ventral and lateral brainstem reticular formation from the rostral pons to the caudal medulla. Those located rostrally project to the spinal cord gray whereas those in the caudal groups project to the brainstem, hypothalamus and basal forebrain.

Histamine

It has been recognized for a number of years that histamine is a likely transmitter.[2] This has been confirmed recently and there are histamine antisera that demonstrate neurons in the caudal hypothalamus with widespread projections, particularly to cerebral cortex.

Glycine

Glycine is an inhibitory transmitter produced by small numbers of spinal and brainstem neurons.[2]

CONCLUSIONS

Understanding of chemical transmission at the synapse is progressing at a rapid pace. It is now evident that the process, on the presynaptic side, involves release of a small molecule transmitter probably with one or more peptides, that interact postsynaptically with receptors that may be directly coupled to channels, initiate a cascade of second messenger systems or activate immediate early genes. The regulation of synaptic transmission, both at the presynaptic and postsynaptic levels, is extremely complex and reminds us that understanding the nervous system at any level, molecular, cellular, system or behavioral is a formidable, but challenging task. Transmitters are segregated to a series of functional systems and the ultimate function of the transmitters is dependent upon the organization and connections of those systems.

REFERENCES

1. BJÖRKLUND, A. & O. LINDVALL. 1984. Dopamine containing systems in the CNS. *In* Handbook of Chemical Neuroanatomy, Vol. 2, Classical Transmitters

in the CNS, Part 1. A. Björklund & T. Hökfelt, Eds. 72–121. Amsterdam. Elsevier.

2. COOPER, J. R., F. E. BLOOM & R. H. ROTH. 1991. The Biochemical Basis of Neuropharmacology, 6th edit. Oxford Press. New York.

3. JACOBS, B. L., E. C. AZMITIA. 1992. Structure and function of the serotonin system. Physiol. Rev. **72**:165–229.

4. MOORE, R. Y. & E. L. GUSTAFSON. 1989. The distribution of dopamine-β-hydroxylase, neuropeptide Y and galanin in locus coeruleus neurons. J. Chem. Neuroanat. **2**:95–106.

5. MOORE, R. Y. & J. P. CARD. 1984. Noradrenaline containing neuron systems. *In* Handbook of Chemical Neuroanatomy. Vol. 2, Classical Transmitters in the CNS, Part 1. A. Björklund & T. Hökfelt, Eds. 123–156. Elsevier. Amsterdam.

6. MOORE, R. Y. 1989. Cranial motor neurons contain either galanin or calcitonin gene-related peptide. J. Comp. Neurol. **282**:512–522.

7. MUGNAINI, E. & W. H. OERTEL. 1985. An atlas of the distribution of GABA ergic neurons and terminals in the rat CNS as revealed by GAD immunohistochemistry. *In* Handbook of Chemical Neuroanatomy, Vol. 4, GABA and Neuropeptides in the CNS. A Björklund, R. T. Hökfelt, Eds. 436. Elsevier. Amsterdam.

8. WOOLF, N. J. & L. L. BUTCHER. 1989. Cholinergic systems: Synopsis of anatomy and overview of physiology and pathology. *In* The Biological Substatus of Alzheimer's Disease. A. B. Scheibel & A. F. Wechsler, Eds. 73–86. Academic Press. New York.

Second Messengers in Neuronal Signaling[a]

BERNARD W. AGRANOFF[b]

Mental Health Research Institute and Departments of Biological Chemistry and Psychiatry, University of Michigan, Ann Arbor, Michigan, USA

ABSTRACT: The past decade has witnessed an enormous increase in our knowledge of the variety and complexity of intracellular signaling events that follow receptor binding on the cell surface. This overview emphasizes the phosphoinositidase C–mediated dual messenger pathway in brain and in brain-derived cells, with special reference to possible significance for research on the dementias.

INTRODUCTION

The metabolic rate of the human brain is high, accounting for some 20–25% of the body's energy consumption at rest, even though it represents only about 2% of total body mass. This remarkable energy requirement is a reflection of the excitable nature of nervous tissue. That is, it is metabolically costly to maintain the ability to rapidly conduct impluses within neurons and to mediate chemically transmitted signals between them. While neurotransmitter synthesis, storage and release all require ATP, some of the brain's metabolic expense can be attributed to the sequence of intracellular signaling events that occur between neurotransmitter binding to extracellular receptors and the ultimate physiological expression of the message, *e.g.,* initiation or block of secretion, of muscular contraction, of nerve impulse generation or of genomic processing. As these intramembrane and cytosolic chemical messengers are identified, convergence on intracellular Ca^{2+} regulation and protein kinases and phosphatases becomes increasingly apparent. A central role in intracellular signaling is evident for the dual pathway initiated by the phosphodiesteratic cleavage of phosphatidylinositol 4,5-bisphosphate (PIP_2) into two moieties, each of which then serves as an intracellular messenger: inositol 1,4,5-trisphosphate (1,4,5-IP_3) and 1,2-diacyl-*sn*-glycerol (DAG). This receptor-stimulated, G-protein-mediated cleavage is catalyzed by a phosphoinositide-specific phospholipase C (phosphoinositidase C; PLC). One turn of the "phosphoinositide cycle" whereby PIP_2 is regenerated consumes at least

[a] Research presented here was supported by the Wiley T. Buchanan Research Fund.

[b] *Send correspondence to:* B. W. Agranoff, Neuroscience Laboratory Building, University of Michigan, 1103 E. Huron Street, Ann Arbor, MI 48104-1687 USA; TEL: (313) 764-4214; FAX: (313) 936-2690.

TABLE 1.[a] Neural Receptors That Activate Phosphoinositidase C-mediated Cleavage of PIP_2

Muscarinic cholinergic (M_1 and M_3)
  Brain slices, retina, cochlea, primary neuronal cultures, neuroblastoma cells (SK-N-SH and SH-SY-5Y), astrocytoma cells (1321N1), glioma cells (C_6), neuroepithelioma cells (SK-N-MC), pheochromocytoma cells (PC-12)
Adrenergic (α_{1A} and α_{1B})
  Brain slices, primary neuronal and primary glial cultures, SK-N-MC cells, C_6 cells
Histaminergic (H_1)
  Primary glial cultures, neuroblastoma cells (NIE-115), C_6 cells
Serotonergic ($5HT_2$ and $5HT_{1C}$)
  Brain (in vivo), brain slices, primary neuronal cultures, pituitary tumor cells (P11), C_6 cells
Glutamatergic (metabotropic)
  Brain slices, retina, synaptoneurosomes, primary glial cultures
Endothelin
  Brain slices, primary neuronal and primary glial cultures, glial cells (C_6 and A_{172}), SK-N-MC cells

Above, brain receptor ligands that mediate a robust stimulation of phosphoinositide turnover in neural tissues, generally demonstated by means of preincubation of the listed preparations with ^3H-inositol, and measurement of accumulated labeled inositol phosphates following further incubation in the presence of the ligand and Li^+. Somewhat reduced stimulation is evoked in neural tissues by a number of additional ligands, for which principal evidence of a phosphoinositide-linkage comes from studies in non-neural tissues. They include: purinergic (P_2), thromboxane (A_2), nerve growth factor, prostaglandin (E_2), bradykinin (B_2), vasopressin (V_1), cholecystokinin, neuropeptide Y, neurotensin, gastrin-releasing peptide, bombesin, substance P, oxytocin, eledoisin, neurokinin, vasointestinal peptide, angiotensin, gonadotropin-releasing hormone, platelet activating factor, and thyrotropin releasing hormone.

---

[a] From ref. 1, in which specific literature references for each example may be found.

5 high energy phosphate equivalents. Given the large and growing list of ligands shown to bind to receptors that utilize the ligand-stimulated PLC pathway (TABLE 1), we may consider that operation of the pathway and its associated cellular functions likely accounts for a significant fraction of total brain metabolism. This complex dual pathway is of great interest, not only because its elucidation will lead to a better understanding of normal brain function, but also for the possibility that such understanding will then lead to the discovery of correlates of the dementias.

BIOCHEMICAL ASPECTS OF THE PHOSPHOINOSITIDE CYCLE

The three phosphoinositides, phosphatidylinositol (PI), phosphatidylinositol 4-phosphate (PIP) and PIP_2 are a family of quantitatively minor components of eukaryotic membrane lipids, of which PI, the metabolic precursor of PIP and PIP_2, is by far the most prevalent. The phosphoinositides are the most acidic of the phospholipids and are synthesized by the cytidine diphosphodiacylglycerol (CDP-DAG) pathway, as are the phosphatidylglycerol series of mitochondrial lipids. The cyclic sequence of reactions whereby phosphoinositide is broken down and regenerated is catalyzed by six enzymes, two of which are unique to the stimulated turnover, while the remaining four also mediate *de novo* synthesis. The latter are CDP-DAG synthase, PI synthase, PI kinase, and PI 4-kinase. One of the two turnover-specific steps is catalyzed by PLC, initiating the cycle of breakdown and resynthesis. DAG released upon PIP_2 cleavage is phosphorylated via DAG kinase to phosphatidate (PA), which in turn serves as substrate for CDP-DAG synthesis, thence to PI, PIP and PIP_2, completing the cycle.

Studies in brain and in other tissues indicate the presence of many isoforms of PLC, based upon purification and characterization on the one hand, and upon established amino acid sequence, on the other. The differences in function of various PLC families thus far identified are not yet certain, but it is clear that some isoforms are regulated by G-proteins (and can in turn regulate G-proteins by serving as GTPase-activating proteins), while others are regulated by tyrosine kinases.[2,3]

DAG kinase may regulate the cycle in a number of ways. By phosphorylating DAG, it can serve as an "off" signal that deactivates protein kinase C (PKC). The product, PA, has been reported to stimulate PIP 4-kinase activity.[4] A membrane-bound DAG kinase activity has been described that is highly selective for the 1-stearoyl, 2-arachidonoyl species of DAG that characterizes all six of the phosphoinositide cycle lipids, and may play a crucial role in isolating this unique DAG species from other cellular DAG pools, such as those seen in phosphatidylcholine or phosphatidylethanolamine synthesis and breakdown.[5] We have found that the essential fatty acid arachidonate ($20:4\omega6cis$) is deficient in standard cell culture media[6] and is largely replaced by "Mead" acid ($20:3\omega9cis$). Cells grown on the deficient media appear normal and show no deficit in phosphoinositide signaling. Since the fatty acid composition of the DAGs has generally been found to have relatively little effect on the DAG's activation of PKC, the effects of arachidonate supplementation on such depleted cells may be useful for investigation of the physiological significance of reported interactions of arachidonate metabolites with the PLC-mediated pathway, as well as with cyclic AMP and other second messenger systems.[7] Similarly, dietary restriction of arachidonate should decrease prostanoid production, but as a result of these cell culture studies, is predicted to have little effect on phosphoinositide-mediated signaling. This observation could be of value in dietary approaches to lowering prostanoid formation *in vivo*.

OTHER BRAIN INOSITOL LIPIDS

A variety of proteins are bound to all membranes via a PI anchor, in which the 6-position of inositol is glycosylated. The carbohydrate substituent, containing glucosamine and mannose, is linked to the protein via ethanolamine. While phospholipse C does not act on these lipids, PI anchor-degrading phospholipases have been found in brain.[1]

A family of polyphosphoinositides has been described, primarily in non-neural tissues, in which PI is phosphorylated on the 3 rather than on the 4 position of inositol to form PI3P, PI(3,4)P_2 and PI(3,4,5)P_3. Roles for these trace lipids in neural function have not yet been indicated, but can be anticipated, since brain has proven to be an excellent source of PI 3-kinase.

RELEVANCE TO THE DEMENTIAS

A number of investigations, using animal models, postmortem human brain or cultured human cells have been employed to examine the possible involvement of the stimulated PLC pathway in Alzheimer's disease. Since a quantitatively major fraction of the brain's PLC-linked receptors are thought to be muscarinic cholinergic, and further, since defects in acetylcholine metabolism have long been implicated in Alzheimer's disease, there have been numerous investigations on a possible link between the disease and the stimulated PLC pathway. Recent examples include studies in cells tranfected with human brain muscarinic receptors, in which cholinergic stimulation alters amyloid precursor protein metabolism, presumably via PKC activation.[8] From studies in rats and in GTP$_\gamma$S-supplemented postmortem human brain membranes, Crews *et al.*[9] conclude that amyloid β-protein may selectively block cholinergic and serotonergic PLC-mediated signal transduction. Comparing cultured fibroblasts from Alzheimer's disease patients with those of age-matched control patients, Gibson's laboratory has reported evidence for differences in available intracellular Ca^{2+} pools in the two cell populations, based on bradykinin receptor-stimulated, PLC-mediated release of 1,4,5-IP$_3$, together with the effects of ionophores and of other agents.[10]

Whether these studies will lead to a common causal mechanism, or to biological markers of the disease or of its progression, they may well constitute an important step forward in our understanding of the underlying pathologic process, and put us on firmer ground in proposing possible therapeutic interventions.

REFERENCES

1. FISHER, S. K., A. M. HEACOCK & B. W. AGRANOFF. 1992. Inositol lipids and signal transduction in the nervous system: An update. J. Neurochem. **58**:18–38.
2. COCKCROFT, S. & M. H. THOMAS. 1992. Inositol-lipid-specific phospholipase C isoenzymes and their differential regulation by receptors. Biochem. J. **288**: 1–14.

3. BERRIDGE, M. J. 1993. Inositol trisphosphate and calcium signalling. Nature **361**:315–325.

4. MORITZ, P. N. E. DE GRAAN, W. H. GISPEN & K. W. A. WIRTZ. 1992. Phosphatidic acid is a specific activator of phosphatidylinositol-4-phosphate kinase. J. Biol. Chem. **267**:7207–7210.

5. KANOH, H. K. YAMADA & F. SAKANE. 1990. Diacylglycerol kinase: A key modulator of signal transduction? Trends in Biochem. Sci. **15**:47–50.

6. STUBBS, E. B., JR., R. O. CARLSON, C. LEE, S. K. FISHER, A. K. HAJRA & B. W. AGRANOFF. 1992. Essential fatty acid deficiency in cultured SK-N-SH human neuroblastoma cells. *In* Neurobiology of Essential Fatty Acids. N. G. Bazen, G. Tofanno & M. Murphy, Eds. 171–182. Plenum Publishing Corp. New York.

7. DI MARZO, V., S. H. I. GALADARI, J. R. TIPPINS, H. R. MORRIS. 1991. Interactions between second messenger: Cyclic AMP and phospholipase A_2 and phospholipase C metabolites. Life Sci. **49**:247–259.

8. NITSCH, R. M., B. E. SLACK, R. J. WURTMAN & J. H. GROWDON. 1992. Release of Alzheimer amyloid precursor derivatives stimulated by activation of muscarinic acetylcholine receptors. Science **258**:304–307.

9. CREWS, F. T., P. KURIAN & G. FREUND. 1992. Decreased phosphoinositide signals in Alzheimer's disease: Inhibition by amyloid β-protein may underlie Alzheimer's neurodegeneration. Abstracts, 31st Annual Meeting, Am. Coll. Neuropsychopharmacol, p. 181.

10. GIBSON, G. E., L. TORAL-BARZA. 1992. Characterization of internal calcium stores in cultured skin fibroblasts from Alzheimer and control subjects. Mol. Biol. of the Cell. **3**(Suppl.):145A.

Muscarinic Acetylcholine Receptor Subtypes Associated with Release of Alzheimer Amyloid Precursor Derivatives Activate Multiple Signal Transduction Pathways

CHRISTIAN C. FELDER,[a] ALICE L. MA, EILEEN M. BRILEY, AND JULIUS AXELROD

Laboratory of Cell Biology, National Institutes of Mental Health, Bethesda, Maryland 20892, USA

ABSTRACT: Five subtypes of muscarinic acetylcholine receptors have been identified and designated m1–m5. The m1 and m3 receptors have recently been shown to stimulate APP processing. The m1 and m3 receptors couple to a variety of signal transduction pathways in both tissue slices and a variety of cell lines endogenously expressing either or both subtypes. In contrast, the m2 and m4 receptors have been primarily associated with inhibition of adenylate cyclase. We have transfected all five subtypes of muscarinic receptors into a variety of mammalian cell lines in order to investigate the signaling associated with single receptor subtypes. The m1, m3, or m5 receptors stimulate phospholipase A_2, C, and D, adenylate cylase, receptor-operated calcium channels, and tyrosine kinase activity simultaneously. The m2 or m4 receptor inhibits cAMP accumulation and augments a previously stimulated release of arachidonic acid and calcium influx.

INTRODUCTION

Cholinergic receptor involvement in the etiology of Alzheimer's Disease has been suggested but not fully demonstrated. Recent evidence[1] implicated muscarinic acetylcholine receptors as regulators of normal amyloid precursor protein (APP) processing. This would suggest that deficits in muscarinic receptors or their signaling activity might lead to abnormal APP processing and the deposition of irregular amyloid protein fragments leading to Alzheimer's disease.

[a] *Send correspondence to:* Dr. C. Felder, Laboratory of Cell Biology, Bldg. 36 Rm. 3A-15, National Institute of Mental Health, Bethesda, MD 20892 USA, TEL: (301) 496-9925; FAX: (301) 402-1748.

15

Muscarinic acetylcholine receptors are coded by five separate genes designated m1–m5. Transfection and functional expression of a receptor gene into mammalian cells has provided a means to study how each receptor couples to the activation of transmembrane signaling pathways and regulation of second messenger production. Functional similarity exists between signaling associated with the m1, m3, and m5 receptors and between the m2 and m4 receptors. When expressed in either Chinese hamster ovary cells or A9 fibroblasts the m1, m3, or m5 receptors stimulate multiple transduction pathways including phospholipase A_2, phospholipase C, phospholipase D, adenylate cyclase, receptor-operated calcium channels, and tyrosine kinase activity.[2] In contrast, the m2 and m4 receptors inhibit adenylate cyclase activity and augment previously stimulated phospholipase A_2 and calcium influx.[3]

m1, m3, AND m5 RECEPTORS STIMULATE cAMP

Second messenger production following receptor stimulation can be initiated directly through the activation of specific heterotrimeric G proteins or indirectly by second messengers, independent of G protein involvement. Muscarinic receptor-activated cAMP accumulation was first described in neuroblastoma cells which express endogenous muscarinic receptors.[4] It was not clear which receptor subtype was responsible for the increase in cAMP or the molecular mechanism of the response. Stably expressed m1 receptor-stimulated cAMP generation was shown to be secondary to phospholipase C activation and subsequent IP_3 mediated increases in cytoplasmic calcium.[5] The calmodulin antagonist W7 also blocked the response, suggesting a calcium/calmodulin sensitive adenylate cyclase mediated this effect. Endogenous prostaglandin E_2 receptor activation but not m1 receptor activation increased adenylate cyclase activity in a cell membrane preparation, suggesting that the m1 response was not directly linked to adenylate cyclase through G_s. Taken together, these data suggested that m1-stimulated adenylate cyclase is activated through an indirect mechanism.

m1, m3, AND m5 RECEPTORS STIMULATE PHOSPHOLIPASE A_2, C, AND D

The m1, m3, or m5 receptors stimulate the release of arachidonic acids, inositol phosphates, and phosphatidic acid, an index of phospholipase A_2, phospholipase C, and phospholipase D activity, respectively. Muscarinic receptor-stimulated arachidonic acid and phosphatidic acid release were dependent on both protein kinase C activation and receptor-operated calcium influx. m1, m3, or m5 receptors stimulated phospholipase C-β and phospholipase C-γ simultaneously, phospholipase C-β through direct G protein regulation and phospholipase C-γ through activation of a calcium influx sensitive tyrosine kinase.

m1, m3, and m5 RECEPTORS STIMULATE A RECEPTOR-OPERATED CALCIUM CHANNEL

Calcium plays a central role in the regulation of multiple signaling pathways activated by muscarinic receptors. Calcium influx through receptor-operated calcium channels was initiated at concentrations of carbachol, a muscarinic agonist, two orders of magnitude lower than the release of arachidonic acid, phosphatidic acid, or inositol phosphates and three orders of magnitude lower than cAMP generation. Muscarinic receptor-activated calcium influx was second messenger and intracellular calcium independent, not activated with either cAMP or arachidonic acid, and not affected following activation of protein kinase C.[6] Alterations in receptor structure were used to determine G protein involvement in calcium influx regulation. Studies using m2 and m3 muscarinic receptor chimeras suggested that m3-medicated calcium influx was independent of the third cytoplasmic loop (the primary structural determinant of G protein-coupling selectivity of muscarinic receptors).

WHICH TRANSDUCTION PATHWAY REGULATES APP PROCESSING?

Muscarinic receptor-activated protein kinase C has been suggested as a possible mediator in APP processing.[1] Protein kinase C is activated by diacylglycerol which is generated following m1, m3, or m5 receptor stimulation of phospholipase C. It is also possible that diacylglycerol may arise from muscarinic receptor-activated phosphatidylcholine specific phospholipase C, independent of inositolphospholipid metabolism. The molecular mechanism of muscarinic receptor-mediated activation of APP processing may involve one or more of the transduction pathways associated with the m1, m3 or m5 receptors.

REFERENCES

1. NITSCH, R. N., B. E. SLACK, R. J. WURTMAN & J. H. GROWDON. 1992. Release of Alzheimer amyloid precursor derivatives stimulated by activation of muscarinic acetylcholine receptors. Science **258**:304–307.
2. FELDER, C. C., L. MACARTHUR, A. L. MA, F. GUSOVSKY & E. C. KOHN. 1993.

Tumor suppressor function of muscarinic acetylcholine receptors is associated with activation of receptor-operated calcium influx. Proc. Natl. Acad. Sci. USA. **90:**1706–1710.

3. FELDER, C. C., H. L. WILLIAMS & J. AXELROD. 1991. A transduction pathway associated with receptors coupled to the inhibitory guanine nucleotide binding protein G_i that amplifies ATP-mediated arachidonic acid release. Proc. Natl. Acad. Sci. USA **88:**6477–6480.

4. BAUMGOLD, J. & P. H. FISHMAN. 1988. Muscarinic receptor-mediated increase in cAMP levels in SK-N-SH human neuroblastoma cells. Biochem. Biophys. Res. Commun. **154:**1137–1143.

5. FELDER, C. C., R. Y. KANTERMAN, A. L. MA & J. AXELROD. 1989. A transfected m1 muscarinic acetylcholine receptor stimulates adenylate cyclase via phosphatidylinositol hydrolysis. J. Biol. Chem. **264:**20356–20362.

6. FELDER, C. C., M. O. POULTER & J. WESS. 1992. Muscarinic receptor-operated Ca^{2+} influx in transfected fibroblast cells is independent of inositol phosphates and release of intracellular Ca^{2+}. Proc. Natl. Acad. Sci. USA **89:**509–513.

Neurotransmitters and Second Messengers in Aging and Alzheimer's Disease

PAUL T. FRANCIS[a], M-T. WEBSTER[a], I. P. CHESSELL[a],
C. HOLMES[a], G. C. STRATMANN[a], A. W. PROCTER[a],
ALAN J. CROSS[b], A. R. GREEN[b], AND DAVID M. BOWEN[a,c]

[a]Miriam Marks Department of Neurochemistry, Institute of Neurology,
Queen Square, London, United Kingdom
[b]Astra Neuroscience Research Unit, 1, Wakefield Street, London, United Kingdom

ABSTRACT: A substantial loss of cortical cholinergic nerve endings, along with a much more circumscribed cortical degeneration of pyramidal neurons, almost certainly causes glutamatergic hypoactivity in live Alzheimer's patients. These *selective* pathologies are discussed in terms of therapy. An additional effect of some proposed treatments is emerging as there is evidence that processing pathways for β-amyloid precursor proteins in cortical pyramidal neurons, a target cell for acetylcholine, are affected by neuronal activity.

INTRODUCTION

Some 10 years after the introduction in 1968 of L-dopa therapy for Parkinson's disease, a substantial presynaptic cholinergic abnormality in the brains of patients with Alzheimer's disease (AD) suggested a basis for rational pharmacological treatments. An additional effect of such neurotransmitter replacement is now emerging as processing pathways for β-amyloid precursor proteins (APPs) appear to be regulated by transmitter receptors, at least those coupled to the phosphoinositide (PI) second messenger system such as the acetylcholine m_1 receptor[1], TABLE 1). There is controversy regarding the mechanism by which mismetabolism of APP might cause cell death as it is not certain that β-amyloid protein is toxic in AD brain.[2]

Postmortem biochemical studies of AD, where extensive transmitter deficits may be seen, has led some workers to the pessimistic conclusion that a transmitter-based therapy cannot be successful. However, such studies almost

[c] *Send correspondence to:* Dr. D. M. Bowen, Miriam Marks Department of Neurochemistry, Institute of Neurology, 1 Wakefield Street, London WC1N 1PJ United Kingdom; TEL: 44-71-278, 1562; FAX: 44-71-278-6572.

TABLE 1. Acetylcholinesterase Inhibitors Are Well Known to Be under Development for Treatment of Alzheimer's Symptoms: Will These Also Affect β-Amyloid Precursor Protein?

Nerve growth factor differentiated PC 12 cells treated for 1 h with:	Secreted APP	
	751/770 (% untreated)	695 (% untreated)
Phorbol-12,13-dibutyrate, 100 nM (n = 4)[a]	151 ± 17	161 ± 9[b]
Bradykinin (PI coupled), 500 nM (n = 5)	172 ± 25[b]	202 ± 22[b]

[a] n = number of experiments, each experiment in triplicate.

[b] Significantly higher than untreated (t statistic). APPs (approx. 110–140 apparent kDa) detected with commercial antibody 22C11.[17]

invariably examine the end-stage of this slowly progressing disease and this is rarely acknowledged in the interpretation. It has been possible to study samples removed earlier in the disease as neocortical tissues from AD patients has been occasionally removed surgically for diagnostic purposes. Transmitter changes in neurosurgical (biopsy) samples, and the comparison of these with the corresponding evidence obtained from postmortem studies, has been emphasized in this chapter. The issue of transmitter systems in normal aging brain is a difficult area as it is often unclear whether investigators have had access to suitable human material, in terms of neuropsychological and neuropathological criteria. Moreover, the anatomical/chemical basis of "age-associated memory impairment" has not been defined.

SUBCORTICAL NEUROTRANSMITTERS

In cases of early onset AD studied here, the wet weight and protein content of the caudate nucleus was slightly lower compared with controls of similar age. The caudate nucleus appeared to atrophy with increasing age in controls, but not in patients with AD. Thus in AD of late-onset there was no evidence that the caudate nucleus was more atrophied than in controls of similar age. Therefore, atrophy of the caudate nucleus may not be essential to the production of AD but is probably important in aging.

Transmitter systems in the region of the cell bodies of cholinergic nucleus basalis neurons may provide approaches for ameliorating cholinergic dysfunction in AD.[3,4] An interesting recent observation was that although serotonin (5-HT) and 5-hydroxyindole acetic acid (5-HIAA) concentrations were reduced, an index of 5-HT turnover was increased.[5]

CORTICOPETAL NEUROTRANSMITTERS

By contrast with cholinergic inputs in the brain of AD patients, those using the catecholamines, noradrenaline and dopamine, are relatively unaffected. The situation regarding inputs using 5-HT is complex. Even in autopsy AD brain, half of the many cortical areas assayed had no evidence of a selective reduction in presynaptic 5-HT activity. Hence, deficiency of presynaptic serotonergic activity is probably never widespread, a feature consistent with the preservation of 5-HIAA concentration in ventricular CSF from live AD patients. Indeed, the turnover rate in those 5-HT nerve endings remaining appears to be enhanced in AD patients, based on the increased ratio of 5-HIAA to 5-HT in cortical tissue and the nucleus basalis. Furthermore, 5-HIAA concentration in lumbar CSF positively correlated with the dementia rating in a series of histologically verified AD patients and in another series the mean 5-HIAA value was significantly higher than control.

Neurosurgical samples showed a severe deficiency in acetylcholine synthesis by the midpoint of the disease. Detailed clinical assessments of these patients have been made, and the rating of dementia correlated with synthesis, but not with the transmitters of other corticopetal neurons. Sparing of catecholamines was confirmed.[3]

CORTICAL INHIBITORY NEUROTRANSMITTERS AND NEUROPEPTIDES

The balance of evidence indicates that GABA, glycine, taurine, cholecystokinin, vasoactive intestinal polypeptide, neuropeptide Y and somatostatin are not critically depleted.

HIPPOCAMPAL NEUROTRANSMITTERS

In the hippocampus all the major input and output pathways (except the septohippocampal cholinergic pathway) use L-glutamate (GLU) as transmitter. There was cell loss and tangle formation in the entorhinal cortex and in CA1 in AD patients at postmortem. Indeed, *in vivo* imaging suggests that atrophy of the hippocampus had occurred by the mid-point of the disease process.[6] GLU concentration postmortem in the terminal zone of the perforant pathway was decreased 80% in AD specimens. Consistent with this, decreased GLU staining was observed in the molecular layer of the dentate gyrus. It was noted that GLU and glutaminase immunoreactive pyramidal neurons in the CA fields were decreased in number and the remaining neurons showed irregular shortening and disorganized dendritic fields. Many also showed tangle formation.[7] Thus if the GLU pathways are considered to be involved in memory it follows that the loss of GLU function may contribute to the memory dysfunction in AD. Loss of ChAT activity together with reduced synaptosomal choline uptake indicated that major presynaptic cholinergic pathology was also a feature of the hippocampus in AD.[4]

EXCITATORY NEOCORTICAL NEUROTRANSMITTERS

Three studies indicated that severity of dementia correlated with degeneration of corticocortical pyramidal neurons in association areas.[8–10] Although there are difficulties in separating transmitter GLU from the large metabolic pools, a combination of techniques has provided evidence for a transmitter role for GLU in a number of pathways, including corticocortical pyramidal neurons. The temporal and parietal lobes of AD patients may be major and early sites of pathological changes, as these regions showed reductions in glucose metabolism as assessed by positron emission tomography, a measurement in living brain which is sensitive to atrophy. Psychological test scores correlated with both the positron emission tomography data, the pyramidal cell counts in layer III and number of synapses in layer III. Thus, a clinically relevant shrinkage or loss of association fibers probably occurred from circumscribed (*i.e.,* parietotemporal) areas and this contributed to an overall reduction in glucose metabolism as assessed by scanning.

In summary, there is now evidence accumulating that GLU is the principal transmitter of the corticocortical association fibers and the major hippocampal pathways above. Histological and scanning studies indicate that these pathways degenerate quite early in AD and some neurochemical data support this.[3,4]

CORTICAL NEUROTRANSMITTER RECEPTOR SYSTEMS

Studies on postmortem AD samples have indicated that binding sites for most transmitters are unaltered in the cerebral cortex.[3] The main postsynaptic muscarinic receptor (m_1) seems to be preserved, which should provide a suitable target for acetylcholine (TABLE 1). Nicotinic and m_2 muscarinic receptors (both may be primarily presynaptic) are reduced. Binding sites for 5-HT are not consistently abnormal. Altered populations of binding sites for GLU have been reported in the hippocampus but little change was seen in the neocortex, although reduced GLU binding in cortical layers 1 and 11 has been reported. Apart from reduced sensitivity to modulation by glycine the properties of the NMDA receptor complex seem to be normal but the number of complexes may be reduced, probably due to pyramidal cell loss.[11] Penney and colleagues used quantitative receptor autoradiography to measure m_1, benzodiazepine and various GLU binding sites in sections of the hippocampal region. The binding loss was greater for NMDA sites than for m_1.

Jansen and colleagues, also found reduced NMDA receptors. By contrast [^{3}H] kainate binding was not reduced (and even increased in the neorcortex), as was found by Chalmers, Dewar and colleagues. Quisqualate-dependent GLU binding estimates two sub-types of receptor, one of these, the α-amino-3-hydroxy-5-methyl-4-isoxazolepropanoic acid (AMPA) site was reduced (as reviewed in ref. 3). The other site, metabotropic receptor (but see ref. 12, where subtypes are discussed), was also reduced. 5-HT$_2$ receptors were reduced whereas the 5-HT$_1$ subtypes have not been studied.[3]

Harrison and Pearson have established reliable *in situ* hybridization methods using [^{35}S]-labeled olignonucleotides for the detection and quantitation of the cell type capable of producing a given receptor. In two of the most affected cortical areas the mRNA for the m$_1$ receptor was increased whereas that for one of the receptor's probable G proteins was not affected. Although the amounts of cortical "G protein" are reported to remain unchanged,[3] evidence has been presented by alterations in the functional integrity of some G proteins. This has been studied carefully by Cowburn and colleagues,[13] albeit at the end of point of the disease (*i.e.*, in autopsy samples). Changes also occur in the cerebellum, a region not showing hallmark histological lesions. Moreover, 5-HT$_{1A}$ receptor-G protein interactions were preserved in AD patients as was found for the m$_1$ receptor by Pearce and Potter (but not by Flynn and colleagues). However, the groups studying m$_1$ did not consider factors such as patients immediate preterminal state (as reviewed in ref. 3).

EXPERIMENTAL PYRAMIDAL NEURON LOSS AND RECEPTORS

Unilateral striatal injections of volkensin, a retrogradely transported suicide toxin, produced a loss of infragranular layer V pyramidal cells with preservation of those in the upper (supragranular) layers and preservation of interneurons in all layers. It is proposed that animals with such a cell loss will address the issue as to whether a specific transmitter receptor(s) is enriched on these cells. This could have important implications for the discovery of drugs affecting higher mental function as well as in the development of badly needed markers of pyramidal neurons for *in vivo* brain imaging techniques. Autoradiographic studies of the rat brain sections indicated that not all receptors were associated to the same extent with the affected pyramidal cells. The rank order was 5-HT$_{1A}$ receptor $\gg$ NMDA receptor $>$ m$_1$ receptor, kainate GLU receptor $>$ 5-HT$_2$ receptor (PI coupled like m$_1$), α-adrenoceptors (also PI coupled) and GABA$_A$ receptors (ref. 3 and I. P. Chessell, P. T. Francis, and D. M. Bowen, unpublished data). Corticocortical and corticofugal pyramidal neurons are probably subject to qualitatively similar regulation, irrespective of species. Thus, the present data provide a better understanding of regulation of cortical pyramidal neurons in general.

CONCLUSION: EMERGING APPROACHES TO TREATMENT

Pharmacological treatment of AD is likely to be difficult both because of the presence of multiple transmitter changes and the difficulty of replacing lost transmitter function in a way which mimics normal neuronal release. With regards to the latter problem the introduction of agents which modify the actions of remaining transmitters may be a more effective approach than one based on introduction of direct agonists. Most clinical studies to date have been directed towards the cholinergic deficit but acetylcholinesterase inhibitors (TABLE 1) that are ideal (*i.e.*, long-lasting and non-toxic) have not yet emerged. Muscarinic m_1 receptors help regulate cortical pyramidal neurons, and there is evidence that the receptors affect APPs. Pyramidal neuron counts in human neocortex correlate with apparent $APP_{751/770}$ immuno-reactivity[14] which is particularly high in human brain.[15] Thus, it is important to study APPs with respect to inhibition of acetylcholine breakdown.

It is unclear whether the remaining GLU neurons in AD brain have the same transmitter receptors characteristics as those lost. For example, heterogeneity of the NMDA receptor complex has been suggested. There is evidence that the structures which selectively degenerate are those bearing NMDA receptor complexes with particular sensitivity to glycine.[11] It has been proposed that the partial agonist acting on the glycine site, D-cycloserine, should be tested for clinical efficacy in AD. Improved understanding of the topography of this glycine site may permit the development of other potentially useful drugs of which D-cycloserine appears to be the lead compound but the issue of the saturation of this site by endogenous glycine *in vivo* needs to be addressed.[3,4]

Although a compound acting at the glycine site should facilitate the effect on the NMDA receptor complex of the remaining pool of transmitter GLU it is unlikely to affect responses of other subtypes of GLU receptor. α-Amino-3-hydroxy-5-phenyl-4-isoxazolepropanoate has a similar affinity for the AMPA sub-type of GLU receptor but only 50% of the efficacy of a full agonist and hence is the prototype partial agonist for non-NMDA subtypes of GLU receptors (as reviewed in ref. 3). The status in the volkensin lesioned animals of AMPA and metabotropic GLU receptors, including the PI-linked subtype,[12] has not been established, but suitable probes are beginning to emerge. Martin and colleagues[16] have found a PI-coupled GLU receptor only on many *non*-pyramidal neurons. The value of considering these receptors in terms of treatment is also uncertain, as a direct acting GLU partial agonist is unlikely to replace the temporal features of a fast acting excitatory transmitter such as GLU and will certainly be suspected of causing neurotoxicity.

Another class of drug, the selective $5\text{-}HT_{1A}$ receptor antagonist, should facilitate the effects of the remaining GLU transmitter pool at *all* GLU receptor sub-types by inhibiting the tonic hyperpolarizing action of endogenous

5-HT on pyramidal neurons, thereby compensating for reduced excitatory (GLU) input caused by the degenerative process. The approach is also indicated as the $5\text{-}HT_{1A}$ receptor seems enriched on the appropriate cell, human neocortical layer II/III pyramidal neurons. There is further support, as it has already been argued that the remaining 5-HT nerve endings appear to be of highest activity in the most demented patients, suggesting a greater inhibitory action on pyramidal neurons. Moreover, decreased 5-HT availability can enhance learning and memory and enhancement of 5-HT activity has been reported to impair avoidance responding and discrimination learning. Specifically, the prototypical $5\text{-}HT_{1A}$ partial agonist 8-OH-DPAT, impairs learning (as reviewed, refs. 3,4). Clearly, it is important to establish whether non-PI second messenger systems, such as is coupled to the $5\text{-}HT_{1A}$ receptor, affect APPs.

REFERENCES

1. NITSCH, R. M., B. E. SLACK, R. J. WURTMAN & J. H. GROWDON. 1992. Release of Alzheimer amyloid precursor stimulated by activation of muscarinic acetylcholine receptors. Science **258**:304–307.
2. BOWEN, D. M., P. T. FRANCIS, N. R. SIMS & A. J. CROSS. 1992. Protection from dementia. Science **258**:1422–1423.
3. FRANCIS, P. T., M. N. PANGALOS & D. M. BOWEN. 1992. Animal and drug modelling for Alzheimer synaptic pathology. Prog. Neurobiol. **39**:517–545.
4. FRANCIS, P. T., N. R. SIMS, A. W. PROCTER & D. M. BOWEN. 1993. Cortical pyramidal neurone loss may cause glutamatergic hypoactivity and cognitive impairment in Alzheimer's disease: investigative and therapeutic perspectives. J. Neurochem. **60**:1589–1604.
5. SPARKS, L. D., J. C. HUNSAKER, J. T. SLEVIN, S. T. DEKOSKY, R. J. KRYSCIO & W. R. MARKESBERY. 1992. Monoaminergic and cholinergic synaptic markers in the nucleus basalis of meynert (nbM): Normal age-related changes and the effect of heart disease and Alzheimer's disease. Ann. Neurol. **31**:611–620.
6. KESSLAK, J. P., O. NALCIOGLU & C. W. COTMAN. 1991. Quantification of magnetic resonance scans for hippocampal and parahippocampal atrophy in Alzheimer's disease. Neurology **41**:51–54.
7. KOWALL, N. W. & M. F. BEAL. 1991. Glutamate-, glutaminase-, and taurine-immunoreactive neurones develop neurofibrillary tangles in Alzheimer's disease. Ann. Neurol. **29**:162–167.
8. NEARY, D., J. S. SNOWDEN, D. M. MANN, D. M. BOWEN, N. R. SIMS, B. NORTHEN, P. O. YATES & A. N. DAVISON. 1986. Alzheimer's disease: A correlative study. J. Neurol. Neurosurg. Psychiatry **49**:229–237.
9. DEKOSKY, S. T. & S. W. SCHEFF. 1990. Synapse loss in frontal cortex biopsies in Alzheimer's disease: Correlation with cognitive severity. Ann Neurol. **27**:457–464.
10. TERRY, R. D., E. MASLIAH, D. P. SALMON, N. BUTTERS, R. DETERESA, R.

HILL, L. A. HANSEN & R. KATZMAN. 1991. Physical basis of cognitive alterations in Alzheimer's disease: Synapse loss is the major correlate of cognitive impairment. Ann. Neurol. **30:**572–580.

11. STEELE, J. E., A. J. CROSS & D. M. BOWEN. 1992. N-methyl-D-aspartate receptor-associated ionophores determined in Alzheimer's disease by [^{3}H]MK-801 and N-[1-(2-thienyl)cyclohexyl]-3,4-[^{3}H]piperidine binding. Neurodegeneration **1:**225–230.

12. SCHOEPP, D. D. & R. A. TRUE. 1992. 1*S*,3*R*-ACPD-sensitive (metabotropic) [^{3}H] glutamate receptor binding in membranes. Neurosci. Lett. **145:**100–104.

13. COWBURN, R. F., C. O'NEIL, R. RAVID, I. ALAFUZOFF, B. WINBLAD & C. J. FOWLER. 1992. Adenylyl cyclase activity in postmortem human brain: Evidence of altered G protein mediation in Alzheimer's disease. J. Neurochem. **58:** 1409–1419.

14. HOLMES, C., M.-T. WEBSTER, A. W. PROCTER, P. T. FRANCIS & D. M. BOWEN. 1993. Relationship between β-amyloid precursor protein, pyramidal neurones and astrocytes in human neocortex. Biochem. Soc. Trans. **21:**238S.

15. MOIR, R. D., R. N. MARTIN, A. I. BUSH, D. H. SMALL, E. A. MILWARD, B. A. RUMBLE, G. MULTHAUP, K. BEYREUTHER & C. L. MASTERS. 1992. Human brain βA4 amyloid protein precursor of Alzheimer's disease: Purification and partial characterization. J. Neurochem. **59:**1490–1498.

16. MARTIN, L. J., C. D. BLACKSTONE, R. L. HUGANIR & D. L. PRICE. 1992. Cellular localization of a metabotropic glutamate receptor in rat brain. Neuron **9:**259–270.

17. WEBSTER, M. T., P. T. FRANCIS, B. R. PEARCE & D. M. BOWEN. 1993. β-amyloid precursor protein of PC12 cells: Effect of ATP reduction, chloroquine, growth factor and phosphoinositide breakdown. Biochem. Soc Trans. **21:**239S.

In Vivo Detection of Neurotransmitter Changes in Alzheimer's Disease[a]

AGNETA NORDBERG[b]

Department of Geriatric Medicine, Karolinska Institute, Stockholm, Sweden

ABSTRACT: Alzheimer's disease (AD) is characterized by multiple deficits of neurotransmitters in brain. These observations are mainly based upon studies in postmortem brain material where the disease has reached a terminal state. In order to obtain further insight into the early disturbances of the neurotransmitter activities in AD, new imaging techniques such as positron emission tomography (PET) and single positron emission tomography (SPECT) can be applied *in vivo* for detection of neurotransmitter activity in normal as well as AD brains. Nicotinic receptors have been traced in AD patients by PET and ^{11}C-nicotine at different stages of AD. A lower uptake of $(R)(+)$- compared to $(S)(-)$-^{11}C-nicotine was observed in AD patients while the difference in uptake of the two enantiomeres was less pronounced in normal individuals. A positive correlation has been observed between cognitive function (Mini-Mental-State-Examination) and uptake of $(S)(-)$-^{11}C-nicotine in the temporal cortex of AD patients. ^{11}C-benztropine has been used to measure muscarinic receptors in brain by PET. Oral tacrine treatment (80 mg daily) restore nicotinic receptors in AD patients as visualized by PET and ^{11}C-nicotine. Kinetic analysis indicate increased binding of $(S)(-)$-^{11}C-nicotine after 3 months of treatment with tacrine. The PET data are paralleled by improvement in neuropsychological testings. Intraventricular infusion of nerve growth factor (NGF) to an AD patients for 3 months resulted in an transient increase in uptake and binding of $(S)(-)$-^{11}C-nicotine in the temporal and frontal cortex and a persistent increase in cortical blood flow.

INTRODUCTION

Alzheimer's disease (AD) is by definition a progressive neurodegenerative disease where clinical symptoms vary with different stages of the disorder. An early clinical diagnosis of AD is hampered by the lack of early reliable diagnostic markers. Clinically AD is diagnosed as "possible" or "probably" according to NINCDS-ADRDA criteria.[1] The final diagnosis is based upon

[a] This study was supported by the Swedish Medical Research Council, Loo and Hans Osterman's Foundation, Clas Groschinsky's Foundation Swedish Tobacco Company, Stiftelsen Gamla Tjänarinnor, Åke Wiberg's Foundation.
[b] *Send correspondence to:* Agneta Nordberg, Department of Geriatric Medicine, Karolinska Institute, Huddinge Hospital B56, S-141 86 Huddinge, Sweden; TEL: 46/8/7463897; 46/18/174163; FAX: 46/8/7111751, 46/18/559718.

histopathological investigations in autopsy brain tissue. Some lack of agreement still exists between clinical and histopathological diagnosis which emphasis the need for early *in vivo* diagnostic markers.

Over the past decades, research has focused on neurochemical changes in AD brains. Studies in postmortem brain material, or more seldom in neurosurgical biopsies, have revealed multiple disturbances of neurotransmitters, their metabolites, receptors and enzymes involved in their metabolism. Deficits have been observed for classical transmitter systems like the cholinergic, serotonergic, dopaminergic as well as for excitatoric amino acids and peptides.[2,3] The drawback of information obtained from such studies in autopsy human brain material is that the observed changes represent the final stage of AD. Correlation of neurochemical deficits to dementia states and histopathological findings might have limited value. It might be misleading to base new therapeutic strategies on neurochemical findings in autopsy brain tissue from AD patients. To obtain further insight into the early disturbances of the neurotransmitter activity in AD, imaging techniques such as positron emission tomography (PET) and single photon emission tomography (SPECT) have been applied for detection of *in vivo* neurotransmitter changes.

The cholinergic hypothesis of AD is well established. The cholinergic transmitter system is also the transmitter system that best correlates with cognitive function. This motivated us to use imaging techniques like PET primarily for tracing *in vivo* cholinergic activity in AD brains. This study will primarily deal with investigations which have been performed by PET and SPECT in order to visualize cholinergic nicotinic and muscarinic receptors in normal as well as AD brains. The effect of new putative treatment strategies on the *in vivo* cholinergic activity in AD patients will be illustrated.

IN VIVO DETECTION OF CHOLINERGIC ACTIVITY IN HUMAN BRAIN

[11]C-choline was initially used in PET studies to visualize ^{11}C-acetylcholine synthesis and cholinergic activity in human brain.[4] The efforts were hampered by the low penetration of ^{11}C-choline to brain and the rapid conversion of formed ^{11}C-acetylcholine to other radiolabeled metabolites. An alternative to study transmitter precursor transport would be to measure uptake and binding of labeled receptor ligands in brain. This strategy has been tried for the cholinergic receptors both in animal and man.

Attempts to detect cholinergic nicotinic receptors using ^{11}C-nicotine and PET was initially performed in monkeys[5] and later in humans.[6,7] When ^{11}C-nicotine is injected intravenously to healthy non-smoking volunteers the regional distribution of ^{11}C-radioactivity in brain, measured by PET, agrees fairly well with the distribution of nicotinic receptors measured by *in vitro* binding techinques in autopsy brain tissues.[8] Thus the uptake of ^{11}C-nicotine is high in brain regions as the thalamus, caudate nucleus, putamen, intermediate in the frontal, temporal cortices, cerebellum and low in white matter. The time course of ^{11}C-nicotine in brain differ from the time course observed for the blood flow marker ^{11}C-butanol. Calculation of kinetic constants for ^{11}C-nicotine indicate a binding profile for the compound in brain.[9]

Visualization of muscarinic receptors has been performed in human brain by PET and labeled ligands such as ^{11}C-benztropine[10,11]C-tropanyl benzilate[11] and ^{11}C-scopolamine.[12] [121]I-quinuclidinyl-4-iodobenzilate has been used for tracing muscarinic receptors in human brain with SPECT.[12,13] An age-related decrease in the muscarinic receptors in healthy individuals measured by PET was reported by Dewey *et al.*[10] The findings agree with observations made in postmortem brain tissues.[14]

VISUALIZATION OF NICOTINIC RECEPTORS IN ALZHEIMER BRAINS

Neurochemical studies in postmortem brain tissue from AD patients have revealed consistent marked losses of cortical nicotinic receptors.[8] Furthermore, changes have been measured in the proportion of subtypes of nicotinic receptors in AD brains compared to controls.[8] In attempts to confirm these *in vitro* data *in vivo* PET studies with ^{11}C-nicotine have been performed in AD patients at different stage of the disease. A significant lower uptake of ^{11}C-nicotine to the frontal and temporal cortices was found in AD patients compared to controls.[7] A significant positive correlation is found between cognitive function (Mini-Mental State Examination Score) and uptake of (S)($-$)-^{11}C-nicotine to the temporal cortex of AD brains.[15] Interestingly, a lower uptake of (R)($+$)-^{11}C-nicotine compared to (S)($-$)-^{11}C-nicotine has been noticed in AD patients.[7,9] The two enantiomers of nicotine are known from *in vitro* binding studies to preferentially bind to two different types of nicotinic binding sites in brain.[16] The *in vivo* findings might thus indicate changes in the nicotinic receptor properties in AD. Interestingly, the difference in uptake between the two enantiomers of nicotine can be observed early in the progression of AD[9] and is normalized by tacrine treatment (see below).

VISUALIZATION OF MUSCARINIC RECEPTORS IN ALZHEIMER BRAINS

Numerous studies in postmortem brain tissue indicate a preservation of the muscarinic receptors in AD.[3] This observation is different from the consistent losses in nicotinic receptors and other presynaptic cholinergic markers reported in AD. Studies of muscarinic receptors using SPECT, in a limited number of AD patients, have shown relatively preserved muscarinic receptors.[13,17,18] No PET data concerning muscarinic receptors in AD patients have so far been published. We are presently working on this topic, using ^{11}C-benztropine as muscarinic receptor ligand, with special emphasis on the effect of tacrine treatment to AD patients.

EFFECT OF TACRINE TREATMENT ON NICOTINIC RECEPTORS IN AD

The moderately long-acting cholinesterase inhibitor tacrine (THA) has been tested in several treatment studies performed in AD patients. In a recent study of 468 AD patients, improvements were reported after 12 weeks of treatment as recognized by cognitive measures and ratings performed by the physicians and caregivers.[19] We have experience of tacrine treatment in five AD patients who have been treated with 80 to 160 mg daily for 3 up to 27 months and followed by PET investigations. Two of the AD patients had moderate dementia while the other three had mild dementia. The AD patients has been followed by repeated PET investigations as well as neuropsychological testings during tacrine treatment. The PET studies involve a multitracer system consisting of $(S)(-)$- and $(R)(+)$-^{11}C-nicotine (nicotinic receptors), ^{18}F-fluoro-deoxy-glucose (^{18}F-FDG)(glucose metabolism), ^{11}C-butanol (blood flow) and in some patients also ^{11}C-benztropine (muscarinic receptors). Tacrine treatment has been found to increase the uptake of ^{11}C-nicotine to the brain. A small difference in uptake between the enantiomers $(R)(+)$- and $(S)(-)$-^{11}C-nicotine was observed in the frontal and temporal cortex of AD patient after 3 months of tacrine treatment compared to before start of treatment.[9] Kinetic analysis indicate increased binding of ^{11}C-nicotine in brain compatible with a restoration of nicotinic receptors in brain. Increase in glucose utilization have been observed after 3 months of tacrine treatment. Changes in PET data obtained after tacrine treatment are paralleled by improvement in neuropsychological performance, especially in AD patients with mild dementia. In a 70-year-old AD patient with mild dementia, the restoration of nicotinic receptors and glucose metabolism seen after 3 months of treatment still persists after 27 months of tacrine treatment. These PET studies show *in vivo* induction of neurochemical effects in brain by treatment with tacrine to AD patients. Intervention with tacrine in the early course of the disease might be necessary for significant clinical improvement.

EFFECT OF NGF TREATMENT ON NICOTINIC RECEPTORS IN AD

On the basis of animal studies suggesting that nerve growth factor (NGF) can stimulate central cholinergic neurons, infusion of NGF has been performed into the brain of an AD patient.[20] The AD patient was a 69-year-old woman with moderate dementia and symptoms for 8 years. Intraventricular infusion of 6.6 mg NGF for 3 months resulted in a marked transient increase in uptake and binding of $(S)(-)$-^{11}C-nicotine in the frontal and temporal cortex.[20] An increase in the cortical blood flow, measured by ^{11}C-butanol, still persisted 3 months after the end of NGF treatment. An improvement in verbal episodic memory was observed after 1 month of treatment whereas no improvement was observed in other cognitive tests. The result of this study indicate that NGF treatment may counteract cholinergic deficits in AD patients. Further trials of NGF infusion are now planned in AD patients.

REFERENCES

1. McKann, G., D. Drachman, M. Folstein, R. Katzman, D. Prince & E. M. Stadlan. 1984. Clinical diagnosis of Alzheimer's disease: Report of the NINCDS-ADRDA Work Group under the auspices at the Department of Health and Human Services Task Force on Alzheimer's disease. Neurology **34:** 939–944.
2. Hardy, J., R. Adolfsson, I. Alafuzoff, G. Bucht, J. Marcusson, P. Nyberg, E. Perdahl, P. Wester & B. Winblad. 1985. Transmitter deficits in Alzheimer's disease. Neurochem. Int. **7:**545–573.
3. Nordberg, A. 1992. Neuroreceptor changes in Alzheimer disease. Cerebrovasc. Brain Metab. Rev **4:**303–328.
4. Gauthier, S., M. Diksic, L. Yamamoto, J. Tyler & W. Feindel. 1985. Positron emission tomography with ^{11}C-choline in human subjects. Can. J Neurol. Sci. **12:**214.
5. Nordberg, A., P. Hartvig, H. Lundqvist, G. Antoni, J. Ulin & B. Långström. 1989. Uptake and regional distribution of $(+)(R)$- and $(-)(S)$-methyl-^{11}C-nicotine in brain of rhesus monkey—an attempt to study nicotinic receptors *in vivo*. J. Neural Transm. (P-D Sect.) **2:**215–224.
6. Nybäck, H., A. Nordberg, B. Långström, C. Halldin, P. Hartvig, A. Åhlin, C. G. Swahn & G. Sedvall. 1989. Attempts to visualize nicotinic receptors in the brain of monkey and man by positron emission tomography. Progr. Brain Res. **79:**313–319.
7. Nordberg, A., P. Hartvig, A. Lilja, M. Viitanen, K. Amberla, H. Lundqvist, T. Andersson, J. Ulin, B. Winblad & B. Långström. 1990. Decreased uptake and binding of ^{11}C-nicotine in the brain of Alzheimer patients as visualized by positron emission tomography. J Neural Transm. (P-D Sect.) **2:** 215–224.

8. NORDBERG, A., L. NILSSON-HÅKANSSON, A. ADEM, J. HARDY, I. ALAFUZOFF, Z. LAI, M. HERRERA-MARSCHITZ & B. WINBLAD. 1989. The role of the nicotinic receptors in the pathophysiology of Alzheimer's disease. Progr. Brain Res. **79:**353–362.

9. NORDBERG, A., A. LILJA, H. LUNDQVIST, P. HARTVIG, K. AMBERLA, M. VIITANEN, U. WARPMAN, M. JOHANSSSON, E. HELLSTRÖM-LINDAHL, P. BJURLING, K. J. FASTH, B. LÅNGSTRÖM & B. WINBLAD. 1992. Tacrine restores cholinertic nicotinic receptors and glucose metabolism in Alzheimer patients as visualized by positron emission tomography. Neurobiol. Aging **13:**747–758.

10. DEWEY, S. L., N. D. VILKOW, J. LOGAN, R. R. MACGREGOR, J. S. FOWLER, D. J. SCHLYER & B. BENDRIEM. 1990. Age-related decrease in muscarinic cholinergic receptor binding in the human brain measured with positron emission tomography (PET). J. Neurosci. Res. **27:**569–575.

11. FREY, K. A., R. A. KOEPPE, G. K. MULHOLLAND & D. E. KUHL. 1990. Quantification of regional cerebral muscarinic receptors with the use of [C-^{11}[tropanyl benzilate and positron emission tomography. J. Nucl. Med. **31:**779.

12. FREY, K. A., R. A. KOEPPE, G. K. MULHOLLAND, D. JEWETT, R. HICHWA, R. L. E. EHRENKAUFER, J. E. CAREY, D. E. WIELAND, D. E. KUHL & B. W. AGRANOFF. 1992. In vivo muscarinic cholinergic receptor imaging in human brain with [^{11}C]scopolamine and positron emission tomography. J. Cereb. Blood Flow Metab. **12:**147–154.

13. HOLLMAN, B. L., R. E. GIBSON, T. C. HILL, W. C. ECKELMAN, M. ALBERT & R. C. REBZ. 1985. Muscarinic acetylcholine receptors in Alzheimer's disease-*in vivo* imaging with iodine ^{123}I-labelled-1-quinuclidinyl-4-iodobenzilate and emission tomography. JAMA **254:**3063–3066.

14. NORDBERG, A., I. ALAFUZOFF & B. WINBLAD. 1992. Nicotinic and muscarinic subtypes in the human brain: Changes with aging and dementia. J. Neurosci. Res. **31:**103–111.

15. NORDBERG, A., P. HARTVIG, A. LILJA, H. LUNDQVIST, U. WARPMAN, J. ULIN, B. LÅNGSTRÖM, K. AMBERLA, M. VIITANEN & B. WINBLAD. 1991. Nicotinic receptors in the CNS as visualized by positron emission tomography. *In* Cholinergic Basis for Alzheimer Therapy. K. Becker & E. Giacobini, Eds. 107–115. Boston. Birkhäuser.

16. COPELAND, J. R., A. ADEM, P. JACOB III & A. NORDBERG. 1991. A comparison of the binding of nicotine and nornicotine stereoisomers to nicotinic binding sites in rat brain cortex. Naunyn-Schmiedeberg's Arch. Pharmacol. **343:** 123–127.

17. WEINBERGER, D. R., R. E. GIBSON, R. COPPOLA, D. W. JONES, A. R. BRAUN, U. MANN, K. F. BERMAN, T. SUNDERLAND, T. N. CHASE & R. C. REBA 1989. Distribution of muscarinic receptors in patients with dementia: A controlled study of ^{123}I-QNB and SPECT. J. Cereb. Blood Flow Metab. **9:**(Suppl. 1, S): 537.

18. WYPER, D., J. OWENS, D. BROWN, J. PATTERSON, W. WATSON, R. HUNTER & J. MCCULLOCH. 1992. Abnormalities in cerebral muscarinic acetylcholine receptors measured in-vivo with SPECT in patients with Alzheimer's disease. Neurobiol. Aging **13:**(Suppl. 1, S):23.

19. FARLOW, M., S. I. GRACON, L. A. HERSHEY, K. W. LEWIS, C. H. SADOWSKY & J. A. DOLAN-URENO. 1992. A controlled trial of tacrine in Alzheimer's disease. JAMA **268:**2523-2529.

20. OLSON, L., A. NORDBERG, H. VON HOLST, L. BÄCKMAN, T. EBENDAL, I. ALAFUZOFF, I. AMBERLA, P. HARTVIG, A. HERLITZ, A. LILJA, H. LUNDQVIST, B. LÅNGSTRÖM, B. MEYERSSON, A. PERSSON, M. VIITANEN, B. WINBLAD & A. SEIGER. 1992. Nerve growth factor affects ^{11}C-nicotine binding, blood flow, EEG, and verbal episodic memory in an Alzheimer patient. J Neural Transm. (P-D, Sect.) **4:**79–95.

Hyperactivation of Signal Transduction Systems in Alzheimer's Disease[a]

TSUNAO SAITOH[b], KAREN HORSBURGH, AND ELIEZER MASLIAH

Department of Neurosciences, 0624, University of California/San Diego, La Jolla, California 92093-0624 USA

ABSTRACT: A compromise or deregulation in signal transduction cascades could adversely affect cellular functions and possibly contribute to cell death. In recent years, it has become increasingly apparent that pronounced activation of neuronal signal transduction systems is a characteristic of AD brain. There is evidence that signal transduction systems play a role in the formation or development of these pathological features of AD. Aberrant activity and localization of components of signaling mechanisms (growth factors, their receptors, protein kinases, phosphoprotein phosphatases, and phosphoproteins) are closely associated with the intracellular accumulation of PHF, the extracellular deposition of amyloid, and the formation of neuritic plaques in AD brain. In particular, immunohistochemical studies reveal increased levels of neuronal staining for APP, possibly an important growth factor in AD, both in frontal cortex and hippocampus. Anti-APP immunostaining is also associated with the neuritic component of plaques. Additionally, PKC(βII) immunostaining is increased in the neuronal cell body and neuropil of AD samples, particularly in association with plaques, suggesting a postsynaptic involvement of this enzyme. On the other hand, PKC(βI) immunostaining is associated with axonal staining particularly in the sprouting neurites of plaques. Sprouting neuritic components of plaques are immunopositive with other growth-associated proteins, such as GAP43, MARCKS, and spectrin. Immunoreactivity of other members of signal transduction systems such as Fos and stathmin are all increased in AD hippocampal neurons. On the other hand, several protein kinases and phosphoproteins were immunolocalized to tangles. Thus, the hyperactivation and dysfunction of signal transduction systems could be involved in the pathogenesis of AD.

[a] We have been funded by National Institutes of Health grants AG05131, AG08201, AG08205, and AG10689.

[b] *Send correspondence to:* Dr. Tsunao Saitoh, Department of Neurosciences, 0624, University of California/San Diego, La Jolla, CA 92093-0624 USA; TEL: (619) 534-2545; FAX: (619) 534-5569.

HYPERACTIVATION OF SIGNAL TRANSDUCTION SYSTEMS AS A PATHOLOGICAL FEATURE IN ALZHEIMER'S DISEASE: AN HYPOTHESIS

Many molecules of signal transduction systems are altered in AD. Interestingly, they show the signs of potential hyperactivation instead of hypoactivation. Therefore, neuronal death in AD is unlikely to be the result of a general deterioration in cellular activity. In fact, recent experimental data have established the concept that hyperactivation of components of signal transduction is involved in many cases of cell death. Two of the best studied cases for this type of cell death are excitatory amino acid-induced neuronal death and apoptosis or activation-induced cell death.[1] In both cases, it was shown that the inhibition of activation of signal transduction pathways, especially Ca^{2+}/lipid/PKC cascades, prevents the process of cell death. Although in AD there is no direct evidence for the involvement of glutamate-induced neuronal cell death, the presence of excessive amounts of growth factors or their receptors has been well established. Signals induced by these growth factors are mediated by signal transducing proteins, such as protein kinases, phosphoprotein phosphatases, and their substrate proteins that are shown to be altered in their localization and concentration in AD. These growth factors include interleukin-1, FGF, EGF, and APP. Since APP or its fragments play a central role in the pathogenesis of AD, this hypothetical involvement of APP might also be implicated in neuronal death in AD. Excessive activation of signal transduction systems in AD may also be due to altered energy metabolism in AD, possibly because of mitochondrial malfunction.[2] Energy metabolism in cells is required to maintain high ATP levels and the gradient of ions across the membrane. Failure to do so induces an inflow of Ca^{2+} into the cytoplasm, causing excessive activation of signal transduction systems. Experimentally, the inhibition of mitochondrial function by uncouplers and glucose deprivation in culture medium induces some AD-associated markers, notably the overphosphorylation of cytoskeletal proteins in cultured cells (see Barger *et al.*, this volume).

It is hypothesized that the characteristic neuropathology in AD can be explained by alterations of signal transduction systems. Increased protein kinase activity, triggered by environmental (*e.g.*, head trauma, ischemia, hypoxia) and genetic (*e.g.*, altered APP) factors may, through protein phosphorylation, alter APP levels, metabolism, or compartmentalization. The normal clearance of β/A4-peptide will be disrupted leading to amyloid deposition and ultimately neuritic plaque formation. In parallel, increased kinase activity, possibly one of MAP kinases via tyrosine kinase phosphorylation, may abnormally phosphorylate cytoskeletal proteins, ultimately leading to the formation of PHF and, in addition, causing a breakdown in the cytoskeleton leading to neuronal death. Hyperactivation of protein kinases may also induce the altered phosphorylation of nuclear proteins, such as Fos causing altered gene expression, and possibly induce some built-in molecular mechanism that is similar to apoptosis. Thus, in this model, the senile plaques and amyloid are not considered to be a cause of dementia, although this possibility is not excluded.

APP, A GROWTH FACTOR, MIGHT BE INVOLVED IN NEURONAL HYPERACTIVATION

To date, the causal involvement of growth factor alterations in AD pathogenesis is controversial. On the other hand, recent studies on neurotrophic factors have suggested a "hypertrophic" aspect of AD alterations. In AD, bFGF levels are markedly elevated in neurons and are also found to be elevated in association with neuritic plaques. AD is further characterized by increased levels of cortical β-NGF. Reduction in growth inhibitory factor (GIF) in AD brain might contribute to an increase in neurotrophic activity leading to aberrant sprouting and eventual neuronal death. Importantly, recent studies have indicated that the normal function of APP is as a neurotrophic agent (see Roch *et al.*, this volume). Thus, alteration of APP and/or the production of smaller active fragments of APP itself may accentuate aberrant sprouting and eventual death in AD brain.

The extracellular domain of APP can be phosphorylated and this may alter the trafficking of APP (see Gandy *et al.*, this volume). The expression of APP mRNA can also be regulated by PKC (see Beyreuther *et al.*, this volume). Although the physiological significance of these alterations of APP by kinases and protein phosphorylation in relation to plaque formation is unclear, it is noteworthy that they are able to modulate several aspects of APP biology. Many growth factors, such as NGF, bFGF, EGF, and cytokines can also regulate APP expression, secretion, and splicing pattern through transduction mechanisms (see Nitsch *et al.*, this volume). Studies which address the processing of APP and the mechanism of β/A4 deposition will more clearly define the molecular basis of plaque formation (see Golde *et al.* and Haass *et al.*, this volume).

Alternatively APP, as a growth factor, may directly regulate the state of the intracellular signal transduction machinery in neuronal cells. In other words, alterations in APP may be primarily responsible for aberrant signal transduction in AD. Our semiquantitative immunohistochemical analysis has demonstrated increased APP immunostaining in hippocampal and neocortical pyramidal neurons and in the neuritic component of plaques.[3] Molecular components of transduction systems, such as the kinase substrates spectrin and GAP43, are also found in association with dystrophic neurites. Double-immunolabeling has demonstrated the colocalization of APP in GAP43-immunoreactive sprouting neurites in plaques. Other growth factors are also associated with plaque pathology in AD; the EGF receptor is increased in the neuritic component of plaques whereas bFGF is concentrated in amyloid, possibly by its binding to HSPG. Thus, there is evidence for an important role of signal transduction mechanisms in mediating the neuronal sprouting in AD brain and formation of neuritic plaques.

HYPERACTIVATION OF SIGNAL TRANSDUCTION SYSTEMS SUGGESTED BY PROTEIN KINASES (PKC, CKII, PTK, AND Cdc2)

The alterations in protein kinases and their substrates in AD are potentially involved in the formation of neuritic plaques and neurofibillary tangles. Studies of PKC might be particularly relevant because it is centrally involved in modulating many aspects of synaptic plasticity and neuronal survival. Analysis of four PKC isoforms—α, βI, βII, and γ—demonstrated the complexity of the individual involvement of these isoforms in AD pathology.[1] Immunohistochemical analysis of PKC(βII) staining revealed that, in the frontal cortex of AD brain, neuronal staining was diminished in number and intensity. On the other hand, in the hippocampus of AD brain, neuronal staining by anti-PKC(βII) of CA3–CA4 was more intense than controls. Although similar alterations were observed for PKC(α) and – (βI), they were not as great as those for PKC(βII). In contrast, the concentration and distribution of PKC(γ) was unaltered in AD brain. Of further interest was the differential staining patterns of each PKC isoform in neuritic plaques. Whereas anti-PKC(α) stained entire plaques and the surrounding glial cells, anti-PKC(βI) stained dystrophic plaque neurites, and anti-PKC(βII) stained neuronal membrane apposed to amyloid. Thus, the different isoforms are selectively altered to varying degrees in AD brain and are possibly involved at different stages of AD pathogenesis. Most importantly one of these PKC isoforms, PKC(βII), colocalized with diffuse plaques. Staining by anti-PKC(α), – (βI), and – (γ) was not detected in diffuse plaques. Diffuse plaques are thought to be an early stage of plaque formation. Thus, PKC(βII) may be involved in the early pathological changes in AD. This is supported by the finding that in the cortex of clinically nondemented individuals with diffuse plaques, PKC(βII) levels and the *in vitro* phosphorylation of an endogenous substrate (P86 or MARCKS) are reduced.

Anti-PKC(βII) immunostained the cortical neuropil. The intensity of this immunostaining is altered in AD in a characteristic fashion depending on the proximity to the plaques.[1] The anti-PKC(βII) immunostaining of the neuropil is reduced outside plaques. However, within the diffuse plaques, the anti-PKC(βII) immunoreactivity is elevated. This increased anti-PKC(βII) staining is more pronounced in mature plaques. Although, the high intensity of anti-PKC(βII) immunolabeling does not necessarily indicate a high activity, these results are compatible with the hypothesis that neuronal hyperactivation may be involved in AD neuropathology. Here, to avoid confusion, it is important to note that neuronal cell bodies and their processes in diffuse plaques, and the neuropil (dendrites) as representative of postsynaptic structures are positive with anti-PKC(βII) whereas sprouting neurities (axons) in mature neuritic plaques are positive with anti-PKC(βI) but are not positive with anti-PKC(βII).

While PKC is associated with plaques, another protein kinase, casein kinase II (CKII) is associated with tangles. Anti-CKII immunoreactivity is decreased in non–tangle-bearing neurons of AD frontal cortex compared to normal frontal cortex whereas NFT are strongly stained with anti-CKII.[1] Unlike neocortex, the immunoreactivity is increased in AD hippocampal neurons as was also found in anti-PKC immunoreactivity. Anti-CKII immunoreactivity seems to precede increased accumulation of τ-like immunoreactivity in AD hippocampal neurons. In the AD hippocampus, CKII immunoreactivity is increased both in non–tangle-bearing neurons and tangle-bearing neurons. At the ultrastructural level, anti-CKII was diffusely distributed throughout the cytoplasm of non–tangle-bearing neurons and immunolocalized to PHF in tangle-bearing neurons.[4] The elevated levels of anti-CKII immunoreactivity in neurons vulnerable to PHF neuropathology suggest that neuronal hyperactivation might be involved in the NFT formation.

In AD brain, the activity of protein tyrosine kinases which are of central importance in cellular growth and survival is reduced in the particulate fraction. Yet, in the cytosolic fraction, although there is no change in protein tyrosine kinase activity, the levels of two anti-phosphotyrosine-positive protein bands (55, 60 kDa) are elevated.[1] The function and identity of these bands are yet to be determined. Immunohistochemical techniques have demonstrated an increased anti-phosphotyrosine staining in tangle-bearing neurons as well as in the dystrophic neurities. Thus, altered tyrosine kinases and phosphorylation closely parallel AD pathology.

Although there are many kinases, the elucidation of the majority of their involvement in AD brain pathology awaits clarification. A class of novel protein kinases has recently been identified and may warrant further attention in AD. During the course of our study to identify protein kinases which may be responsible for neuronal hyperactivation in AD, we found that extracts prepared from AD brain contain more "histone kinase" activity than those from control brains. Because a major histone kinase in cultured cells is cdc2 kinase, we quantified anti-cdc2 immunoreactive protein and found that their levels are elevated in AD. More importantly, in the same samples, the levels of this kinase had a positive correlation with the number of NFT. It is interesting to note that τ proteins associated with NFT are excessively phosphorylated at the site preceding proline, which is the site recognized by this cdc2 kinase and MAP kinases (see Mandelkow *et al.*, this volume). Because there are many proline-directed protein kinases, it is premature to draw a definite picture as to the protein kinases involved in NFT formation. It is safe to conclude, however, that AD neurons which develop NFT are hyperactive and contain more protein kinases relative to neurons in normal individuals.

HYPERACTIVATION OF SIGNAL TRANSDUCTION SYSTEMS SUGGESTED BY PHOSPHORYLATION SUBSTRATES (GAP43, FOS, STATHMIN, AND SPECTRIN)

The binding of growth factors or neurotransmitters to receptors activates protein kinases which ultimately leads to protein phosphorylation. There are several phosphoproteins that may be relevant for the consideration of hyperactivation and synaptic pathology in AD.

GAP43, a growth-associated phosphoprotein, is a subtrate for PKC and CKII. Although the exact cellular function(s) of GAP43 is not yet known, the levels of this protein are markedly elevated during axogenesis and in postinjury regeneration, suggesting a functional role for GAP43 in growth and development. In AD neocortex, the levels of GAP43 are reduced, whereas in hippocampal regions and particularly in areas associated with sprouting, such as the periphery of neuritic plaques, GAP43 immunoreactivity is elevated as has been shown for PKC(βI) and CKII.[5]

Fos is a transcriptional factor phosphorylated by PKC. Because its gene location is close to the newly found FAD mutation site on chromosome 14, interest in this protein in AD research has been renewed. Similar to PKC, the levels of Fos are found to be increased in AD hippocampal neurons. Again, we do not know the precise role of this protein in AD pathogenesis. It is interesting to note, however, that Fos is induced in many cases of neuronal injury. Since head trauma and myocardial infarct are risk factors of AD, it is tempting to speculate that Fos plays an important role in the neuronal hyperactivation and degeneration in AD. Because the APP promoter contains Fos/Jun binding site, Fos could be responsible for elevated APP transcription in these pathological cases.

Brain spectrin, a substrate of CKII, is primarily located in presynaptic boutons. The levels of spectrin are reduced in AD particulate fractions whereas in the cytosolic fraction an increase is detected in the breakdown product of spectrin possibly derived from calpain-mediated degradation. Immunolocalization of spectrin in AD cortex demonstrated an increased staining in areas of neurodegeneration and synapse pathology. Alterations in CKII in AD brain may be related to the abnormal spectrin distribution and levels in AD.[1,3]

One phosphoprotein worth discussing here is stathmin. Stathmin has been identified as a protein which is phosphorylated when neuronal cells are stimulated by various growth factors.[6] It is a major substrate for cAMP-dependent protein kinase, and plays a pivotal role in intracellular signal transductions.

Thus, stathmin provides a good marker for cellular activation. The phosphorylation state of stathmin, as determined by the technique of back phosphorylation revealed a highly significant decrease in AD frontal cortex, whereas the mRNA level is increased. This finding differs from that of other proteins, such as GAP43 and Fos, in that the sign of stathmin elevation is found not only in hippocampus but also in neocortex.

CONCLUSION

In this communication, we have developed an hypothesis that is summarized as "hyperactivation-induced pathogenesis in AD." This hypothesis is based on the many signs of hyperactivation of neurons in AD as listed in TABLE 1. There are two aspects of this hypothesis. First, in AD, neuritic pathology is associated with pronounced sprouting reactions which are associated with proteins such as PKC(βI), GAP43, APP, and spectrin. These changes are most remarkable in AD hippocampus. The second aspect of our hypothesis does not specifically involve plaque neurites. Increased levels of PKC(βII), Fos, stathmin, spectrin, phosphotyrosine, and APP are found in neuronal cell bodies and often in AD frontal cortex. In this hypothesis, APP is proposed to be a growth factor. Alterations in APP in AD may trigger cellular hyperactivation. These features are reminiscent of programmed cell death, apoptosis, which is triggered by excessive activation of cellular signal

TABLE 1. Alteration of Molecules of Signal Transduction in AD

Markers	Neocortex	Hippocampus	Plaque Association	Tangle Association
PKC(βI)	↓	↑	+	−
PKC(βII)	↓	↑	+	−
CKII	↓	↑	+	+
Cdc2	↑	↑	−	+
GAP43	↓	↑	+	−
Fos	↓	↑	−	−
Stathmin	↑	↑	−	+
Spectrin	↑	↑	+	−
APP	↑	↑	+	−
PTyr	↑	↑	+	+

Arrows in the table indicate the alteration of the intensity of neuronal cell body immunostaining for each molecular marker. It should be noted that neuropil staining or Western blot staining does not necessarily follow this pattern of change. Plaque association indicates the sprouting neurite (axon) staining except for PKC(βII) that stains cell body and processes (dendrites) aposed to amyloid in plaques. Tangle association indicates the tangle immunostaining except for stathmin that is immunodetected in tau-positive (as tangle marker) neurons without colocalization with tangles.

transduction systems. As yet, the relevance of this idea to AD neurodegeneration awaits future verification.

ACKNOWLEDGMENTS

We thank Robert Davignon and Isabelle Hafner for editorial help in preparing this paper.

REFERENCES

1. SAITOH, T., E. MASLIAH, L-W. JIN, G. M. COLE, T. WIELOCH & I. P. SHAPIRO. 1991. Biology of disease. Protein kinase and phosphorylation in neurologic disorders and cell death. Lab. Invest. **64:**596–616.
2. BLASS, J. P. & G. E. GIBSON. 1991. The role of oxidative abnormalities in the pathophysiology of Alzheimer's disease. Rev. Neurol. **147:**513–525.
3. MASLIAH, E., M. MALLORY, N. GE & T. SAITOH. 1992. Protein kinases and growth associated proteins in plaque formation in Alzheimer's disease. Rev. Neurosci. **3:**99–107.
4. MASLIAH, E., D. S. IIMOTO, M. MALLORY, T. ALBRIGHT, L. HANSEN & T. SAITOH. 1992. Casein kinase II alteration precedes tau accumulation in tangle formation. Am. J. Pathol. **140:**263–268.
5. MASLIAH, E., M. MALLORY, L. HANSEN, M. ALFORD, R. DeTERESA, R. TERRY, J. BAUDIER & T. SAITOH. 1992. Localization of amyloid precursor protein in GAP-43 immunoreactive aberrant sprouting neurities in Alzheimer's disease. Brain Res. **574:**312–316.
6. SOBEL, A. 1991. Stathmin: A relay phosphoprotein for multiple signal transduction? Trends Biochem. Sci. **16:**301–305.

Changes in G Protein-mediated Signal Transduction in Aging and Alzheimer's Disease

J. A. JOSEPH,[a] R. CUTLER, AND G. S. ROTH

Gerontology Research Center, NIA/NIH, Baltimore, Maryland 21224 USA

ABSTRACT: Previous reports have shown that there are age-related reductions in muscarinic receptor (mAChR) sensitivity to agonist stimulation. Our research has elucidated the mechanisms involved in this loss. These studies have shown that this decline is the result of decreases in mAChR concentration, reductions in the number of neuronal cells, and altered phosphoinositide (PI)-mediated signal transduction (ST). The decrements in PI-mediated ST are observed as a reduced ability of muscarinic (m) agonists to enhance K^+-evoked release of DA (K^+ERDA) from striatal slices from old rats. Additional experiments indicated that the locus of the ST deficits appears to be at the mAChR-G protein interface, since attempts to bypass this interface reduced m-enhanced K^+ERDA deficits in the striata from old rats. Moreover, it appears that the ability of mAChR to decouple from their respective G proteins is reduced as a function of age, since carbachol-stimulated low K_M GTPase activity was found to be reduced in hippocampal and striatal tissue obtained from old rats. Similar findings were observed in this parameter in AD hippocampus and basal ganglia. Further reductions were seen in carbachol-stimulated low K_M GTPase as a function of the duration of the disease. Results are discussed in terms of structural membrane alterations in aging and disease that may lead to reductions in the efficacy of receptor-G protein coupling/uncoupling.

INTRODUCTION

We have been examining the nature of the loss in muscarinic agonist stimulation that occurs during normal aging and is exaggerated in AD. The results of this work indicate that this loss may be the result of altered neuronal signal transduction in the phosphoinositide (PI) system. Beginning at the first step in signal transduction processing, the ligand-receptor interface, we have shown that the decrements in responsiveness of central cholinergic systems to stimulation in senescent rats are the result of decreases in muscarinic receptor (mAChR) concentrations[1] without corresponding decreases in mRNA concentrations.[2] In addition, this decrement in responsiveness is the result of an

[a] *Send correspondence to:* Dr. J. A. Jospeh, Gerontology Research Center INIA/NIH, 4940 Eastern Avenue, Baltimore, MD 21224 USA; TEL: 410-558-8178; FAX: 410-558-8323.

age-related reduction in the processing and transducing of a signal that begins upon the stimulation of the mAChR and proceeds through several steps to activate Ca^{2+}. These deficits appear to be quite specific, such that if the receptor is bypassed and signal transduction activated at later points in the pathway, the age deficit in PI responsiveness disappears.[3] Further investigations described below indicate that these alterations are the result of structural changes (*e.g.,* fluidity) in receptor-containing membranes that lead to decrements in receptor-G protein coupling/uncoupling and that these deficits are also observed in AD brains. These findings could explain the failure of cholinergic replacement therapies to improve cognitive function in AD and senescence, since increases in the ACh availability would not result in improvements in mAChR-G protein coupling/uncoupling. They suggest that future therapeutic efforts to restore cognitive function should focus on elucidating membrane structural alterations and enhancing subsequent steps in signal transduction.

mAChR-G PROTEIN COUPLING/UNCOUPLING

G proteins are composed of three subunits, α, β, and γ. The binding of an agonist to the receptor facilitates an exchange of GTP for GDP on the α subunit in the presence of Mg^{2+}. The activated α_{GTP} subunit dissociates from $\beta\gamma$ subunits to interact with effectors such as phospholipase C. An intrinsic low K_M GTPase activity of the α subunit hydrolyzes GTP to GDP to end the activation cycle. Assessment of carbachol-stimulated low K_M GTPase is, therefore, a direct method of assessing the receptor-G protein coupling/uncoupling efficacy. In our initial experiment[4] we examined low K_M GTPase activity in crude membrane preparations in the hippocampi and striata obtained from rats 6 and 24 months of age (and analyzed according to the methods of Cassel and Selinger 5). The results indicated that there was an approximately 40% decline in carbachol-stimulated low K_M GTPase activity (delta G activity in pmoles/mg protein) in the old rats at each carbachol concentration (10^{-3}–10^{-5}). In a subsequent experiment we examined this parameter in human brain tissue obtained from the Institute for Biogerontology, Sun City, Arizona (mean ages: young-51.4 $\pm$ 15.9 years; aged-75.4 $\pm$ 4.7 years; AD-77.8 $\pm$ 4.8 years. The tissue was shipped in dry ice and maintained at $-70°C$ until the membranes were prepared. Results showed that there were significant reductions in carbachol-stimulated low-K_M GTPase activity in the basal ganglia in aged (40%) and AD (75% at 10^{-3} carbachol). Similar trends were observed in the hippocampal tissue. However, perhaps the most striking findings were that there were significant negative correlations between disease duration and carbachol-stimulated low K_M GTPase activity in both the basal ganglia ($r = -0.833, p < 0.05$) and hippocampus (r $= -0.70$, $p < 0.05$). This finding may be important, since it is the first time that a change seen in this devastating disease has also been observed in a normal aged rodent. The finding suggests that there may be at least some aspects of synaptic transmission that show similar changes in the aged rodent and human and are exaggerated in AD. If this is the case, it might be important to ask what common mechanism might exist among these species and conditions that would produce such similar alterations in coupling? One hypothesis is described in the next section.

ALTERATIONS IN MEMBRANE FLUIDITY

Our present working hypothesis is that this loss of responsiveness mAChR may be the result of changes in membrane structure (*e.g.*, fluidity). Using a striatal slice superfusion system in which we assessed oxotremorine enhancement of K^+-ERDA release, we have been able to increase mAChR sensitivity in tissue from old animals by over 200% when the slices were preincubated in *S*-adenosyl-L-methionine (SAM). Conversely, mAChR sensitivity in striatal tissue from young animals can be decreased to below baseline (*i.e.*, HiKCl alone) by preincubation the slices with cholesterol (CHO). Determinations of membrane viscosity by fluorescence depolarization using 1,6-diphenyl 1,3,5-hexatriene (DPH) indicated that striatal membranes obtained from young animals were more fluid than those from old and that SAM exposure significantly increased fluidity in the striatal membranes prepared from the old animals. Exposure to CHO had the opposite effects, but only in young animals. Indeed, in a subsequent preliminary study, these procedures also respectively increased and decreased low KM GTPase activity, suggesting that alterations in the structural integrity of the receptor-containing membranes may alter receptor-G protein interactions. Additional investigations have suggested that these age-related membrane alterations may be the consequence of oxidative damage. These considerations are being examined further.

REFERENCES

1. BLAKE, M. J., N. M. APPEL, J. A. JOSEPH, C. A. STAGG, M. ANSON, E. B. DE SOUZA & G. S. ROTH. 1991. Muscarinic acetylcholine receptor subtype mRNA expression and ligand binding in the aged rat brain. Neurobiol. Aging **12:** 193–199.
2. YAMAGAMI, K., J. A. JOSEPH & G. S. ROTH. 1991. Muscarinic receptor concentrations and dopamine release in aged rat striata. Neurobiol. Aging **13:**51–56.
3. JOSEPH, J. A., T. K. DALTON, G. S. ROTH & W. A. HUNT. 1988. Alterations

in muscarinic control of striatal dopamine, autoreceptors in senescence: A deficit at the ligand-muscarinic receptor interface. Brain Res. **454:**149–155.

4. YAMAGAMI, K., J. A. JOSEPH & G. S. ROTH. 1992. Decrement of muscarinic receptor-low K_M GTPase in striatum from the aged rat. Brain Res. **576:**327–331.
5. CASSEL, D. & Z. SELINGER. 1976. Catecholamine-stimulated GTPase activity in turkey erythrocyte membranes. Biochem. Biophys. Acta **452:**538–551.

Aberrant Phosphoinositide Metabolism in Alzheimer's Disease[a]

SHUN SHIMOHAMA,[b,h] SADAKI FUJIMOTO,[c] NANCY TRESSER,[e]
PEGGY RICHEY,[e] GEORGE PERRY,[e] PETER J. WHITEHOUSE,[f]
YOSHIMI HOMMA,[f] TADAOMI TAKENAWA,[f] TAKASHI
TANIGUCHI,[d,g] TOSHIHIKO SUENAGA,[b] AND JUN KIMURA[b]

[b] *Department of Neurology, Faculty of Medicine, Kyoto University,*
Kyoto 606 Japan
[c] *Departments of Biochemistry and* [d] *Neurobiology,*
Kyoto Pharmaceutical University, Kyoto 607 Japan
[e] *Division of Neuropathology, Institute of Pathology,* [f] *Department of Neurology,*
University Hospitals of Cleveland, Case Western Reserve University,
Cleveland, Ohio 44106-4901 USA
[g] *Department of Biosignals, Tokyo Metropolitan Institute of Gerontology,*
Tokyo 173 Japan

ABSTRACT: Since phosphoinositide-specific phospholipase C (PLC) is one of
the key molecules in signal transduction, its involvement was assessed in Alzheimer's disease (AD). The phosphatidyl-inositol (PI)-specific PLC activity in the
Alzheimer cytosolic and particulate fractions was not significantly different from
that in the control fractions. The PI-specific PLC activity as a function of the
free Ca^{2+} concentration was also similar between control and Alzheimer brains.
These results suggest that the PI-specific PLC activity is not altered in AD. Immunostaining of a specific antibody against the PLC isozyme, PLC-δ, demonstrated that this enzyme was abnormally accumulated in neurofibrillary tangles
(NFT), the neurites surrounding senile plaque (SP) cores, and neuropil threads
in AD brains. Western blot analysis confirmed that PLC-δ was concentrated in
the paired helical filament (PHF)-rich fraction of AD brains. PLC-δ marked the
same neurons containing τ immunoreactivity and yet τ and PLC-δ often marked
different structures within the same neuron, with τ more clearly on NFT and
PLC-δ covering it superficially. The double stain with PLC-δ and basic fibroblast
growth factor (bFGF) binding suggest that PLC-δ is an intracellular marker,
showing little overlap with bFGF binding, an extracellular marker. All of this
was consistent with the electron microscopy, with PLC-δ being NFT associated.

[a] This work was supported by Grants-in-Aid for Scientific Research on Priority Areas
(04268206, 05261206), a Grant-in-Aid for Encouragement of Young Scientists (04770495)
from the Ministry of Education, Science and Culture, Japan, and by grants from Yamanouchi
Foundation for Research on Metabolic Disorders, National Institutes of Health Grants (AG-
07552, AG-09287) and Sandoz Foundation for Gerontological Research.

[b] *Send correspondence to:* Dr. Shun Shimohama, Department of Neurology, Faculty of Medicine,
Kyoto University, 54 Shogoin-kawaharacho, Sakyo-ku, Kyoto 606 Japan; TEL: 81-75-751-
3767; FAX: 81-75-761-9780.

Antibodies to other PLC isozymes did not produce positive immunostaining of these pathologic structures. Moreover, diffuse and amorphous deposits of PLC-δ were found to precede the accumulation of fibrillary deposits. These results suggest that PLC-δ accumulation plays a possible role in the formation of intraneuronal inclusions in AD.

The characteristic lesions of Alzheimer's disease (AD) consist of senile plaques (SP) and neurofibrillary tangles (NFT). NFT are also found in the brains of patients with a variety of other diseases, suggesting that they represent a reactive change imposed on neurons by various causes. An important question is: what is the signaling responsible for the formation of NFT?

Evidence is mounting that inositol phospholipid-specific phospholipase C (PLC) is a key molecule in signal transduction. PLC catalyzes the three phosphoinositides, phosphatidylinositol (PI), phosphatidylinositol 4-monophosphate (PIP), and phosphatidylinositol 4,5-biphosphate (PIP_2), to generate diacylglycerol and three inositol phosphates, among which diacylglycerol and inositol 1,4,5-trisphosphate serve as intracellular messengers for protein kinase C (PKC) activation and intracellular Ca^{2+} mobilization.[1,2] We have already reported the alterations of muscarinic cholinergic, α-adrenergic, and glutamatergic receptors that trigger the activation of PLC,[3–5] and have demonstrated the involvement of PKC in AD pathology.[6] These findings have suggested a crucial role for PLC in the aberrant signaling that occurs in AD brains. To examine the involvement of PLC in the pathogenesis of AD, we investigated the change of PI-specific PLC activity in AD brains, and used four antibodies against different PLC isozymes to immunostain PLC isozymes in AD brain tissues.

The PI-specific PLC activity was measured according to the method of Hofmann and Majerus.[7] Specific antibodies against four PLC isozymes were independently prepared using each type of PLC protein produced by *E. coli* expression systems.[8] Antibodies to τ and basic fibroblast growth factor (bFGF) were also used.

The PI-specific PLC activity in the Alzheimer brain cytosolic and particulate fractions was not significantly different from that in the control fractions. The PI-specific PLC activity as a function of the free Ca^{2+} concentration also showed no significant difference between control and Alzheimer brains.[9]

PLC-δ immunostaining of AD brains with the anti-PLC-δ antibody was specifically localized to 1) intraneuronal NFT, 2) dystrophic neurites in SP, and 3) curly fibers in the neuropil. Preabsorption of the anti-PLC-δ antibody with purified mammalian PLC-δ prevented the positive immunostaining of these structures. The reduction in NFT staining was proportional to the amount of antigen used to preabsorb the antibody, indicating its specificity. This antibody also immunostained non–NFT-bearing neurons. Positive

PLC-δ immunoreactivity in these neurons appeared as either small discrete granules in the cell body or as large coalescing granules that completely filled the cytoplasm. NFT, dystrophic neurites in SP and curly fibers in the neuropil in AD brains were not stained by antibodies to other PLC isozymes (PLC-β, -γ₁, and -γ₂), indicating the specific involvement of PLC-δ in AD.[10]

In comparisons with bFGF binding, an extracellular marker,[11] only a few were marked by both PLC-δ and bFGF binding. PLC-δ marked the same neurons containing τ immunoreactivity and yet τ and PLC-δ often marked different structures within the same neuron, with τ more clearly on NFT and PLC-δ covering it superficially. All of this is consistent with the electron microscopy, with PLC-δ being NFT associated.

The present study revealed that the PI-specific PLC activity in Alzheimer brains was not significantly different from that in controls, and that the PI-specific PLC activity as a function of free Ca^{2+} was also similar in both groups of brains, indicating that the PI-specific PLC activity is not significantly altered in the Alzheimer brain.

Several PLC isozymes have been demonstrated by protein purification and cDNA cloning.[2] Our present results suggest that PLC-δ might be closely associated with paired helical filaments (PHF). At present, τ and ubiquitin are the only definite components of PHF identified by chemical studies.[12,13] However, it is unlikely that the anti-PLC-δ antibody used in this study recognized either τ or ubiquitin, because it did not react with polypeptides at 45-70 kDa or 8 kDa in Western blotting. Indeed PLC-δ marked the same neurons containing τ immunoreactivity and yet τ and PLC-δ often marked different structures within the same neuron, with τ more clearly on NFT and PLC-δ covering it superficially. The double stain with PLC-δ and bFGF binding suggest that PLC-δ is an intracellular marker, showing little overlap with bFGF binding, an extracellular marker.[11] The brains from age-matched nondemented subjects did not contain abundant NFT, but instead demonstrated "diffuse" or "amorphous" deposits that were immunopositive for this anti-PLC-δ antibody. These deposits may represent one of the earliest detectable changes observed in the aging brain before the appearance of NFT. Thus, the finding of "diffuse" or "amorphous" deposits before the accumulation of fibrillary deposits may indicate that PLC-δ accumulation is one of the crucial intracellular changes contributing to the formation of NFT.

PLC is a key enzyme in signal transduction between the extracellular and intracellular compartments. Therefore, alterations in PLC-δ in AD brains suggested by the unusual PLC-δ staining may be related to key features such as the neurofibrillary degeneration and aberrant axonal architecture seen in AD.

REFERENCES

1. BERRIDGE, M. J. & R. F. IRVINE. 1984. Inositol trisphosphate, a novel second messenger in cellular signal transduction. Nature **312**:315–321.

2. RHEE, S. G., P. G. SUH, S. H. RYU & S. Y. LEE. 1989. Studies of inositol phospholipid-specific phopholipase C. Science **244:**546–550.

3. SHIMOHAMA, S., T. TANIGUCHI, M. FUJIWARA & M. KAMEYAMA. 1986. Changes in nicotinic and muscarinic cholinergic receptors in Alzheimer-type dementia. J. Neurochem. **46:**288–293.

4. SHIMOHAMA, S., T. TANIGUCHI, M. FUJIWARA & M. KAMEYAMA. 1986. Biochemical characterization of α-adrenergic receptors in human brain and changes in Alzheimer-type dementia. J. Neurochem. **47:**1294–1301.

5. NINOMIYA, H., T. TANIGUCHI, M. FUJIWARA, S. SHIMOHAMA & M. KAMEYAMA. 1990. [^{3}H]N-[1-(2-Thienyl(cyclohexyl]-3,4-piperidine ([^{3}H]TCP) binding in human frontal cortex: Decreases in Alzheimer-type dementia. J. Neurochem. **54:**526–532.

6. MASLIAH, E., G. COLE, S. SHIMOHAMA, L. HANSEN, R. DETERESA, D. T. TERRY & T. SAITOH. 1990. Differential involvement of protein kinase C isozymes in Alzheimer's disease. J. Neurosci. **10:**2113–2124.

7. HOFMANN, S. L. & P. W. MAJERUS. 1982. Identification and properties of two distinct phosphatidylinositol-specific phospholipase C enzymes from sheep seminal vesicular glands. J. Biol. Chem. **257:**6261–6469.

8. HOMMA, Y., Y. EMORI, F. SHIBASAKI, K. SUZUKI & T. TAKENAWA. 1990. Isolation and characterization of a γ-type phosphoinositide-specific phospholipase C (PLC-γ2). Biochem. J. **269:**13–18.

9. SHIMOHAMA, S., S. FUJIMOTO, T. TANIGUCHI & J. KIMURA. 1992. Phosphatidylinositol-specific phospholipase C activity in the postmortem human brain: No alteration in Alzheimer's disease. Brain Res. **579:**347–349.

10. SHIMOHAMA, S., Y. HOMMA, T. SUENAGA, S. FUJIMOTO, T. TANIGUCHI, W. ARAKI, Y. YAMAOKA, T. TAKENAWA & J. KIMURA. 1991. Aberrant accumulation of phospholipase C-δ in Alzheimer brains. Am. J. Pathol. **139:**737–742.

11. SIEDLAK, S. L., P. CRAS, M. KAWAI, P. RICHEY & G. PERRY. 1991. Basic fibroblast growth factor binding is a marker for extracellular neurofibrillary tangles in Alzheimer disease. J. Histochem. Cytochem. **39:**899–904.

12. MORI, H., J. KONDO & Y. IHARA. 1987. Ubiquitin is a component of paired helical filaments in Alzheimer's disease. Science **235:**1641–1644.

13. WISCHIK, C. M., M. NOVAK, H. C. THOGERSEN, P. C. EDWARDS, M. J. RUNSWICK, R. JAKES, J. E. WALKER, C. MILSTEIN, M. ROTH & A. KLUG. 1988. Isolation of a fragment of τ derived from the core of the paired helical filament of Alzheimer disease. Proc. Natl. Acad. Sci. USA **85:**4506–4510.

NMDA Receptor Status in Elderly Normal Individuals and Those with Alzheimer's Disease[a]

R. H. P. PORTER,[b] P. J. ROBERTS,[b,d] AND R. S. J. BRIGGS[c]

[b] *Department of Physiology & Pharmacology, University of Southampton, Southampton United Kingdom*
[c] *Department of Geriatric Medicine, University of Southampton General Hospital, Southampton United Kingdom*

ABSTRACT: The status of NMDA receptors in the brains of normal aged individuals and those with Alzheimer's disease was investigated. The binding of [³H]3-((±)-2-carboxypiperazin-4-yl)propyl phosphonic acid ([³H]CPP) to NMDA antagonist-preferring sites on frontal and temporal cortical synaptic membranes was assessed. Binding could be resolved into two components, one of high and the other of low affinity. Pharmacologically, the two sites were qualitatively similar. Considerable intersubject variation in binding parameters was detected, but no significant differences were found between the mean values for the control and Alzheimer's disease groups. This study indicates that, when changes in receptor integrity occur in individual patients, these may be occluded because of the large variations between individuals.

Alzheimer's disease, which is the most common cause of dementia in the elderly, is characterized histopathologically by neuronal cell death and accumulation of neurofibrillary tangles and neuritic plaques, particularly within the hippocampus and parahippocampal gyrus.[1] While the aetiology of Alzheimer's disease has still not been elucidated, there is good evidence to implicate glutamate (or a related excitatory amino acid, EAA) in the pathophysiology of the disease. Glutamate is likely to be the major neurotransmitter of the cortico-cortical association, corticofugal and hippocampal pyramidal neurons,[2–4] and a dysfunction of these systems might be directly involved in neuronal cell loss via an excitotoxic process, and/or contribute to the deterioration in cognitive functions seen in Alzheimer's disease.

Severe losses of cortical and hippocampal glutamatergic terminals have

[a] We thank Research into Aging, The Wellcome Trust, and the Wessex Medical Trust for support.
[d] *Send correspondence to:* P. J. Roberts, Department of Pharmacology, University of Bristol, University Walk, Bristol B58ITD United Kingdom.

50

been reported to occur in Alzheimer's disease as evidenced by decreased high-affinity uptake and sodium-dependent binding of D-[^{3}H]aspartate,[5–7] together with reduced tissue glutamate concentrations.[8] In contrast to these widely accepted decrements in presynaptic glutamatergic function, considerable controversy exists concerning the status of postsynaptic EAA receptors. Many studies have focused on the NMDA receptor, in view of its proposed involvement in learning and memory—processes that are strikingly compromised in Alzheimer's disease. Some studies have reported that NMDA receptors are lost from cortical and hippocampal areas,[9,10] while other studies have found hippocampal NMDA receptors to be relatively stable, except in those cases where very severe cell loss is evident.[11,12]

In a previous study, we reported that the binding of L-[^{3}H]glutamate to the agonist-preferring state of the NMDA receptor on synaptic membranes from hippocampus, frontal-temporal- and parietal-cortex indicated no loss of NMDA receptors in Alzheimer's disease brain, while D-[^{3}H]aspartate binding was severely reduced.[13] In this study, we have examined the binding of [^{3}H]3-(($\pm$)-2-carboxypiperazin-4-yl)propyl-1-phosphonic acid ([^{3}H]CPP) to the antagonist-preferring site of the NMDA receptor in Alzheimer's disease and control brain groups.

Briefly, tissue was obtained at autopsy from patients clinically diagnosed as having Alzheimer's disease, and from control patients without neurological or psychiatric disease. The two groups were closely matched for age (77–80 years) and postmortem delay (~20h). Brains were dissected, frozen in 0.32M buffered sucrose and stored at $-70°C$. Following thawing in 0.32M sucrose in Tris-acetate buffer at 37°C, synaptic membranes were isolated and extensively washed with buffer. Binding assays of [^{3}H]CPP were carried out at 20°C in microfuge tubes, routinely for 30 min. Assays were terminated by microcentrifugation, the pellets solubilized and radioactivity determined by liquid scintillation spectrometry. Specific binding was determined in the presence of unlabeled CPP or ($-$)2-amino-5-phosphonopentanoate.

[^{3}H]CPP was found to bind to both high- and low-affinity components on cortical synaptic membranes (high-affinity site: K_d = 85.7 nM, B_{max} = 0.30 pmol/mg protein; low-affinity site: K_d = 5.3μM, B_{max} = 11.8 pmol/mg protein; determined for frontal cortex). These results are in accord with molecular cloning studies indicating multiple forms of the NMDA receptor. They are also analogous to our findings with rat membranes and another recently published study,[14] where CPP was similarly found to recognize two NMDA binding sites of high- and low-affinity respectively on cerebral cortex membranes). Pharmacologically, we have not detected any obvious qualitative pharmacological differences in sensitivity of the two binding sites to NMDA agonists or antagonists.

Saturation analysis was carried out for the binding of [^{3}H]CPP to membranes from Alzheimer's and control brain membranes. Two areas of the brain were examined: the gyrus temporalis medius and gyrus frontalis medius. The former area shows severe pathology in Alzheimer's disease, while the latter is less severely affected. Binding was best resolved into two components by LIGAND analysis of the data. Within each group of brains, there was considerable variation in the values for both K_d and B_{max}. However, no significant differences were detected in either parameter between the two regions of brain studied. Furthermore, no differences were detected between the mean values for control and Alzheimer disease tissue. Our results confirm recent studies from Cotman's group[15] that there is marked intersubject variability in NMDA receptor status both in controls and Alzheimer's disease brains. Assessment of mean values for groups is likely to obscure significant declines that may occur in some individual patients.

REFERENCES

1. MANN, D. M. A., P. O. YATES & B. MARCYNIUK. 1985. Some morphometric observations on the cerebral cortex and hippocampus in presemile Alzheimer's disease, senile dementia of Alzheimer type and Down's syndrome in middle age. J. Neurol. Sci. **69:**139–159.
2. COTMAN, C. W., D. T. MONAGHAN, O. P. OTTERSEN & J. STORM-MATHISEN. 1987. Anatomical organization of excitatory amino acid receptors and their pathways. TINS **10:**273–280.
3. FONNUM, F. 1984. Glutamate: A neurotransmitter in mammalian brain. J. Neurochem. **42:**1–11.
4. FONNUM, F. & I. WALAAS. 1978. The effect of intrahippocampal kainic acid injections and surgical lesions on neurotransmitters in hippocampus and septum. J. Neurochem. **31:**1173–1181.
5. COWBURN, R. F., J. A. HARDY, P. J. ROBERTS & R. S. J. BRIGGS. 1988. Presynaptic and postsynaptic glutamatergic function in Alzheimer's disease. Neurosci. Lett. **86:**109–113.
6. CROSS, A. J., P. SLATER, J. M. CANDY, E. K. PERRY & R. H. PERRY. 1987. Glutamate deficits in Alzheimer's disease. Ann. Neurol. Neurosurg. Psychiatry **50:**357–358.
7. HARDY, J. A., R. F. COWBURN, A. BARTON, G. REYNOLDS, E. LOFDAHL, A. M. O'CARROLL, P. WESTER & B. WINBLAD. 1987. Region-specific loss of glutamate innervation in Alzheimer's disease. Neurosci. Lett. **50:**356–357.
8. HYMAN, B. T., G. W. VAN HOESEN & A. R. DAMASIO. 1987. Alzheimer's disease: Glutamate depletion in the hippocampal perforant pathway zone. Ann. Neurol. **22:**37–40.
9. GREENAMYRE, T. J., J. B. PENNY, A. B. YOUNG, C. J. D'AMATO, S. P. HICKS & I. SHOULSON. 1985. Alterations in L-glutamate binding in Alzheimer's and Huntington's diseases. Science **227:**1496–1499.
10. GREENAMYRE, T. J., J. B. PENNY, C. J. D'AMATO & A. B. YOUNG. 1987. Dementia of the Alzheimer's type: Changes in hippocampal L-[^{3}H]glutamate binding. J. Neurochem. **48:**543–551.

11. GEDDES, J. W., H. CHANG-CHUI, S. M. COOPER, I. T. LOTT & C. W. COTMAN. 1986. Density and distribution of NMDA receptors in the human hippocampus in Alzheimer's disease. Brain Research **399**:156–161.
12. MONAGHAN, D. T., J. W. GEDDES, D. YAO, C. CHUNG & C. W. COTMAN. 1987. [^{3}H]TCP binding sites in Alzheimer's disease. Neurosci. Lett. **73**: 197–200.
13. COWBURN, R., J. HARDY, P. ROBERTS & R. BRIGGS. 1988. Regional distribution of pre- and postsynaptic glutamatergic function in Alzheimer's disease. Brain Res. **452**:403–407.
14. VAN AMSTERDAM, F. T. M., A. GIBERTI, M. MUGNAINI & E. RATTI. 1992. 3-[(±)-2-carboxypiperazin-4-yl]propyl-1-phosphonic acid recognizes two N-methyl-D-aspartate binding sites in rat cerebral cortex membranes. J. Neurochem. **59**:1850–1855.
15. ULAS, J., L. C. BRUNNER, J. W. GEDDES, W. CHOE & C. W. COTMAN. 1992. N-methyl-D-aspartate receptor complex in the hippocampus of elderly, normal individuals and those with Alzheimer's disease. Neuroscience **49**:45–61.

X-Ray Diffraction Analysis of Brain Lipid Membrane Structure in Alzheimer's Disease and β-Amyloid Peptide Interactions[a]

R. PRESTON MASON,[b] WILLIAM J. SHOEMAKER, LYDIA
SHAJENKO, AND LEO G. HERBETTE

*Departments of Radiology, Medicine, Biochemistry, and Psychiatry,
The Travelers Center on Aging, Neurobiology Laboratory,
Biomolecular Structure Analysis Center, University of Connecticut Health Center,
Farmington, Connecticut 06030-2017 USA*

ABSTRACT: Small angle x-ray diffraction analysis of Alzheimer's disease (AD) lipid membranes reconstituted from cortical gray matter showed significant, reproducible structure changes relative to age-matched control samples.[1] Specifically, there was an average 4 Å reduction in the lipid bilayer width and marked changes in membrane electron density profiles of AD cortical samples. There were no significant structure differences in the membrane bilayers isolated from an unaffected region (cerebellum) of the AD brain. Lipid and protein analysis of six AD and six age-matched controls showed that the phospholipid:protein mass ratio was unchanged, but that the unesterified chlolesterol:phospholipid (C:PL) mole ratio decreased by 30% in the AD temporal gyrus relative to age-matched controls. The C:PL mole ratio was not significantly different for samples prepared from cerebellum of AD versus control patients. X-ray diffraction analysis of a cholesterol-enriched AD sample demonstrated a virtual restoration of the normal membrane bilayer width and electron density profile, suggesting that the cholesterol deficit played a major role in the AD lipid membrane structure perturbation. Addition of β-amyloid peptide to bovine brain phospholipid membranes signficantly changed the electron density associated with the hydrocarbon core. Alterations in the composition and structure of the membrane bilayer may play an important role in the pathophysiology of AD by altering the activity and catabolism of membrane-bound proteins, including the β-amyloid precursor protein.

[a] This work was supported by the American Health Assistance Foundation (L.G.H., W.J.S., R.P.M.), the John A. Hartford Foundation (R.P.M.), American Federation for Aging Research Award (R.P.M., L.S.) and University of Connecticut Health Center Research Advisory Committee (R.P.M.).

[b] *Send correspondence to:* R. Preston Mason, Biomolecular Structure Analysis Center, University of Connecticut Health Center, Farmington, CT 06030-2017 USA; TEL: 203-679-4419; FAX: 203-679-1989.

INTRODUCTION

To explore possible biophysical and chemical changes specific to Alzheimer's disease, we examined lipid membrane bilayers using small angle x-ray diffraction. Membranes were isolated from the temporal gyrus and cerebellum of brains affected by AD and Parkinson's disease (PD) as well as from age-matched controls (AD: 5 males, 4 females; control: 5m, 4f; PD: 5m).

The postmortem delay was not significantly different (AD: 3.20 ± 3.01 h; control: 2.28 ± 0.84 h; PD 3.25 ± 1.30 h). We correlated the structure data with measurements of protein, phospholipid, and unesterified cholesterol in the same brain membranes. Results of this study show significant, reproducible changes in the structure and composition of membranes isolated from affected regions of AD brain. These changes may play an important role in the pathophysiology of AD. We also examined the interaction of β-amyloid (1–40) with bovine brain phosphatidylcholine membranes and observed significant changes in membrane structure.

RESULTS

Analysis of Membrane Protein, Cholesterol, and Phospholipid Content

The protein, phospholipid, and unesterified cholesterol content of brain membranes from the gray matter of superior temporal gyrus and cerebellum were measured and compared. The results of the analysis demonstrated a significant decrease ($p < 0.01$, Wilcoxon two-sample rank test, two-tailed, n = 12) of 30% in the C:PL mole ratio of AD temporal gyrus ($0.46:1 \pm 0.08$) versus age-matched controls ($0.66:1 \pm 0.05$). By contrast, the C:PL mole ratio in the cerebellum did not change significantly ($0.45:1$ for AD versus $0.50:1$ for control). Moreover, the mass ratio of protein to phospholipid was not significantly perturbed in either the temporal gyrus or the cerebellum of AD and control tissue. As a further control, we analyzed brain samples from five age-matched PD brains. The C:PL mole ratios from the temporal gyrus (0.57 ± 0.10) and cerebellum (0.48 ± 0.06) of PD brains were not significantly different from the controls.

Small Angle X-ray Diffraction

There were significant differences ($p < 0.01$, Student's two-tailed t-test) in the membrane bilayer width of reconstituted lipid membranes from AD temporal gyrus but not cerebellum. The unit cell width (D-space), which includes the width of the lipid bilayer plus associated water layers, decreased from 62.6 ± 1.2 Å for control to 58.7 ± 0.4 Å for AD samples. There was a correlation between the C:PL content of the lipid extracts and membrane bilayer width that was independent of the brain location of the sample. To test this correlation, free cholesterol was added to the organic phase of an AD lipid extract from the superior temporal gyrus prior to vesicle formation. The amount of free cholesterol added brought the AD C:PL mole ratio to a level similar to that of the control. Multilayers were then prepared for x-ray diffraction. Analysis of the diffraction pattern showed an increase in the AD membrane bilayer width of 3.9 Å (from 58.3 Å to 62.2 Å) following the addition of unesterified cholesterol. The difference in the average membrane bilayer width of control and AD samples were 4 Å. Thus, addition of free cholesterol by the amount observed to be lacking to AD membranes from temporal gyrus was able to account for the difference in membrane bilayer width between control and AD membranes.

Effect of β-Amyloid on Membrane Structure

The interaction of β-amyloid with bovine brain phosphatidylcholine membranes (0.6:1 C:PL mole ratio) was examined using small angle x-ray diffraction. The peptide had a significant, dose-dependent disordering effect on the membrane hydrocarbon core. The disordering effect of β-amyloid was evident over a wide temperature range (5°C–37°C). This is consistent with the hypothesis that the amphipathic peptide is intercalating into the membrane lipid bilayer and disrupting acyl chain packing parameters.

DISCUSSION

Molecular structure changes were observed in lipid membranes reconstituted from the gray matter of autopsy-confirmed AD patients relative to age-matched controls and PD subjects. The biochemical basis for these differences may, in part, be related to a significant decrease in the C:PL mole ratios measured in the lipid extracts. For example, a direct relationship between the C:PL mole ratio and membrane bilayer width was observed. Adding cholesterol back to the AD samples, to levels similar to control, restored the membrane bilayer width. This is consistent with the known effect of cholesterol on ordering the acyl chain region in the hydrocarbon core, which results in increased overall membrane bilayer width. The addition of β-amyloid (1–40) to brain lipid bilayers altered the membrane structure, as evidenced by a broad change in hydrocarbon core electron density. These data suggest that the β-amyloid molecule has significant membrane structure effects and

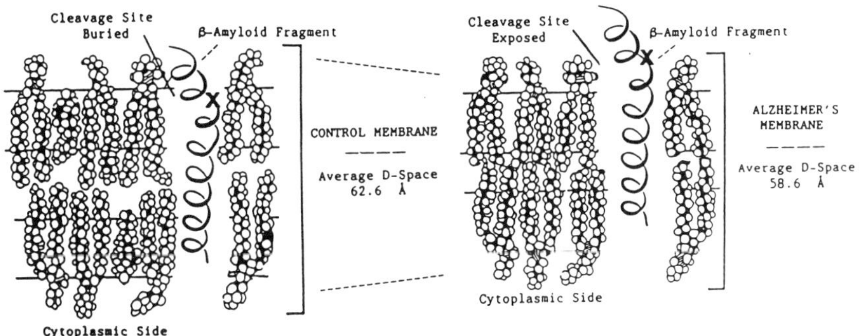

FIGURE 1. This figure is Figure 1 from Mason *et al.*[1]

may remain associated with the plasma membrane following cleavage from APP.

Changes in the composition and structure of AD brain membrane may affect cleavage of the amyloid precursor protein (APP), resulting in elevated levels of β-amyloid.[2,3] Mutagenesis studies have demonstrated that APP cleavage is more dependent on the peptide's conformation and orientation with respect to the plasma membrane than its primary sequence.[4] Thus, alterations in AD membrane structure (*e.g.*, a decrease in membrane bilayer width) may alter the tertiary structure of APP and increase the probability for proteases to gain access to the β-amyloid cleavage site. FIGURE 1 (from Mason *et al.*[1]) shows a molecular model based on the x-ray diffraction data to illustrate how alterations in membrane structure may result in exposure of the βA cleavage site. The putative βA site indicated in the figure as an "X" is buried within the lipid bilayer under normal cholesterol conditions (Frame A) but is exposed in AD brain membranes (Frame B) whose lower cholesterol content may produce the decreased membrane bilayer width (D-space). The changes in membrane cholesteral content may be related to alterations in cholesterol metabolism, as reported elsewhere in this volume by Goldgaber and colleagues. Further structure analysis on the APP protein will determine where the β-amyloid cleavage site is located with respect to the membrane lipid bilayer derived from AD tissue.

ACKNOWLEDGMENT

We are grateful to Joseph Rogers, Ph.D. of the Institute for Biogerontology Research (Sun City, AZ) who provided the frozen samples of human brain tissue for these studies.

REFERENCES

1. MASON, R. P., W. H. SHOEMAKER, L. SHAJENKO, T. E. CHAMBERS & L. G. HERBETTE. 1992. Evidence for changes in the Alzheimer's disease brain cortical membrane structure mediated by cholesterol. Neurobiol. Aging **13:**413–419.
2. PETTEGREW, J. W. 1989. Molecular insights into Alzheimer's disease. Ann. N.Y. Acad. Sci. **568:**5–29.
3. NITSCH, R. M., J. K. BLUSZTAJN, A. G. PITTAS, B. E. SLACK, J. H. GROWDON & R. J. WURTMAN. 1992. Evidence for a membrane defect in Alzheimer disease brain. Proc. Natl. Acad. Sci. USA **89:**1671–1675.
4. SISODIA, S. S. 1992. β-Amyloid precursor protein cleavage by a membrane-bound protease. Proc. Natl. Acad. Sci. USA **89:**6075–6079.

Synaptic Pathology of Alzheimer's Disease[a]

H. LASSMANN,[b,e] P. FISCHER,[c] AND K. JELLINGER[d]

[b] *Research Unit for Experimental Neuropathology, Austrian Academy of Sciences and Neurological Institute, University of Vienna, Vienna, Austria*
[c] *Department of Psychiatry, University of Vienna, Vienna, Austria*
[d] *Ludwig Boltzmann Institute of Clinical Neurobiology, Vienna, Austria*

ABSTRACT: Prospective clinico-pathological studies on dementia in Alzheimer's disease (AD), performed during the past decades, revealed a relatively poor correlation between the degree of clinical deficit and the severity of the typical neuropathological lesions of AD, the amyloid plaques and the neurofibrillary tangles. More recent data, obtained by electron microscopy, immunocytochemical as well as immunochemical techniques indicate that synaptic loss may be a better structural correlate of dementia than other brain lesions. Synaptic pathology is reflected by a loss of all major components of small synaptic vesicles and most peptides, stored in large dense cored vesicles. The significant increase of chromogranin A proprotein, a major component of large dense cored vesicles, may rather represent a defect of protein processing than preservation of a specific synaptic subpopulation. Within the brain of AD patients, the degree of synaptic loss is uneven. Most prominent reduction of synapses is found in the outer parts of the dentate gyrus molecular layer, possibly reflecting the destruction of neurons, located in the layer 2 of the entorhinal cortex. However, within the neocortex, no preferential loss of synapses in any of the cortical layers has been found. Cerebral amyloid deposition in diffuse plaques has little effect on synapse density and structure. However, within the dense amyloid core of a classical plaque, synapses are completely lost. In the surrounding neuritic portion of the plaques, synaptophysin reactivity is frequently increased, due to enlargement of synaptic boutons and to accumulation of synaptophysin in dystrophic axons. Although the reason for synapse loss in AD is yet unknown, most results suggest that it may reflect degeneration of neurons, projecting into the respective cortical areas.

CORRELATES OF DEMENTIA IN ALZHEIMER'S DISEASE

Amyloid plaques and neurofibrillary tangles are the hallmark of neuropathological lesions in Alzheimer's disease. Indeed, in early studies on clinicopathological correlation in AD a strong correlation was found between the

[a] The study was partially funded by a project of the Bundesministerium für Wissenschaft und Forschung, Austria.

[e] *Send correspondence to:* H. Lassmann, Research Unit for Experimental Neuropathology, Austrian Academy of Sciences and Neurological Institute, University of Vienna, Schwarzspanierstrasse 17, A-1090, Wien, Austria; TEL: (222) 40 48 02 56; FAX: (222) 40 34 077.

severity of dementia and either neocortical plaques[1] or neurofibrillary tangles.[2] However, more recent prospective clinico-pathological studies revealed several aspects that question the significance of previous correlations (refs. 3 and 4; Fischer *et al.*, in preparation). Highly significant correlations are only obtained when undemented controls and a high number of the most severely demented AD patients are included. Exclusion of these two groups of patients results in the loss of significant correlations. This may be partly explained by the fact that there is a sharp increase in the density of neurofibrillary tangles and amyloid plaques in the end stages of AD dementia, which contributes to a large degree to the significance of the correlations. Furthermore, intellectually normal patients above 90 years of age may contain much higher numbers of plaques in their neocortex compared to demented, younger AD patients.[5] Thus, from all these data it can be safely concluded that there is no direct relation between cognitive dysfunction in AD and the presence or absence of neurofibrillary tangles and amyloid plaques in the brain.

Recent electron microscopical,[6] immunocytochemical,[4] and immunochemical data[7] suggest that synapse loss may be more directly related to dementia than other structural brain lesions.

BIOCHEMICAL ALTERATIONS OF SYNAPTIC MARKERS IN ALZHEIMER'S DISEASE

Ultrastructural studies revealed a loss of presynaptic elements in the neocortex of AD patients.[6] This was later confirmed by quantitative confocal laser microscopy, using synaptophysin as a marker for synapses. In these studies, too, a reduction of the density of synaptic profiles was noted.[8] By using immunochemical techniques, it became clear that not only synaptophysin, but also other markers for small synaptic vesicles, such as SV2 and p65 proteins, are lost in AD in comparable degree as synaptophysin.[7] A similar pattern of synaptic loss is also found in Pick's disease.[9] Markers for large dense cored vesicles of synapses, overall, revealed similar results than those for small vesicles. Nevertheless, the distribution and loss of neuropeptides in AD cortex indicates some more specific involvement of different transmitter systems.[7] Contrary to other neuropeptides, however, chromogranin A accumulates in the neocortex of AD and Pick's disease patients.[7,9,10] Immunocytochemically, chromogranin reactivity was found in the perikarya of cortical neurons, within the neuropil and especially enriched in dystrophic neurites within plaques. The alterations appeared specific for chromogranin A, since they were not found for two other, closely related proteins, chromogranin B and C. Since chromogranin A has a very wide distribution within different nerve cell populations of the central nervous system, this increase in chromogranin A cannot be explained on the basis, that specific nerve cell populations escape destruction in the course of AD pathogenesis. This view is further supported by the observation that chromogranin C, a peptide which is generally colocalized with chromoganin A in the same vesicles, is not enriched in AD lesions. Thus, the present findings rather suggest a defect in the processing of chromogranin A proprotein, that may interfere with subsequent degradation.[7]

STRUCTURAL CHANGES OF SYNAPSES IN ALZHEIMER'S DISEASE

A surprising aspect of synaptic loss in Alzheimer's disease is that it is associated only with minor structural alterations at the synaptic level. As determined by confocal laser imaging the number of synapses per area of neocortical tissue is reduced but the average size and synaptophysin reactivity of individual synapses appear to be unchanged.[8] This finding is in some disagreement with earlier electron microscopic data, showing an increased size of the remaining synapses in AD cortex.[11] The relation of synapse pathology to β-amyloid deposition is of special interest since it may shed some light on the mechanisms of synaptic damage in AD. There is good agreement, that in the amyloid center of classical compound plaques synaptophysin reactivity is lost. Furthermore, enlarged nerve terminals and irregular, synaptophysin reactive, dystrophic neurites can consistently be found in neuritic plaques. Synapse pathology in diffuse plaques, however, is still controversial. No differences in synaptophysin reactivity was found between diffuse plaques and periplaque tissue by Masliah *et al.*[12] On the other hand, Probst *et al.*[13] described dilated presynaptic terminals with increased synaptophysin reactivity colocalized with β-amyloid in diffuse plaques. In our own material both, increased synaptophysin reactivity and synaptic enlargement was restricted to plaques which, by Bielschowsky silver impregnation, showed at least some degree of axonal dystrophy. Diffuse deposits of amyloid in the neuropil revealed the same synaptophysin reactivity compared to the surrounding tissue. However, dystrophic neurites prominently expressed synaptophysin within plaques but also when diffusely dispersed in the neuropil.

Although a significant correlation between the diminuation of synaptic markers and the density of neurofibrillary tangles and neuropil threads was obvious in our material,[7] by imunocytochemistry in accordance with other studies[8] we found no evidence for a spatial relation between synapse density in the neuropil and neurofibrillary pathology in pericarya and dendrites.

TOPOGRAPHICAL DISTRIBUTION OF SYNAPTIC PATHOLOGY IN ALZHEIMER'S DISEASE

Judging from immunochemical data, synapse loss appears to be most prominent in the hippocampus, followed by the temporal cortex.[7,14] The changes were less pronounced in the frontal cortex, and no significant reduction in the synaptophysin content was found in the occipital cortex and in the caudate nucleus. These results differ from those obtained by confocal laser microscopy, where the frontal and parietal neocortex appeared to be more severely affected than the temporal cortex and hippocampus.[15] There is good agreement between different studies that in the neocortex synaptophysin content in severely demented cases may amount 35–50% of control levels.[4,7,14] It is yet an unresolved question to what extent the regional distribution of synapse loss allows conclusions regarding the destruction of specific anatomical pathways in Alzheimer's disease. One consistent pattern is the synaptic loss in the outer molecular layer of the hippocampal dentate gyrus.[14,16,17] This loss may be related to degeneration of nerve cells in layer II of the entorhinal cortex.[17] Within the neocortex, however, an even reduction of synapse density is found throughout all layers,[15] thus arguing against a defect in a single cortical input system.

CONCLUSION

Synapse loss in the neocortex and the hippocampal formation is an important structural feature of the brain lesion in Alzheimer's disease. This observation raises several questions intimately related to the etiology and pathogenseis of the disease. The following questions have to be addressed:

Is synaptic loss the primary correlate of dementia in Alzheimer's disease? Although this is a very attractive hypothesis, current available evidence is insufficient for such a conclusion. Studies up to now are based on a very small sample of patients. Furthermore, several technical points, related to the design of the studies cast doubt on the interpretation of the findings. They relate to inclusion/exclusion criteria of patients, the time interval between neuropsychological testing and neuropathological analysis and inconsistencies between different studies on the question, what brain regions are mostly affected by synapse loss in AD.

What is the relation between synaptic loss in Alzheimer's disease and β-amyloid protein deposition in the brain? Since the amyloid β-A4 precursor protein is localized in synapses and may play a role in synapse function, pathological processing of this protein may lead in parallel to synapse degeneration and amyloid deposition.[18] However, most studies on synaptophysin localization in AD cortex agree that there is no spatial relation between amyloid deposition in diffuse plaques and synapse pathology. Such a colocalization should be expected when either synapse degeneration would provoke amyloid deposition or when amyloid deposition would induce synapse destruction and/or dysfunction.

What is the relation of synaptic pathology to neurofibrillary tangles? Since the synaptic input to neurons may influence the degree of phosphorylation of cytoskeletal elements,[19] chronic synaptic deprivation could lead to over-phosphorylation of cytoskeletal elements, in particular tau proteins. Such a mechanism could explain the high correlation between the density of neurofibrillary tangles and synaptic loss in the neocortex.[7] However, within the cortex itself, no spatial coincidence between synaptic loss and tangle formation in individual nerve cell pericarya or dendrites has been noted up to now.[8]

Does synaptic loss just reflect degeneration of neurons in Alzheimer's disease? The extensive loss of synapses in the molecular layer of the hippocampal dentate gyrus may reflect degeneration of neurons in layer II of the entorhinal cortex. In the neocortex, however, synaptic loss may be due to a summation of loss of intracortical connections, cortico-cortical projections and afferents from the brain stem and hippocampus.

REFERENCES

1. BLESSED, G., B. E. THOMLINSON & M. ROTH. 1968. The association between quantitative measures of dementia and of senile change in the cerebral grey matter of elderly subjects. Br. J. Psychiatry **114:**797–811.
2. WILCOCK, G. K. & M. M. ESIRI. 1982. Plaques, tangles and dementia. A quantitative study. J. Neurol. Sci. **56:**343–356.
3. DELAERE, P., C. DUYCKAERTS, J. P. BRION, V. POULAIN & J. J. HAUW. 1989. Tau, paired helical filaments and amyloid in the neocortex: A morphometric study of 15 cases with graded intellectual status in ageing and senile dementia of Alzheimer type. Acta Neuropathol. 77:645–653.
4. TERRY, R. D., E. MASLIAH, D. P. SALMON, N. BUTTERS, R. DE THERESA, R. HILL, L. A. HANSEN & R. KATZMAN. 1991. Physical basis of cognitive alterations in Alzheimer's disease: Synaptic loss is the major correlate of cognitive impairment. Ann. Neurol. **30:**572–580.
5. MIZUTANI, T. & H. SHIMADA. 1992. Neuropathological background of twenty-seven centenarian brains. J. Neurol. Sci. **108:**168–177.
6. DE KOSKY, S. T. & S. W. SCHEFF. 1990. Synapse loss in frontal cortex biopsies in Alzheimer's disease: Correlation with cognitive severity. Ann. Neurol. **27:** 457–464.
7. LASSMANN, H., R. WEILER, P. FISCHER, C. BANCHER, K. JELLINGER, E. FLOOR, W. DANIELCZYK, F. SEITELBERGER & H. WINKLER. 1992. Synaptic pathology in Alzheimer's disease: Immunological data for markers of synaptic and large dense core vesicles. Neuroscience **46:**1–8.
8. MASLIAH, E., M. ELLISMAN, B. CARRAGHER, M. MALLORY, S. YOUNG, L. HANSEN, R. DE THERESA & R. D. TERRY. 1992. Three dimensional analysis of the relationship between synaptic pathology and neuropil threads in Alzheimer's disease. J. Neuropath. Exp. Neurol. **51:**404–414.
9. WEILER, R., H. LASSMANN, P. FISCHER, K. JELLINGER & H. WINKLER. 1990. A high ratio of chromogranin A to synaptin/synaptophysin is a common feature of brains in Alzheimer and Pick disease. FEBS. Lett. **263:**337–339.

10. MUNOZ, D. G. 1991. Chromogranin A like immunoreactive neurities are major constituents of senile plaques. Lab. Invest. **64:**283–286.
11. DAVIES, C. A., D. M. MANN, P. Q. SUMPTER & P. O. YATES. 1987. A quantitative morphometric analysis of the neuronal and synaptic content of the frontal and temporal cortex in patients with Alzheimer's disease. J. Neurol. Sci. **78:** 151–164.
12. MASLIAH, E., R. D. TERRY, M. MALLORY, M. ALFORD & L. HANSEN. 1990. Diffuse plaques do not accentuate synapse loss in Alzheimer's disease. Am. J. Pathol. **137:**1293–1297.
13. PROBST, A., D. LANGUI, S. IPSEN, N. ROBAKIS & J. ULRICH. 1991. Deposition of β/A4 protein along neuronal plasma membranes in diffuse senile plaques. Acta Neuropathol. **83:**21–29.
14. HONER, W. G., D. W. DICKSON, J. GLEESON & P. DAVIES. 1992. Regional synaptic pathology in Alzheimer's disease. Neurobiol. Ageing **13:**375–382.
15. MASLIAH, E., R. D. TERRY, M. ALFORD, R. DE THERESA & L. A. HANSEN. 1991. Cortical and subcortical patterns of synaptophysinlike immunoreactivity in Alzheimer's disease. Am. J. Pathol. **138:**235–246.
16. HAMOS, J. E., L. J. DEGENNARO & D. A. DRACHMAN. 1989. Synaptic loss in Alzheimer's disease and other dementias. Neurology **39:**355–361.
17. LIPPA, C. F., J. E. HAMOS, D. PULASKI-SALO, L. J. DEGENNARO & D. A. DRACHMAN. 1992. Alzheimer's disease and ageing: Effects on perforant pathway perikarya and synapses. Neurobiol. Ageing **1:**405–411.
18. SCHUBERT, W., R. PRIOR, A. WEIDEMANN, H. DIRCKSEN, G. MULTHAUP, C. L. MASTERS & K. BEYREUTHER. 1991. Localization of Alzheimer beta A4 amyloid precursor protein at central and peripheral synaptic sites. Brain Res. **563:**184–194.
19. AOKI, C. & P. SIEKEVITZ. 1985. Ontogenetic changes in the cyclic adenosine 3′,5′-monophosphate-stimulatable phosphorylation of cat visual cortex proteins, particularly of microtubule-associated protein 2 (MAP2): Effects of normal and dark rearing and of the exposure to light. J. Neurosci. **5:**2465–2483.

Protease Inhibitors and Indolamines Selectively Inhibit Cholinesterases in the Histopathologic Structures of Alzheimer's Disease[a]

CHRISTOPHER I. WRIGHT, CHANGIZ GEULA, AND M.-MARSEL MESULAM[b]

Harvard Department of Neurology, Beth Israel Hospital,
Boston, Massachusetts 02215 USA

ABSTRACT: Neurofibrillary tangles and amyloid plaques express acetylcholinesterase (AChE) and butyrylcholinesterase (BChE) activity in Alzheimer's disease. We had found that traditional AChE inhibitors such as BW284C51, tacrine and physostigmine were more potent inhibitors of the AChE in normal axons and cell bodies than of the AChE in plaques and tangles (1). We now report that the reverse pattern is seen with indolamines, carboxypeptidase inhibitor, and the nonspecific protease inhibitor bacitracin. These substances are more potent inhibitors of the cholinesterases in plaques and tangles than of those in normal axons and cell bodies. These results show that the enzymatic properties of plaque and tangle-associated cholinesterases diverge from those of normal axons and cell bodies. The selective susceptibility to bacitracin and carboxypeptidase inhibitor indicates that the catalytic sites of plaque and tangle-bound cholinesterases are more closely associated with peptidase or protease-like properties than the catalytic sites of cholinesterases in normal neurons and axons. This shift in enzymatic affinity may lead to the abnormal protein processing which is thought to play a major role in the pathogenesis of AD. The availability of pharmacological and dietary means for altering brain indolamines raises novel therapeutic possibilities for inhibiting the abnormal cholinesterase activity associated with Alzheimer's disease.

INTRODUCTION

Light and electron microscopic studies have demonstrated that neurofibrillary tangles and neuritic plaques contain histochemically and immunohistochemically definable acetylcholinesterase (AChE) and butyrylcholinesterase

[a] This article is modified from: Wright, C.I., C. Geula & M.M. Mesulam. 1993. Protease inhibitors and indoleamines selectively inhibit cholinesterases in the histopathologic structures of Alzheimer disease. Proc. Natl. Acad. Sci. USA **90:**683–686.

[b] *Send correspondence to:* M. Marsel Mesulam, Harvard Department of Neurology, Beth Israel Hospital, Boston, MA 02215 USA: TEL: 617-735-2075; FAX: 617-735-5216.

(BChE), and that these Alzheimer's disease (AD)-related cholinesterases (ADChE's) have different histochemical properties from the cholinesterases associated with intact neuronal cell bodies and axons.[1–6] Specifically, the ADChE's are more resistant to traditional cholinesterase (ChE) inhibitors,[7,8] require more substrate for inhibition,[9] and are histochemically more intensely reactive at a lower pH than the AChE of normal cells and fibers.[4]

We have searched for modifiers of ChE function that may act preferentially on the ADChE's. One set of modifiers that we have investigated are the indolamine derivatives, based on evidence that these substances can inhibit an acetylcholine hydrolyzing esterase from several mammalian sources,[10–14] and on information that there is an aryl-acylamidase activity associated with purified ChE's that is inhibited by indolamines.[15–17] We have also examined protease inhibitors, since AChE may be associated with a protease function.[18–19]

RESULTS AND DISCUSSION

Our experiments showed that traditional anti-ChE substances such as BW284C51, tacrine and physostigmine are more potent inhibitors of normal axonal and perikaryal AChE whereas indolamines (5-hydroxytryptophan [5-HTP] and serotonin [5-HT]), carboxypeptidase inhibitor (CPI) and the non-specific peptidase inhibitor bacitracin (but not tyrosine, tyramine, glycine, or pepstatin A) inhibit the *in situ* cholinesterase activity of plaques and tangles but not of normal perikarya and axons. These experiments definitively show that the enzymatic properties of ChE's detected within the histopathologic structures of AD differ from those normally found in neuronal perikarya and cortical fibers. The plaque and tangle associated ChE activity could originate from altered remnants of premorbid ChE's, from the *de novo* synthesis (or deposition) of variant molecular forms, or from the peripheral circulation.

The potential peptidase activity of cholinesterases has been claimed by some and denied by others.[18] There is evidence that an AChE-associated protease can cleave the β-amyloid precursor protein, albeit at a non-amyloido-genic site,[19] and that a 5-HT inhibitable aryl-acylamidase activity is associated with purified AChE and BChE.[16,17] The presence of the aryl-acylamidase activity and the esterase activity could give the ChE's the potential to act as proteases since these two activities may be used for protein bond cleavage.[15]

The selective inhibition of the ADChE's by carboxypeptidase inhibitor and bacitracin suggests that the ChE's of plaques and tangles are more closely associated with protease-like activity than the AChE found in normal fibers and perikarya. This property of the ADChE's could participate in the altered protein processing and therefore pathogenesis of AD. Our results have also identified substances that may have a preventive or therapeutic potential through the selective inhibition of the ChE's that accumulate within the histopathological structures of AD. This is particularly pertinent to indolamines whose levels in the brain can be altered pharmacologically (*e.g.*, by fenfluramine or fluoxetine) or by the dietary intake of L-tryptophan.

REFERENCES

1. MESULAM, M. M. & C. GEULA. 1990. Shifting patterns of cortical cholinesterases in Alzheimer's disease: Implication for treatment, diagnosis and patholgenesis. Adv. Neurol. **51:**235–240.
2. FRIEDE, R. L. 1965. Enzyme histochemical studies of senile plaques. J. Neuropath. Exp. Neurol. **24:**477–491.
3. PERRY, R. H., G. BLESSED, E. K. PERRY & B. E. TOMLINSON. 1980. Histochemical observations on the cholinesterase activities in the brains of elderly normal and demented (Alzheimer-type) patients. Age Aging **9:**9–16.
4. MESULAM, M. M. & A. MORAN. 1987. Cholinesterases with neurofibrillary tangles of aging and Alzheimer's disease. Ann. Neurol. **22:**223–228.
5. CARSON, K. A., C. GEULA & M. M. MESULAM. 1991. Electron microscopic localization of cholinesterase activity in Alzheimer brain tissue. Brain Res. **40:** 204–208.
6. GEULA, C., S. BRIMIJOIN & M. M. MESULAM. 1992. Immunocytochemical detection of cholinesterases in Alzheimer's plaques and tangles. Neurology. **41**(Suppl.):376.
7. MESULAM, M. M., C. GEULA & A. MORAN. 1987. Anatomy of cholinesterase inhibition in Alzheimer's disease: Effect of physostigmine and tetrahydroaminoacridine on plaques and tangles. Ann. Neurol. **22:**683–691.
8. GEULA, C. & M. M. MESULAM. 1989. Special properties of cholinesterases in the cerebral cortex of Alzheimer's disease. Brain Res. **498:**185–189.
9. SCHATZ, C., C. GEULA & M. M. MESULAM. 1990. Competitive substrate inhibition in the histochemistry of cholinesterase activity in Alzheimer's disease. Neurosci. Lett. **117:**56–51.
10. ODERFELD-NOWAK, B., J. R. SIMON, L. CHANG & M. H. APRISON. 1979. Interactions of the cholinergic and serotonergic systems. Gen. Pharmacol. **11:** 37–45.
11. APRISON, M. H. 1960. Effect of 5-hydroxytryptamine on cholinesterase activity. Fed. Proc. Fed. Am. Soc. Exp. Biol. **19:**275.
12. ZSIGMOND, E. K., F. F. FOLDER & V. M. FOLDER. 1961. The *in vitro* inhibitory effect of LSD, its cogners and 5-hydroxytryptamine on human cholinesterases. J. Neurochem. **8:**72–80.
13. MOHAMMED, Y. S., M. Y. OSMAN & Y. GABR. 1975. Inhibition of cholinesterase by 5-hydroxytryptamine. Arzmein-Forsch./Drug Res. **25:**1714–1715.
14. OSMAN, M. Y., M. M. MAHFOUZ, A. E. EL-HABET & H. EL-SHERBINI. 1982. Inhibition of erythrocyte and plasma cholinesterase by 5-hydroxytryptamine. Arzneim-Forsch./Drug Res. **32:**1120–1122.
15. BALASUBRAMANIAN, A. S. 1984. Have cholinesterases more than one function? TINS 467–468.

16. OOMEN, A. & A. S. BALASUBRAMANIAN. 1977. The inhibition of brain aryl-acylamidase by 5-hydroxytryptamine and acetycholine. Biochem. Pharmacol. **26:**2163–2167.
17. GEORGE, S. T. & A. S. BALASUBRAMANIAN. 1980. The identity of the serotonin-sensitive aryl c\acylamidase with acetylcholinesterase from human erythrocytes, sheep basal ganglia, and electric eel. Eur. J. Biochem. **111:**511–524.
18. SMALL, D. H., Z. ISMAEL & I. W. CHUBB. 1987. Acetylcholinesterase exhibits a trypsin-like and metalloexoperoxidase-like activity in cleaving a model peptide. Neuroscience **21:**991–995.
19. SMALL, D. H., R. D. MOIR, S. H. FULLER, S. MICHAELSON, A. I. BUSH, Q-X. LI, E. MILWARD, C. HILBICH, A. WEIDERMAN, K. BEYREITHER & C. MASTERS. 1991. A protease activity associated with acetylcholinesterase releases the membrane bound form of the amyloid precursor of Alzheimer's disease. Biochemistry **30:**10795–10799.

Transmitters in the Developing and Senescent Human Brain

ELAINE K. PERRY,[a,c] MARGARET A. PIGGOTT,[a] JENNIFER A. COURT,[a] MARY JOHNSON,[a] AND ROBERT H. PERRY[b]

[a] *Medical Research Council Neurochemical Pathology Unit and*
[b] *Department of Neuropathology, Newcastle General Hospital,*
Newcastle upon Tyne, United Kingdom

ABSTRACT: During development and throughout adult life, modeling of CNS structure and function occurs as a result of experience. Transmitters play a central role in this mechanism both directly and indirectly (through control of neurotrophin expression) by governing synapse formation, elimination or consolidation. Cholinergic and excitatory amino acid transmitter system activities have been examined in postmortem human brain obtained from normal individuals varying from the prenatal period to old age. Whereas glutamate NMDA receptor binding (measured using MK801) was not substantially altered across the postnatal period, dramatic and differing patterns of choline acetlytransferase (ChAT) activity were evident. Thus, in the cerebellum, ChAT activity was 10-fold higher in fetal compared to adult individuals whereas in the hippocampus there was little or no activity in the fetus and activity rose postnatally to reach a maximum in middle age and then declined to half that level by the tenth decade. Acetylcholinesterase (AChE) histochemical reactivity paralleled the developmental pattern for ChAT in the hippocampus and adjacent cortex with respect to fiber reactivity. These findings indicate that cholinergic synaptic plasticity may be restricted to the prenatal period in cerebellum but occur in both the postnatal period and throughout adult life in the hippocampus and cortex, a concept consistent with the temporal and regional expression of cholinoneurotrophins (NGF and related peptides). Vulnerability of the hippocampus and cortex to age-related pathology such as β-amyloidosis and neuritic plaque formation may relate to the extended period of cholinergic synaptic sculpting in these areas.

According to Aristotle[1]: "Infants and very old persons have bad memories owing to the amount of movement going on within them, for the latter are in the process of rapid decay, the former in the process of vigorous growth." Whether or not rapid growth and decay can be related to memory, there is no doubt that understanding the mechanisms of synaptic generation during development will contribute to the explanation and treatment of degenerative

[c] *Send correspondence to:* E. K. Perry, MRC Neurochemical Pathology Unit, Newcastle General Hospital, Westgate Road, Newcastle upon Tyne, NE4 6BE, United Kingdom; TEL: 44-091-273-5251; FAX: 44-091-272-5291.

changes associated with senescence and disease. Amongst various forms of learning in the CNS, cognitive memory in humans is remarkable for its progressive formation postnatally and partial decline in old age. Cholinergic activity in the human hippocampus during development and senescence parallels this pattern of change and contrasts with that in the cerebellum and also with the pattern of glutamate (NMDA) receptor binding.

FIGURE 1 illustrates the strikingly different patterns of ChAT activity in the human hippocampus and cerebellum of 37-65 normal individuals varying in age from 24 gestational weeks to 94 years. In the hippocampus, both ChAT and AChE-positive axons were absent prenatally, appeared after birth, reached a maximum between the 3rd–5th decades, and declined substantially thereafter. AChE in the multipolar cells of the denatate hilus were, however, positive throughout life.[2] In the cerebellum, ChAT was 10-fold higher in the fetal compared with adult groups, and AChE appeared transiently and then declined in the Purkinje cell layer perinatally, although it intensified in the molecular layer up to adulthood. The periods of maximum ChAT activity coincided with those in which NGF receptor immunohistochemistry was most intense in both human brain areas (Kerwin *et al.*, unpublished)—consistent with previous reports on non human species.[3] In contrast to these cholinergic patterns, glutamate NMDA receptor binding detected using MK801, was relatively unchanged with the exception of a 4-fold perinatal increase in the cerebellum.

In interpreting these results in terms of synaptic plasticity, two important aspects of the cholinergic system are worth considering: 1) proliferation of cholinergic neuronal processes is governed by specific trophic factors such as NGF[4]; and 2) acetylcholine itself has neurotrophic activity which may be controlled by the balance between synthesis (ChAT) and catabolism (AChE) of the transmitter.[5,6] The data so far available suggest that extension of cholinergic processes into the cerebellum occurs during a restricted perinatal period, after which the innervation remains constant, whereas cholinergic innervation of the hippocampus primarily occurs postnatally and continues up to middle age, after which it declines. This pattern is likely to be governed by neurotrophins, the synthesis of what is controlled by physiological activity.[7] Thus, in adult life, the cholinergic input to the hippocampus (but to a lesser extent cerebellum) is likely to be continually modeled by experience. The trophic role of AChE[8] in, for example, controlling the influence of acetylcholine in the architectural modeling of postsynaptic components is an intriguing area for further enquiry in view of the differential developmental patterns of enzyme reactivity associated with cholinergic and non-cholinergic systems. Moreover, since high AChE activity is intimately associated with βA4 peptide deposition in senile plaques,[9] acetylcholine may play a direct role in aberrant neurite formation in the plaque region. Therapeutic manipulation of AChE in dementia may be relevant not only in terms of the neurotropic but also neurotrophic action of acetylcholine.

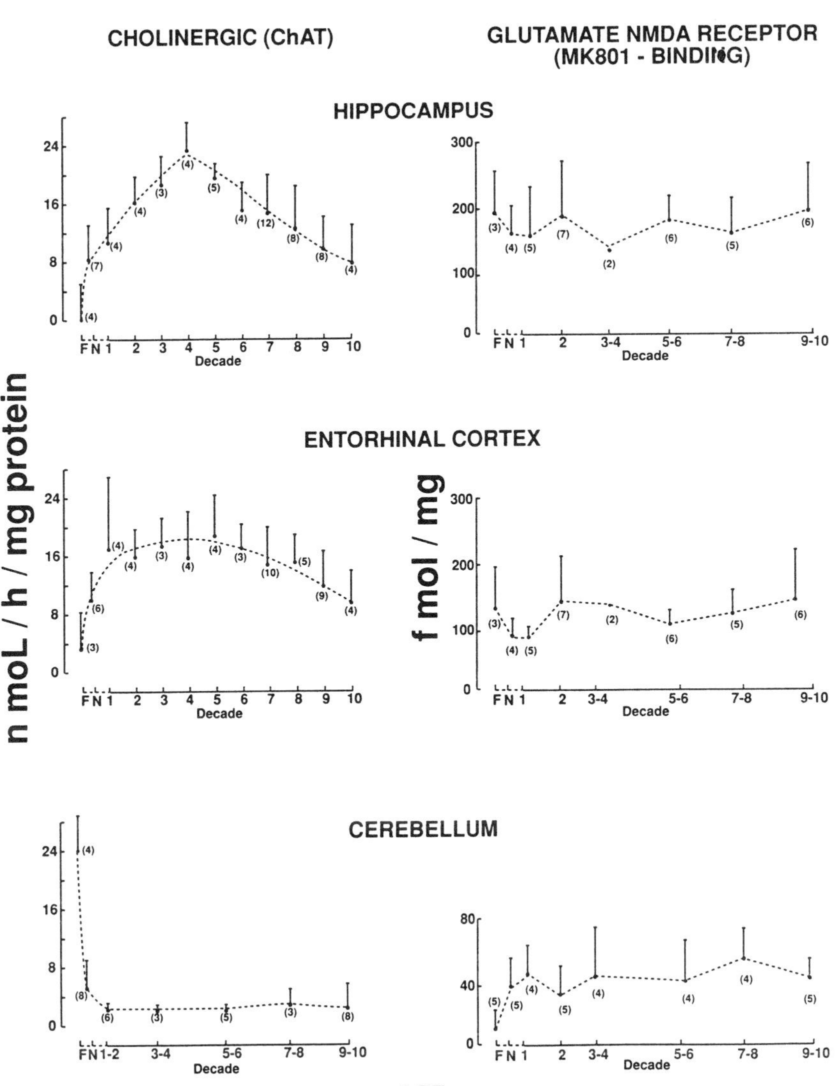

FIGURE 1. Cholinergic and glutamate activities in human brain across the age range from fetal (F) and neonatal (N) to adulthood and old age. Points represent mean values (for n individuals, numbers in parentheses) and bars are standard deviations.

REFERENCES

1. ROSS, R. N. 1928. The works of Aristotle translated into English. Oxford University Press. Oxford.
2. PERRY, E. K., M. JOHNSON, J. M. KERWIN, M. A. PIGGOTT, J. A. COURT, P. J. SHAW, P. G. INCE, A. BROWN & R. H. PERRY. 1992. Convergent cholinergic activities in aging and Alzheimer's disease. Neurobiol. Aging **13:**393–400.
3. SCHATTEMAN, G. C., L. GIBBS, A. A. LANAHAN, P. CLAUDE & M. BOTHWELL. 1988. Expression of NGF receptor in the developing and adult primate central nervous system. J. Neurosci. **8:**860–873.
4. PERRY, E. K. 1990. Nerve growth factor and the basal forebrain cholinergic system: A link in the etiopathology of neurogenerative dementias? Alz. Dis. Assoc. Disord. **4:**1–13.
5. MATTSON, M. P. 1988. Neurotransmitters in the regulation of neuronal cytoarchitecture. Brain Res. Rev. **13:**179–212.
6. SCHWARTZ, J. P. 1991. Neurotransmitters as neurotrophic factors: A new set of functions. Int. Rev. Neurobiol. **54:**1–23.
7. GALL, C. M. 1992. Regulation of brain neurotrophin expression by physiological activity. Trends Pharmacol. Sci. **13:**401–403.
8. LAYER, P. G., S. ROMMEL, H. BÜLTHOFF & R. HENGSTENBERG. 1988. Independent spatial waves of biochemical differentation along the surface of chicken brain as revealed by the sequential expression of acetylcholinesterase. Cell Tissue Res. **251:**587–595.
9. ULRICH, J., W. MEIER-RUGE, A. PROBST, E. MEIER & S. IPSEN. 1990. Senile plaques: Staining for acetylcholinesterase and A4 protein. Acta. Neuropathol. **80:**624–628.

Free Radicals in the Genesis of Alzheimer's Disease[a]

J. STEVEN RICHARDSON[b]

*Departments of Pharmacology and of Psychiatry, College of Medicine,
University of Saskatchewan, Saskatoon, SK. S7N 0W0 Canada*

ABSTRACT: As part of an ongoing investigation of the role of oxygen free radicals in Alzheimer's disease (AD), the formation of peroxidation products, the activities of free radical defense enzymes, and the level of total iron were determined in autopsy brain tissue from donors with AD and from age-matched non-demented donors. Calcium uptake was also investigated in mitochondria harvested from fibroblasts grown in tissue culture from skin samples taken from brain donors.

Compared to controls, homogenates of AD frontal cortex produced elevated levels of peroxidation products and this difference was amplified in a dose-dependent manner by iron (1 to 200 μM). Peroxidation produced by 200 μM iron was reduced dose dependently by the lazaroid U-74500A. The IC_{50} was 10 μM in AD cortex and 2.5 μM in controls.

Superoxide dismutase (SOD), one of the free radical defensive enzymes, was reduced by 25 to 35% in AD frontal cortex, hippocampus and cerebellum. In other brain areas, SOD did not differ between AD and control. The activities of catalase and glutathione peroxidase were the same in AD and control samples. Endogenous iron levels were higher in AD frontal cortex (2.5 nmol/mg protein) than in controls (1.5 nmol/mg protein).

Calcium uptake by AD fibroblast mitochondria is 50% lower than in controls under basal conditions. Following exposure to 200 μM iron, mitochondrial calcium uptake is increased by 58% in AD and by 38% in controls. Pretreatment with 200 μM U-74500A or 1 mM deferoxamine, prior to exposure to 200 μM iron, gave complete protection to control mitochondria but gave only partial protection to AD mitochondria.

These studies indicate that in AD, both CNS and peripheral cells show increased sensitivity to oxygen free radicals. The source of this increased sensitivity has not yet been identified but could reflect either reduced free radical defenses or increased free radical formation or both. Work is underway using electron paramagnetic resonance spectrometry to determine *in vivo*, premortem free radical activity in AD patients.

---

[a] The work discussed in this paper was in large part performed by my past and present Postdoctoral Fellows, Drs. K. V. Subbarao, L. Chen, and U. Kumar. These studies were supported in part by Grants PRG-90-025 (David Finkle) and IIRG-91-092 from the Alzheimer's Association (USA), by a grant from the Upjohn London Neuroscience Program and by donations from the Saskatchewan Alzheimer's Society and from private individuals.

[b] *Send correspondence to:* Dr. J. Steven Richardson, Department of Pharmacology, College of Medicine, University of Saskatchewan, Saskatoon, SK. S7N 0W0 Canada; TEL: (306) 966-6301; FAX: (306) 966-6220.

INTRODUCTION

In addition to neuritic plaques, neurofibrillary tangles, amyloid deposits, and other classic neuropathological signs in the brain, the membranes of various central and peripheral cells from AD patients show increase permeability, and brain samples show reduced gene expression and increased cell death. These latter characteristics are consistent with the expected actions of free radicals on biological tissue. Free radicals are any atoms or molecules with an unpaired electron in the outer orbital. This unpaired electron makes them unstable and highly reactive and they will change the structure and function of nearby molecules by donating or extracting electrons.[1] Oxygen free radicals are generated by many biological processes and are normal, although hazardous, members of the cellular environment. They are produced by oxidases and other enzymes, by cytochrome P450 electron transfer, by white blood cells during the respiratory burst after engulfing a bacteria, and by the Fenton reaction in which the formation of hydroxyl radicals from hydrogen peroxide is catalyzed by transitional metals such as iron, copper or manganese. Cellular protection against free radicals is provided by the enzymes superoxide dismutase (SOD), catalase and glutathione peroxidase, by antioxidants such as vitamin E, vitamin C (at low concentrations) and β-carotene, and by binding transitional metals to proteins so they cannot catalyze the formation of hydroxyl radicals. In excessive concentrations, free radicals can damage membrane lipids and proteins, thus altering membrane permeability and the regulation of ions, can impair mRNA formation by producing nicks and breaks in DNA strands, and can induce cell death by a variety of mechanisms. The similarity of these actions of free radicals to the characteristics of AD tissue, suggests that the study of free radicals might provide clues regarding the neuropathological etiology of AD.

METHODS

All assays were performed with tissue samples prepared from autopsy specimens taken within 24 hours of death from clinically well documented donors. Brain samples were quickly frozen and stored at $-86°C$. Skin samples were minced and plated and outgrowth cultures of fibroblasts were established in standard tissue culture conditions. All brains were examined histologically by Dr. L. C. Ang, Pathology, Royal University Hospital, Saskatoon, and evaluated according to the NIA/AARP criteria to confirm the diagnosis of Alzheimer's or control.

Peroxidation product formation was determined by a modified TBAR assay.[2] Superoxide dismutase,[3] catalase[4] and glutathione peroxidase[5] were measured by spectrophotometric methods. The uptake of calcium by mitochondria harvested from fibroblasts was monitored by using tracer amounts of ^{45}calcium. Statistical analysis was done using appropriate analyses of variance and post hoc tests contained in the SPSS-X statistical package.

RESULTS

The basal level of peroxidation product formation (TBAR) was significantly higher in homogenates of Alzheimer's cortex than in controls, and this difference was increased further in a dose-dependent manner by iron. Peroxidation of cortical homogenates induced by 200 μM iron was reduced dose dependently by the lazaroid U-74500A, with the IC$_{50}$ being 4 times higher in Alzheimer's samples (10 μM) than in samples from controls (2.5 μM). Superoxide dismutase activity was 27% to 35% lower than controls in Alzheimer's cortex, hippocampus, and cerebellum. There were no differences in catalase or glutathione peroxidase between Alzheimer's and control samples. Total iron levels were significantly higher in Alzheimer's frontal cortex samples (2.5 nmoles/mg protein) than in controls (1.5 nmoles/mg protein). Under basal conditions, the uptake of calcium by Alzheimer's fibroblast mitchondria was significantly lower (55 pmoles/min/mg protein) than that of controls (124 pmoles/min/mg protein). Pretreatment with 200 μM iron significantly increased calcium uptake by 58% in Alzheimer's mitochondria and by 38% in controls. When the iron exposure was done in the presence of 200 μM U-74500A or 1mM desferoxamine, calcium uptake by Alzheimer's mitochondria was increased only 34% and 32% respectively, while uptake by control mitochondria was the same as that under basal conditions.

DISCUSSION

Taken together, these observations indicate that, compared to samples from age-matched non-demented controls, autopsy samples of frontal cortex from Alzheimer's patients have higher basal peroxidation, show a greater increase in peroxidation activity when exposed to iron, have a higher antioxidant requirement, and contain greater amounts of iron. Moreover, mitochondria from Alzheimer's fibroblasts in tissue culture have reduced ability to take up calcium compared to control fibroblast mitochondria, but show a greater increase in calcium uptake following an iron-induced peroxidation challenge. Compared to controls, both CNS and peripheral tissue from Alzheimer's donors show increased sensitivity to the effects of free radicals and require greater amounts of antioxidants to protect against a standard peroxidation challenge induced by 200 μM iron. The source of this increased sensitivity to free radicals and the consequence of it to the Alzheimer's patient have not been identified. It also remains to be established that Alzheimer's patients *in vivo* have a higher free radical burden than non-demented people. Research is underway using the electron paramagnetic resonance with spin trapping technique to determine free radicals in premortem samples from AD patients.

ACKNOWLEDGMENT

The stenographic expertise of Mrs. E. Habbick is greatly appreciated.

REFERENCES

1. HALLIWELL, B. 1992. Reactive oxygen species and the central nervous system. J. Neurochem. **59:**1609–1623.
2. BRAUGHLER, J. M., L. A. DUNCAN & R. L. CHASE. 1986. The involvement of iron in lipid peroxidation. Importance of ferric ratios in initiation. J. Biol. Chem. **261:**10282–10289.
3. YOANAGUI, Y. 1984. Reevaluation of assay methods and establishment of kit for superoxide dismutase activity. Anal. Biochem. **132:**290–296.
4. AEBI, H. 1974. Catalase. Methods in Enzymatic Analysis, Vol. 2. Academic Press. New York. Pp. 673–680.
5. PAGLIA D. E. & W. N. VALENTINE. 1967. Studies on the quantitative and qualitative characterization of erythrocyte glutathione peroxidase. J. Lab. Clin. Med. **70:**158–169.

Abnormalities in Brain Glucose Utilization and Its Impact on Cellular and Molecular Mechanisms in Sporadic Dementia of Alzheimer Type

SIEGFRIED HOYER[a]

*Department of Pathochemistry and General Neurochemistry,
University of Heidelberg, W-6900 Heidelberg, Germany*

ABSTRACT: Brain glucose utilization and ATP formation were found to be reduced to 54% and 81%, respectively, of control values in incipient sporadic dementia of Alzheimer type, causing reduced availability of the glucose-derived neurotransmitter acetylcholine. With respect to energy shortage, impacts on energy-dependent processes such as synaptic transmission, ion homeostasis, protein processing and degradation, extracellular transmission, and extracellular phosphorylation may be expected. Normal processing of the amyloid precursor protein was demonstrated to occur via a muscarinergic acetylcholine M1 and M3 receptor-mediated signal transduction pathway. Since both the muscarinergic acetylcholine receptors on pyramidal neurons and G proteins were found to be unaltered in DAT, the possibility is discussed that the diminution of glucose utilization and the energy shortage in DAT brain may contribute considerably to abnormal amyloid precursor protein processing and thus to secondary amyloid formation.

INTRODUCTION

Glucose is essential for the mature, healthy mammalian brain to obtain acetylcholine[1–3] and energy in the form of ATP.[4,5] Acetylcholine mediates learning, memory, and cognition,[6,7] while ATP is necessary for several basic cellular and molecular processes, such as synaptic transmission,[8] ion homeostasis,[9] protein processing,[10] extracellular transmission[11] and protein phosphorylation.[12] Any abnormality in glucose supply to the brain or in glucose utilization by the cell can thus be expected to cause reductions in both acetylcholine synthesis and ATP formation. In incipient sporadic dementia of the Alzheimer type (DAT), global cerebral glucose metabolism was found to be

[a] *Send correspondence to:* Siegfried Hoyer, Department of Pathochemistry and General Neurochemistry, University of Heidelberg, W-6900 Heidelberg, Germany; TEL: 49-6221-562618; FAX: 49-6221-563328.

severely diminished to 55% of control,[13,14] as was the formation rate of acetylcholine to 47% of control.[3] This report deals with the ATP formation rate in incipient sporadic DAT and discusses the impact of glucose diminution and energy shortage on acetylcholine signal transduction.

SUBJECTS AND METHODS

Eleven patients aged from 61 to 78 years were diagnosed as having incipient late-onset (sporadic) DAT. A group of eleven physically and mentally intact subjects aged 29 to 60 years acted as a control group (HMAC). Global cerebral blood flow and the cerebral metabolic rates of oxygen, CO_2, glucose and lactate were investigated. These results have been detailed earlier, as have the diagnostic criteria and age-related aspects.[13] ATP formation was calculated from the cerebral metabolic rates of oxygen, glucose and lactate.[5]

RESULTS

The results are seen in TABLE 1. Consideration of the values recorded in the two groups reveals that in DAT, glucose utilization had fallen to 54% of control, whereas ATP had dropped only to 81% of control.

DISCUSSION

It is suggested that the disproportion between the more severe reduction in glucose utilization and the less severe reduction in ATP formation was due to a substitutional utilization of endogenous amino acids, in particular glutamate, or free fatty acids, or both.[5,15] Since ammonia, the source of which may be glutamine[16] and purine bodies,[17] was also generated in the brain, the neuron can be assumed to be subject to extreme stress. Recently, clear evidence has emerged that stimulation of the muscarinergic M1 and M3 receptor

TABLE 1.

	CMR of Glucose		ATP Formation
	(μmol/g $\times$ min)		
	Total	Oxidized	
HMAC	0.28	0.26	9.36
Incipient sporadic DAT	0.15[a]	0.14[a]	7.62[a]

[a] $p \leq 0.05$.

sub-types increases the basal release of amyloid precursor protein (APP) derivatives.[18] In DAT, persistence of muscarinergic acetylcholine receptors on pyramidal neurons was found,[19] as was the preservation of G proteins.[20] Otherwise, protein kinase C levels were found to be diminished in DAT,[21] which may be due to the perturbed signal transduction resulting both from severely reduced ligand availability to muscarinergic receptors and from ATP reduction. As a consequence, APP processing may be abnormal and this may be accentuated by the enhanced cellular ammonia concentration[16,22] and by the reduced proteolytic capacity resulting from energy shortage.[23]

REFERENCES

1. GIBSON, G. E. & J. P. BLASS. 1976. Inhibition of acetylcholine synthesis and of carbohydrate utilization by maple-syrup-urine disease metabolites. J. Neurochem. **26:**1073–1078.

2. GIBSON, G. E. & J. P. BLASS. 1976. Impaired synthesis of acetylcholine in brain accompanying mild hypoxia and hypoglycemia. J. Neurochem. **27:**37–42.

3. SIMS, N. R., D. M. BOWEN & A. N. DAVISON. 1981. [^{14}C]acetylcholine synthesis and [^{14}C] carbon dioxide production from [U^{-14}C] glucose by tissue prisms from human neocortex. Biochem. J. **196:**867–876.

4. ERECINSKA, M & I. A. SILVER. 1989. ATP and brain function. J. Cereb. Blood Flow Metab. **9:**2–19.

5. HOYER, S. 1992. Oxidative energy metabolism in Alzheimer brain. Studies in early-onset and late-onset cases. Mol. Chem. Neuropathol. **16:**207–224.

6. DEUTSCH, J. A. 1973. The cholinergic synapse and the site of memory. *In* The Physiological Basis of Memory. J. A. Deutsch, Ed. :59–76. Academic Press. New York.

7. GOLD, P. E. & S. F. ZORNETZER. 1983. The mnemon and its juices: Neuromodulation of memory processes. Behav. Neural Biol. **38:**151–189.

8. HUGANIR, R. L. & P. GREENGARD. 1990. Regulation of neurotransmitter receptor desensitization by protein phosphorylation. Neuron **5:**555–567.

9. SIESJÖ, B. K. 1981. Cell damage in the brain: A speculative synthesis. J. Cereb. Blood Flow Metab. **1:**155–185.

10. GETHING, M. J. & J. SAMBROOK. 1992. Protein folding in the cell. Nature **355:**33–45.

11. BURNSTOCK, G. 1990. Purinergic mechanisms. Ann. N. Y. Acad. Sci. **603:**1–17.

12. EHRLICH, Y. H., T. B. DAVIS, E. BOCK, E. KORNECKI & R. H. LENOX. 1986. Ecto-protein kinase activity on the external surface of neural cells. Nature **320:**67–70.

13. HOYER, S., R. NITSCH & K. OESTERREICH. 1991. Predominant abnormality in cerebral glucose utilization in late-onset dementia of the Alzheimer type: A cross-sectional comparison against advanced late-onset and incipient early-onset cases. J. Neural Transm. (P-D Sect.). **3:**1–14.

14. MIELKE, R., K. HERHOLZ, M. GROND, J. KESSLER & W. D. HEISS. 1991. Differences of regional cerebral glucose metabolism between presenile and senile dementia of Alzheimer type. Neurobiol. Aging **13:**93–98.

15. HOYER, S. & R. NITSCH. 1989. Cerebral excess release of neurotransmitter amino acids subsequent to reduced cerebral glucose metabolism in early-onset dementia of Alzheimer type. J. Neural. Transm. **75:**227–232.

16. HOYER, S., R. NITSCH & K. OESTERREICH. 1990. Ammonia is endogenously generated in the brain in the presence of presumed and verified dementia of Alzheimer type. Neurosci. Lett. **117:**358–362.

17. DEGRELL, I. & F. NIKLASSON. 1988. Purine metabolites in the CSF in presenile and senile dementia of Alzheimer type, and in multi-infarct dementia. Arch. Gerontol. Geriatr. **7:**173–178.

18. NITSCH, R. M., B. E. SLACK, R. J. WURTMAN & J. H. GROWDON. 1992. Release of Alzheimer amyloid precursor derivatives stimulated by activation of muscarinic acetylcholine receptors. Science **258:**304–307.

19. SCHRÖDER, H., E. GIACOBINI, R. G. STRUBLE, P. G. M. LUITEN, E. A. VAN DER ZEE, K. ZILLES & A. D. STROSBERG. 1991. Muscarinic cholinoceptive neurons in the frontal cortex in Alzheimer's disease. Brain Res. Bull. **27:** 631–636.

20. MCLAUGHLIN, M., B. M. ROSS, G. MILLIGAN, J. MCCULLOCH & J. T. KNOWLER. 1991. Robustness of G proteins in Alzheimer's disease: An immunoblot study. J. Neurochem. **57:**9–14.

21. COLE, G., K. R. DOBKINS, L. A. HANSEN, R. D. TERRY & T. SAITOH. 1988. Decreased levels of protein kinase C in Alzheimer brain. Brain Res. **452:** 165–174.

22. CAPORASO, G. L., S. E. GANDY, J. D. BUXBAUM & P. GREENGARD. 1992. Chloroquine inhibits intracellular degradation but not secretion of Alzheimer beta/A4 amyloid precursor protein. Proc. Natl. Acad. Sci. USA **89:**2252–2256.

23. OKADA, M., M. ISHIKAWA & Y. MIZUSHIMA. 1991. Identification of a ubiquitin- and ATP-dependent protein degradation pathway in rat cerebral cortex. Biochim. Biophys. Acta **1073:**514–520.

Dopamine D2 Receptors in Normal Human Brain: Effect of Age Measured by Positron Emission Tomography (PET) and [^{11}C]-Raclopride[a]

ANGELO ANTONINI[b] AND KLAUS L. LEENDERS

Paul Scherrer Institute, PET Department, Villigen, Switzerland

ABSTRACT: Human post-mortem and animal experimental results suggest a decline of the cerebral dopaminergic neuronal system with age. In this study, the radiotracer [^{11}C]raclopride (dopamine D2 antagonist) and positron emission tomography were applied to determine the effect of age on striatal dopamine D2 receptors in 32 healthy volunteer subjects (age range 21–68 years). Subjects were divided in two age groups on the basis of median age (31 years). An index for specific tracer uptake was calculated for caudate nucleus and putamen. Uptake indices in the older group of subjects were reduced on average 26% in putamen and 20% in caudate nucleus. The decline appeared to be steep until 30 years, but slower afterwards. After 30 years of age the decline of specific raclopride binding was found to be 0.6% per year. These results suggest that dopamine D2 receptor binding sites (mainly post-synaptically located) decrease as a consequence of normal aging in parallel with the decline of the pre-synaptic nigrostriatal dopa-minergic system.

INTRODUCTION

A progressive decline of the nigrostriatal dopaminergic system with age has been reported by human post-mortem and animal studies. A reduction with age of the dopamine D2 receptor density in striatum was suggested in mice, rats, monkeys and humans.[1] The question of the effect of normal aging on the nigrostriatal system in man can be directly addressed *in vivo* by positron emission tomography (PET) using radiolabeled tracers.

Human striatal dopamine D2 receptor density was specifically studied in

[a] Part of the work reported in this study was supported by the Swiss National Research Foundation (No 31-28816.90).

[b] *Send correspondence to:* Dr. A. Antonini, PET Department, Paul Scherrer Institute, CH-5232 Villigen, Switzerland; TEL: 41-56-993682; FAX: 41-56-993294.

healthy volunteer subjects with the tracer [¹¹C]methyl-spiperone.[2] In that study, a significant decline of tracer uptake with age was found. Although methyl-spiperone and the other spiperone derivatives are ligands with high affinity for dopamine D2 receptors, they additionally bind to S2 serotonin and α1-adrenergic receptor sites. In recent years, [¹¹C]-raclopride has been developed as PET tracer to investigate cerebral D2 dopamine receptors. This ligand is a neuroleptic of the class of benzamides which binds, as an antagonist, selectively to dopamine D2 receptors and has a different tracer kinetic from spiperone derivates. Also, the application of [¹¹C]methyl-spiperone and [¹¹C]raclopride in clinical studies has led to conflicting results.

In view of the scarcity of available PET data and on the basis of the above mentioned differences between tracers, we set out to investigate the effect of normal aging using [¹¹C]raclopride.

METHODS

Thirty two healthy volunteer subjects (5 females and 27 males) were investigated. The age range was from 21 to 68 years (median: 31 years). Selection criteria were: no history of psychiatric or neurological disease; no abnormal signs at general medical and neurological examination; no signs of drugs or alcohol abuse. All subjects older than 30 years were investigated with a MRI scan and, in addition, with a set of neuropsychological tests to check normality of cognition. None of them showed signs of brain atrophy or vascular lesions at the MRI. Scoring for cognitive performances was in the normal range for all subjects.

[¹¹C]raclopride was infused intravenously, in a volume of 10 ml of physiological saline, over a period of 3 minutes using a constant volume infusion pump. At the beginning of tracer infusion a dynamic scan sequence was started, consisting of 20 time frames from 1 minute gradually increasing to 5 minutes duration. Total scanning time after tracer application was 58 minutes. Regions of interest (ROI's) were placed by visual inspection, using an anatomy atlas as reference, in a standard template arrangement over the head of caudate, putamen and cerebellum for each brain hemisphere. An index for specific tracer uptake was calculated for each subject using the ratio: (Target ROI-Cerebellum)/Cerebellum. Mean index values for every ROI were calculated between 35 and 58 minutes after tracer administration, when equilibrium between specifically bound and free radioligand concentration has occurred. Values of left and right hemisphere of each subject were pooled. Subjects were also divided in two age groups on the basis of the median age (31 years). Seventeen subjects were in the first group (mean age 25.1 ± 3.1 SD) and fifteen in the second (mean age 52.4 ± 10.6 SD).

RESULTS

A significantly lower specific uptake was found in putamen ($p < .0001$ t-test two-tailed, unpaired) and in caudate nucleus ($p < .004$ t-test, two-tailed, unpaired) comparing the second with the first group of subjects. The putamen

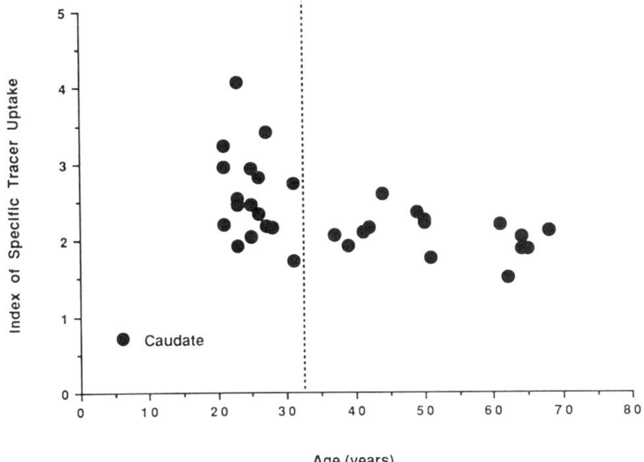

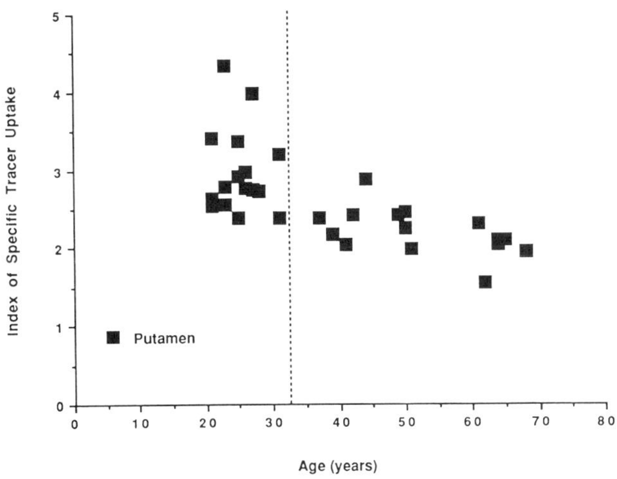

FIGURE 1. Scatter diagram of the index for specific [^{11}C]raclopride uptake in caudate nucleus and putamen versus age in all subjects (n = 32). The broken vertical line indicates the median age (31 years).

indices of the second group showed on average a 26% lower value than the first group. For caudate nucleus the mean decrease was 20%. In FIGURE 1, the indices of specific uptake in putamen and caudate nucleus are plotted as a function of age. Putamen and caudate uptake indices showed a significant decline over the total age range (n = 32 subjects, $p < .001$ for putamen and $p < .002$ for caudate, Spearman rank). When considering only the second group of subjects (n = 15), a correlation with age was found in putamen ($p < .05$ Spearman rank) but not in caudate nucleus (n.s. Spearman rank). The decrease of the index appeared to be steep until 30 years and slower afterwards. The slope of the linear regression line for the second group was -0.014 ± 0.007 (95% confidence limits) in putamen and -0.008 ± 0.006 (95% confidence limits) in caudate nucleus. The total decline from 37 to 68 years was 19% in putamen and 12% in caudate nucleus. This corresponds to a decrease of uptake of 0.6% per year in putamen and 0.4% per year in caudate nucleus in the age range between 37 and 68 years.

CONCLUSION

Our results show a significant decrease with age of specific [^{11}C]raclopride binding in human striatum. They are consistent with the results of the authors who applied spiperone derived radiotracers.[2] In spite of the different pharmacological and binding properties of the two radioligands, striatal dopamine D2 receptor binding was found to decrease with age in all PET studies reported so far. Human post-mortem studies differ concerning their conclusions about the effect of age on D2 receptor density. A decrease as well as no change have been reported. It seems most likely that the pre-synaptic nigrostriatal dopaminergic neuronal system is reduced with normal aging. In turn, under normal circumstances, the post-synaptic dopamine D2 receptors seems to follow this decline in parallel, possibly through internal cellular regulatory mechanisms. Recent evidence from our laboratory indicates, that under pathological circumstances, as in Parkinson's disease, the post-synaptic dopaminergic receptor response contrasts with that in normal aging.[3]

ACKNOWLEDGMENT

Manufacturing of tracer precursor and pharmacological support by Ciba-Geigy, Ltd. are gratefully acknowledged.

REFERENCES

1. SEVERSON, J. A., J. MARCUSSON, B. WINBLAD & C. E. FINCH. 1982. Age-correlated loss of dopaminergic binding sites in human basal ganglia. J. Neurochem. **39:**1623–1631.

2. WONG, D. F., H. WAGNER, R. DANNALS, *et al.* 1984. Effects of age on dopamine and serotonin receptors measured by positron tomography in the living human brain. Science **226:**1391–1395.

3. LEENDERS, K. L. & A. ANTONINI. 1991. Pathophysiology of Parkinson's disease and positron emission tomography (PET). *In* Basic and Clinical Approaches. Basal Ganglia and Movement Disorders, Vol 3. New Issues in Neurosciences. A. Bignami, Ed.: 143–148. Georg Thieme Verlag. Stuttgart.

Comparative Effects of Aging Process on Phosphatidylcholine Biosynthesis Pathway: A Key Role for CTP-Phosphocholine Cytidylyltransferase?

J. M. LEPAGNOL[a] AND V. HEIDET

Institut de Recherches Servier, Suresnes, France

ABSTRACT: The effects of aging on phosphatidylcholine (PtdCho) biosynthesis were investigated in liver and brain subcellular fractions of the rat, by studying the activity and regulation of CTP phosphocholine cytidylyltransferase (CT), the rate limiting enzyme in PtdCho biosyntheses. With both tissues, CT activity was present in cytosolic and microsomal fractions, but in brain, CT activity seemed to escape to an inhibiting feed back mechanism. In brain, CT activity was greater in the microsomal fraction, whilst in liver, a higher CT activity was seen in the cytosolic fraction.

In liver fractions of aged animals, there was no significant change in CT activity or its sensitivity to negative feedback regulation, as compared to young animals. In contrast, a progressive age related decline in CT activity was observed in the brain microsomal fraction. Furthermore, the incorporation of newly formed CDPCho into PtdCho was also reduced in aged animals, and paralleled the decreased incorporation of choline in PtdCho. The age-related decrease in CT activity cannot be explained by product feed back inhibition or decreased diacylglycerol levels.

Since PtdCho is a major membrane lipid, the reduction in CT activity may lead to a decreased membrane integrity and fluidity during the aging process, and these effects may be greater in neuronal cells.

Recent progress in biochemical characterization of cerebral aging and Alzheimer's disease (AD) has led to the proposal of different hypotheses for the etiology of progressive neuronal cell death. Among these hypothesis, the role of β-amyloid (β/A4) formation, toxicity and/or deposit seems to be of great importance.[1] On the other hand, the most extensively explored therapeutical target for AD treatment has been cholinergic neurotransmission, since the release of acetylcholine (ACh) decreases during the aging process[2] and since

[a] *Send correspondence to:* Dr. J. M. Lepagnol, Institut de Recherches Servier, Department of Cerebral Pathology, 11, rue des Moulineaux, 92150 Suresnes, France; TEL: 33-1-41182200; FAX: 33-1-41182430.

the cholinergic neurons are the most vulnerable in AD.[3] It has been suggested that the selective vulnerability of the cholinergic neuron could be due to a unique property of these cells, namely their use of choline for two purposes: acetylcholine and membrane phosphatidylcholine (PtdCho) synthesis. Thus, membrane PtdCho could be considered as the potential reservoir of choline for ACh synthesis,[4] which in aging and AD situations, could be maintained by excessive PtdCho catabolism and depletion, leading to cholinergic neuronal death. This hypothesis has been called "autocannibalism"[5] and suggests that a deficit in PtdCho synthesis capability could jeopardize both the membrane integrity and the neuronal resistance to cumulative aggressive stimuli, as in aging process. We have aimed at determining if this could be the case.

For this purpose, our studies have mainly concerned the rate limiting step in PtdCho biosynthesis, *i.e.*, the conversion of phosphocholine to CDP-choline by CTP: phosphocholine cytidylyltransferase (CT; EC 27715). This enzyme has been extensively studied in peripheral organs but surprisingly never in brain tissue. In lung and liver, CT has been reported to exist in two forms: one inactive phosphorylated cytosolic form (enzyme reservoir) and one active unphosphorylated microsomal form. By a reversible translocation of CT between cytosol and membrane, cells have an easy and rapid mechanism for regulating PtdCho biosynthesis, and many studies have demonstrated a close correlation between microsomal CT activity and the rate of PtdCho synthesis.[6]

We have compared rat brain and liver CT activation capacities in cytosolic and microsomal fractions by using a new HPLC technique based on rapid measurement of neosynthetized methyl [^{14}C] CDP-choline after incubation of the fractions with [^{14}C] choline and CTP. We then studied the influence of the aging process on CT activation, and tried to correlate it with the age-related changes in PtdCho synthesis by using a TLC analysis of final radiolabeled compounds (PtdCho).

RESULTS AND DISCUSSION

Comparison of Brain and Liver CT Activation

CT activation appeared to differ between brain and liver tissues, both quantitatively and qualitatively. In brain, CT activation resulted in a synthesis of CDP-choline 10-fold greater than in liver. CDP-choline synthesis in brain was predominantly located in the microsomal fraction, thus showing a high requirement of neuronal membrane for rapid phospholipid turn-over.

In both organs, the kinetic profiles of CT activation were quite different between cytosolic and microsomal fractions: in cytosol, the amount of neosynthesized CDP-choline accumulated continuously during more than 1 hour, but in microsomes, it reached a maximum level after 10–15 minutes, then stabilized in liver tissue but decreased significantly in brain tissue, reflecting, in this latter case, a fast (and necessary) transformation of CDP-choline into PtdCho.

In both organs, CT activity was regulated by an inhibitory feedback mechanism exerted by the final compound of the enzymatic reaction, CDP-choline. However, the needed concentration of CDP-choline, for such a feedback mechanism was 50-fold higher in brain as compared with liver (IC50 = 10 μM and 0.2 μM respectively). Consequently, it has been calculated that in liver microsomes this feedback thereby could explain the physiological arrest of CDP-choline synthesis after 10 minutes of CT activation, which absolutely could not be the case in brain microsomes. Thus, brain CT appeared not to be influenced by a feedback regulation, which was, once more, in good accordance with the high phospholipid turn-over necessity in neuronal cells.

Comparative Effects of Aging Process on Brain and Liver CT Activity

In F344 rats, the influence of aging process appeared to be radically different between brain and liver (FIG. 1—left and right, respectively). Indeed, in livers of 22-month-old rats, CT activation appeared to be more important than in 3-month-old rats and the maximal amount of neosynthesized CDP-choline was twofold higher (0.25 and 0.12 nmoles/mg, respectively). This

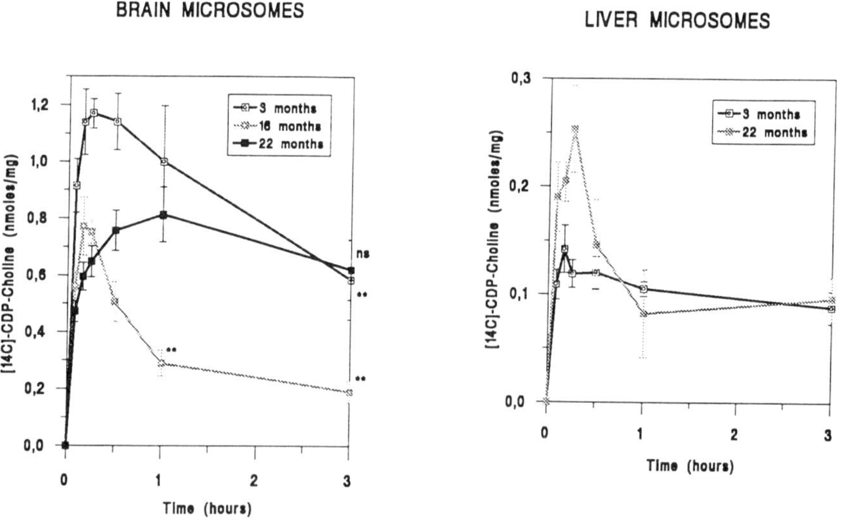

FIGURE 1. Comparative effects of aging process on CT activation in rat brain and liver.

significant increase was only transient (less than 1 hour) and could represent a useful pool of CDP-choline for PtdCho synthesis in old hepatocytes.

In brain tissue, however, aging process was accompanied by a progressive decline of CT activation and CDP-choline utilization. Thus, in 16-month-old rats the maximal amount of synthetized CDP-choline was decreased by 40% as compared with young animals (0.8 and 1.2 nmole/mg respectively) but the initial rate of CT activation remained the same in both groups. Surprisingly, an intense and significant utilization (disappearance) of CDP-choline took place during the following 2 hours (proof of neuron "vitality"). This was not the case in aged 22-month-old rat. Indeed, although the same 40% decrease in maximal CDP-choline amount was observed, it took place much more slowly in 1 hour and no significant utilization followed.

It is noteworthy that, by measuring the final amount of neosynthetized PtdCho, a similar 40% decrease was observed in old animals as compared with young rats. This clear-cut similarity conferred a strong pathophysiological relevance to the age-related deficit in CT activation. Neither excessive feedback mechanism by CDP-choline nor decrease of diacylglycerol level for the following step of PtdCho biosynthesis pathway could explain the age-related CT deficiency.

In view of the classically described CT regulation by the cellular kinase-phosphatase equilibrium, it has been observed that okadaic acid (OKA)-induced inhibition of PtdCho synthesis (pmol/mg tissue) was much more dramatic in young, than in old brains:

Young control: 1.9   Old control: 1.15

Young OKA: 0.9   Old OKA: 0.8

Although, in young and old rat, okadaic acid induced a 50% decrease in PtdCho synthesis, the final amount of PtdCho was the same in both groups. Thus, the influence of aging process seemed to act in the same way than the phosphatase inhibition and considering CT deficiency, aging could potentially be accompanied by a dysfunction of the kinase-phosphatase system.

CONCLUSION

These results show clearly for the first time, that in brain CTP-phosphocholine cytidylyltransferase activation exhibits a specific behavior as compared with liver CT. The higher basal CT activity and the absence of CDP-choline induced feedback inhibition are in good accordance with the physiological need for elevated PtdCho turnover for adequate neuronal plasticity and function.

The close relationship between CT activation and PtdCho synthesis deficits during the aging process, confers to the CT deficiency a key-role in progressive neuronal loss, especially in well-known vulnerable neurons. Looking back to the β-amyloid protein hypothesis in AD, it must be remembered that because of the partly intramembranar location of the β/A4 protein, eventual changes in membrane composition and plasticity could expose the neuronal membraneous proteins to abnormal cleavage by proteases and facilitate both the β/A4 extracellular deposit and intracellular toxic effect. However, it remains to be verified that CT activation deficiency can be observed in aged and/or demented human brain.

REFERENCES

1. BANNER, C. 1990. Toward a molecular etiology of Alzheimer's Disease. Int. Psychogeriatrics **2**:135–147.
2. WEILER, M. H. 1990. Acetylcholine release from striatal slices of young adult and aged fischer 344 rats. Neurobiol. Aging **11**:401–407.
3. BOWEN, D. M., P. WHITE, J. A. SPILLANE, M. J. GOODHARDT, G. CURZON, P. IWANGOFF, W. MEIER-RUGE & A. N. DAVISON. 1979. Accelerated ageing or selective neuronal loss as an important cause of dementia? Lancet: 11–14.
4. BLUSZTAJN, J. K. & R. J. WURTMAN. 1983. Choline and cholinergic neurons. Science **221**:614.
5. WURTMAN, R. J. 1992. Choline metabolism as a basis for the selective vulnerability of cholinergic neurons. TINS **15**:117–122.
6. VANCE, D. E. 1991. Phospholipid metabolism and cell signalling in eucaryotes. *In* Biochemistry of Lipids, Lipoproteins and Membranes. D. E. Vance & J. Vance, Eds. 205–240. Elsevier.

Regulation and Expression of the Alzheimer's β/A4 Amyloid Protein Precursor in Health, Disease, and Down's Syndrome[a]

KONRAD BEYREUTHER,[b,d] PETER POLLWEIN,[b]
GERD MULTHAUP,[b] URSULA MÖNNING,[b] GERHARD KÖNIG,[b]
THOMAS DYRKS,[b] WALTER SCHUBERT,[b]
AND COLIN L. MASTERS[c]

[b] *ZMBH, Center for Molecular Biology, Heidelberg, University of Heidelberg,
D-69120 Heidelberg Germany*
[c] *The Department of Pathology, University of Melbourne and Mental Health
Research Institute of Victoria, Parkville, Victoria 3052 Australia*

ABSTRACT: A four- to fivefold overexpression of the gene for the Alzheimer β/A4 amyloid precursor protein (APP) in individuals with Down's Syndrome (DS) appears to be responsible for the fifty year earlier onset of Alzheimer's disease (AD) pathology in DS compared to the normal population. It is therefore likely that a deregulated overexpression of the APP gene is a risk factor for the β/A4 amyloid formation. To test this hypothesis and to get a better understanding of how APP expression is regulated, we studied the 5′ control region of the human APP gene, alternative splicing of the 19 APP exons, and APP biogenesis, metabolism and function. The analysis of the APP promoter revealed its similarity with those of housekeeping genes by the presence of a GC-rich region around the transcription start site and the lack of a TATA box. Gene transfer experiments showed this GC-rich region to contain overlapping binding sites for different transcription factors whose binding is mutually excluded. An imbalance between these factors may cause APP overexpression and predispose to AD pathology. Another putative risk factor for AD is regulation of splicing of exon 7 in APP mRNA's which changes in brain during aging. This is relevant for APP processing since exon 7 codes for a Kunitz protease inhibitory domain. Investigation of further splicing adjacent to the β/A4 exons 16 and 17 which might also

[a] This work was supported by funds from the Deutsche Forschungsgemeinschaft (DFG) through Sonderforschungsboreich (SFB) 317 and 258, the Bundesminister für Forschung und Technologie (BMFT project 3016001A), the Fonds der Chemischen Industrie, the Metropolitan Life Foundation and the Boehringer Ingelheim Fonds. C.L.M. is supported by grants from the National Health and Medical Research Council of Australia, the Victorian Health Promotion Foundation and the Aluminum Development Corporation.
[d] *Send correspondence to:* Konrad Beyreuther, ZMBH, Center for Molecular Biology Heidelberg, Im Neuenheimer Feld 282, D-69120 Heidelberg, Germany; TEL: 49-6221-566845; FAX: 41-6221-565891.

interfere with APP processing led to the identification of the leukocyte-derived (L-APP) splice forms which lack exon 15. In brain this splicing occurs in activated astrocytes and microglia. The localization of APP at synaptic sites in brain suggests that APP regulation and expression are critical determinants of a potential and early impairment of central synapses. This may be the case during pathological evolution of AD and DS when β/A4 derived from synaptic APP is converted to β/A4 amyloid by radical generation.

It is less than a decade since the molecular basis of the Alzheimer's disease lesions started to become apparent. This was the case when it was shown that the β/A4 protein is the amyloid component of cerebral amyloid angiopathy and senile plaques in AD and Down's Syndrome (DS).[1,2] Subsequently, the human gene for the β/A4 amyloid precursor protein (APP) was identified by cDNA sequencing and suggested to play a central role in the development of Alzheimer's disease.[3] This APP gene maps to the long arm of human chromosome 21 and consists of 19 exons which are alternatively spliced into different products, named APP or L-APP and according to their length in amino acids.[4] APP's are ubiquitously expressed isoforms whereas L-APP's are the first splice products of the APP gene for which a restricted expression pattern has been established.[4,5] The amino acid sequences of these APP and L-APP isoforms show the characteristic features of typical membrane glycoproteins. The single transmembrane domain of these proteins is encoded by exon 17. The β/A4 amyloid subunit is a polypeptide of 39–43 residues and derived in part from this domain since it is encoded within exons 16 and 17 of the APP gene. The N-terminal 28 residues of the β/A4 region are located within its extracellular part and the C-terminal 11-14 residues within the transmembrane domain of APP and L-APP. Secreted forms of APP and L-APP are generated by APP secretase or APPase which cleaves within this amyloidogenic β/A4 region. The β/A4 protein was identified in soluble form in the media of neural and non-neural cell cultures and in body fluids of AD patients and of controls suggesting that the cleavage of APP into βA does occur normally and not cause amyloid deposition.[6] We were able to demonstrate that the aggregation of β/A4 does not occur spontaneously at physiological concentrations but depends on additional factors.[7] We identified these factors as radical generation systems which are capable of transforming soluble β/A4 into insoluble and aggregating molecules. We were also able to demonstrate inhibition of this process by radical scavengers.[7]

RISK FACTORS OF β/A4 AMYLOID PATHOLOGY RELATED TO APP

Up to now, there are five risk factors known which predispose to the onset of AD pathology (FIG. 1), one of which is, in some rare familial forms (FAD),

FIGURE 1. The known risk factors for Alzheimer's disease β/A4 pathology include Trisomy of the APP gene of chromosome 21 in Down's Syndrome (APP-DOWN SYNDROME), alternative splicing of exon 7 which codes for the Kunitz protease inhibitory domain (KPI-AGE) in APP becomes prominent in brain during aging, mutation of the β/A4 amyloid protein precursor in familial Alzheimer's disease which clusters at the borders of the β/A4 region and proximal to the APPase cleavage site (FAD-MUTATIONS), and shearing of nerve terminal by microtrauma (HEAD-TRAUMA).

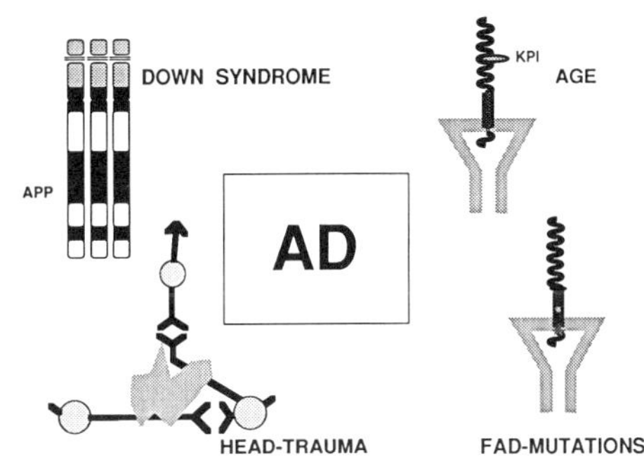

a mutation in the APP gene. The FAD mutations so far described for the APP gene are clustered at the borders of the β/A4 part of APP and within β/A4 proximal to the APP secretase site.[8] The second risk factor is a mutation in a hitherto unknown gene on chromosome 14[9] and therefore not included in the scheme outlined in FIGURE 1. The third risk factor is an additional copy of this gene in individuals with DS. The trisomy of the APP gene does not simply cause a fifty percent increase in APP expression. Instead, a four- to fivefold overexpression of the APP gene in DS brain has been demonstrated at both the mRNA and the protein level. This is suggested to increase the risk for the earlier onset of β/A4 amyloid pathology in DS which was determined to occur fifty years earlier than in the normal population.[9] The fourth and most prominent risk factor is advancing age[10] and the fifth may be head trauma,[11] which both are proposed to act at the level of APP expression, biogenesis and turnover. Aging brings about a change in alternative splicing of APP in favor of those APP isoforms that include the Kunitz protease inhibitory domain (KPI$^+$ APP's) which has the specificity to inhibit APPase activity. Head trauma which leads to shearing of nerve terminals may interfere with APP regulation and compartmentation and thus increase APP expression and/or alter APP turnover. It is therefore proposed that these five risk factors influence amyloid formation at different levels of the pathway summarized in FIGURE 2.

It becomes now more and more accepted that a fundamental component of the molecular aetiology of Alzheimer's disease (AD) may lie in the expression of APP, its biogenesis and turnover since the induction of the pathway leading to β/A4 amyloid formation will depend on the amount of APP or β/A4 present at a pathognomonic site. That the load of β/A4 released normally from neural cells is altered by FAD mutations of the APP gene has already been shown.[6] Equally important is the normal function of this β/A4 amyloid precursor protein and its subcellular localization within the nervous system. Both are determinants for the site of β/A4 deposition.[5,12]

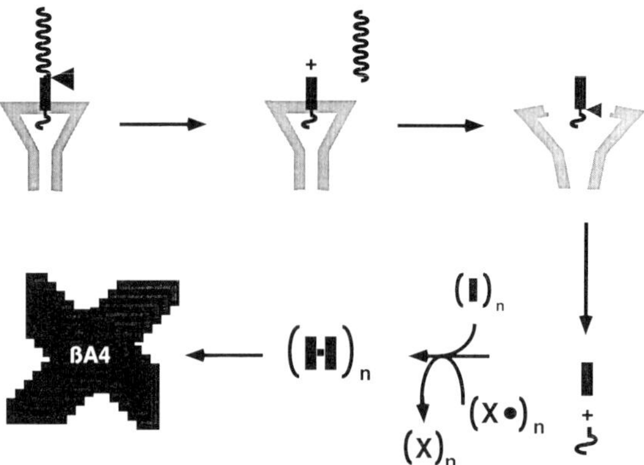

FIGURE 2. Hypothetical model for the release of β/A4 from synaptic amyloid protein precursor molecules by two different proteases (*arrow heads*) and β/A4 aggregation by radical generating systems. According to this model a protease cleaves APP on the amino-site of β/A4 to generate the fragment A4CT.[7] A second protease then releases the non-aggregating soluble β/A4 peptide. In the presence of oxidative stress (radical generating systems X•) preexisting β/A4 dimers and higher aggregates which are unstable become cross-linked and initiate amyloid formation.

In this chapter, we will therefore summarize our studies on the control of the human APP gene expression, the regulation of alternative splicing of APP exons in human cells, the APP biogenesis and metabolism, its function, its localization in brain, and the regulation of the amyloidogenicity of the β/A4 amyloid subunit.

REGULATION OF APP TRANSCRIPTION

The APP promoter is active in a variety of organs and its expression is highest in neuronal cells, especially in the central nervous system. In neurons, APP mRNA may account for up to 0.2% of total mRNA and the number of APP molecules in neurons was estimated to exceed one million. It has also been shown that APP expression can be induced in different cell types by a variety of agents such as interleukin-1 and other cytokines, TPA, NGF, FGF, retinoic acid and phytohemagglutinin.

According to the scheme outlined in FIGURE 2, APP gene expression is considered to be a risk factor for AD pathology. To get a better understanding of how APP gene expression is regulated at the transcriptional level, the 5′ control region of the human gene was isolated. This analysis revealed the promoter of the human APP gene to have the same structure as those of housekeeping genes which are characterized by the lack of a canonical TATA box and the presence of a GC-rich region. The APP promoter sequence was found to include numerous concensus sequencers for known regulatory transcription factors.[14] It was proposed that the putative AP-1, Hox 1.3-binding sites, and the GC-rich elements contribute to the specific expression pattern of the APP gene.

A 5′ deletion analysis of the APP promoter allowed the identification of an activating DNA fragment (Ac-fragment). This Ac-fragment consists of at least two elements, A and C.[13] Element A is located proximal to the transcriptional start site. Element C lies more distal to this site. Both elements have a high GC content and contribute to the transcriptional activation potential of the entire Ac-fragment.

Element A was characterized in more detail because of its close proximity to the transcriptional start site of the APP gene.[15] This analysis revealed the presence of a binding site for the transcription factor Sp1 (FIG. 3). Methylation interference experiments showed the guanosines in the core sequence GGGTGGG to be involved in Sp1 binding. This binding motif is also present in the regulatory regions of other genes, like c-myc, the globin genes and one of the T cell receptor V genes. Furthermore, the sequence of this motif is very similar to that of the retinoblastoma control element (RCE). The RCE is also present in the promoters of the gene for c-fos and TGF-β1 both of which are shown to be regulated by the retinoblastoma gene product. Further analysis of the APP promoter element A revealed the binding of a second transcription factor, termed CA2 in FIGURE 3, in electrophoretic mobility shift assays with nuclear extracts from brain. The sequence recognized by CA2 resembles that for transcription factors AP-1 and AP-4. However, since competition experiments failed to show specificity for AP-1 and AP-4, the identity of the transcription factor remains to be determined which protects the palindromic sequence CAGCTG of site CA2.

The binding sites for Sp1 and CA2 of the APP promoter have the special feature of overlapping recognition sequences (FIG. 3). The involvement of both binding sites in transcriptional activation of the APP promoters was assessed by transient gene transfer experiments with APP promoter fragments containing mutated binding sites for Sp1 and CA2. Transcriptional activity was determined by measuring the activity of the reporter luciferase.

Sp1 is a member of a large family of transcription factors recognizing GC- and GT-elements having high homology in both, the transactivation domain and DNA-binding zinc-finger domains. RNA analysis and immunohistochemistry of different organs in mouse have shown an ubiquitous expression of Sp1, however with substantial variation in different cell types and during development. The low levels of Sp1 detected in different brain regions also suggest that binding site CA2 contributes to the high expression of the APP in neural cells. This was confirmed since nuclear extracts from rat brain showed binding to CA2 but not to the Sp1 binding site. Overlapping binding sites for different transcription factors as it is found for the APP promoter (FIG.

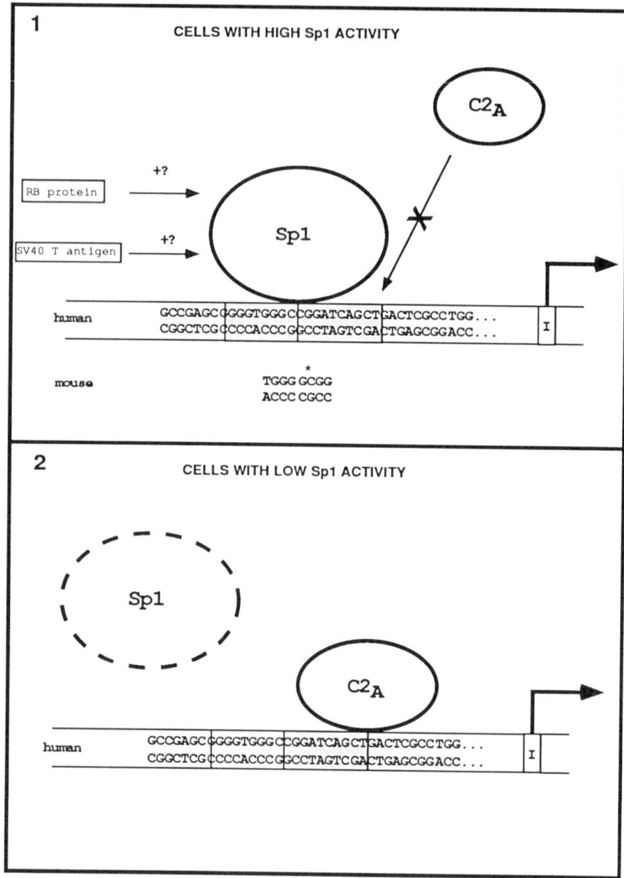

FIGURE 3. Schematic representation of two possible regulatory pathways responsible for APP gene expression. 1: Cells with high levels of Sp1 regulatory transcription factor. 2: Cells with low levels of Sp1 protein.

3) are known to be important for differential gene expression. A deregulated overexpression of the APP gene in brain might simply be brought about by a local increase of the activity of Sp1. The SV40 T Antigen is one known factor that can function as activator for Sp1. The T Antigen is not only able to increase the level of Sp1 mRNA and protein but can also alter the transcriptional activity of Sp1 by posttranslational modification. In some cases the retinoblastoma gene product was shown to increase the activity of Sp1 and to influence directly the activity of promoters through its binding site RCE which is very similar to the core sequence of element A (FIG. 3). It is therefore proposed that an imbalance between different regulatory pathways

for APP gene expression caused by a mutation in the APP promoter or by altered expression of transcription factors in brain might be a risk factor for the development of Alzheimer's disease.

REGULATION OF APP SPLICING

The KPI domain of APP is encoded by exon 7. The exon 7-containing APP mRNA isoforms are predominantly expressed in the periphery, whereas APP695 mRNA is the predominant splice form in neurons. A number of studies have indicated that alternative splicing of exons 7 and 8 in APP mRNA's is changed in brain during aging and possibly during AD.[16] It has already been reported that overall expression of APP mRNA is much higher in fetal brain than in adult differentiated brain. Taken together these results suggest that in the fully developed brain the APP695 transcript is more strongly down-regulated than are the two longer transcripts.

In fetal human brain, APP695 mRNA (KPI$^-$ mRNA) is dominant, making up more than 90% of the total, whereas the KPI$^+$ mRNA's of APP751 and APP770 account for approximately 9% and less than 1%, respectively. A totally different situation is observed in differentiated brains of adult individuals. In all samples that we examined the relative amount of APP751 increases to 50% and more, becoming the dominant splice form in the temporal cortex. In contrast, the relative amount of APP695 mRNA decreases in all older subjects to approximately 40% or less of total APP transcripts. The younger ones aged 31 and 47 years show approximately equal amounts of APP695 and APP751 mRNA. The relative increase of APP770 mRNA with age is roughly two- to eightfold and thus follows that of APP751 mRNA. This means that in human brain the ratios of APP695 to APP751 mRNA and APP695 to APP770 mRNA change drastically with development in favor of the two longer transcripts which include the KPI domain. Given the general involvement of proteases and protease inhibitory domains in tissue repair and homeostasis it is suggested that APP participates in these processes. Furthermore the increase in KPI$^+$ APP isoforms in the aging brain may alter APP turnover and thus directly influence APPase activity. The consequence of which would be an increased amount of intact APP molecules which, in turn, would increase the risk for amyloid formation according to FIGURE 2.

If one assumes specific trans-acting splicing factors to be responsible for the inclusion of exons 7 and 8, giving rise to APP751 and APP770 mRNA, one could envisage a situation in the developing fetal brain in which these factors are expressed at a low level, resulting in a high proportion of the APP695 transcript. According to this model, neurons increase the amount of specific trans-acting splicing factors later in development, thereby generating more of the APP mRNA's including exons 7 and 8 alone and together. Alternatively and less likely (see below), a general reduction of APP mRNA in the adult developed state would also lead to a higher relative amount of the longer APP splice forms, assuming a constant expression of the trans-acting splice factors throughout development.

To study the alternative splicing during development we used a model system, the human neuroblastoma cell line SY5Y, which can be induced to differentiate in cell culture upon exposure to several agents. If we induced this differentiation with retinoic acid (RA) total APP mRNA increased by a factor of 10 after 4 days of treatment. At this time no change in alternative splicing and in cellular phenotype was observed. However, a significant change in the splicing pattern in favor of the APP695 transcript was found to be associated with a sprouting of the cells which occurred 8 days after RA induction. We concluded that RA treatment of cultured SY5Y cells leads to changes in APP expression and splicing that vary both in quantitative and qualitative terms. The switching to a more fetal brain specific splicing pattern is not directly correlated with up-regulation of the APP expression. This suggests that neurons do not simply titrate *trans*-acting splicing factors but are able to regulate the amount of specific *trans*-acting splicing factors during the formation of synaptic contacts.

We have also studied alternative splicing involving exon 15 which is located immediately adjacent to the β/A4 protein encoding exons 16 and 17. This splicing event occurs in leukocytes, activated brain microglia and astrocytes and fuses exon 14 to exon 16, thereby excluding the 54-bp large exon 15.[4] These leukocyte-derived APP isoforms are termed L-APP's. Expression of L-APP677, L-APP733, and L-APP752 and of the corresponding ubiquitous APP forms APP695, APP751, and APP770 appears to be correlated with the functional state of leukocytes. L-APP is high in nonadherent and low in adherent leukocytes. This regulation of alternative splicing might be necessary to allow the rapid transition of the dual functions of nonadherence and adherence in the immune system since it has been proposed that APP's play a role in cell-cell interactions and cellular growth.

Activation of microglial cells during neuro-degeneration in the brain results in active production of APP and L-APP. In the light of the proposed role of microtrauma and redox potential as possible factors for the induction of β/A4 amyloidogenesis (FIGS. 1 and 2), we suggested that microglial cells are an attractive brain cell to study APP regulation, biosynthesis and degradation pathways in more detail.[4,5]

REGULATION OF APP BIOGENESIS AND METABOLISM

Recently, we have examined the expression of APP/L-APP during immune-mediated responses in freshly isolated leukocytes since these cells offer several advantages over other cells for the analysis of APP biogenesis and turnover.[5] We have also examined APP expression in different cells of the nervous system and compared their APP-specific biosynthetic behavior to that of T-lymphocytes. From these studies we conclude that APP is associated with defense mechanisms in the central nervous system involving the intrinsic immune system.

Kinetic experiments with regard to APP maturation by lymphocytes using the lymphoid CD4[+] T-cell line H9 indicated that APP of lymphocytes primarily has a function as secretory APP. This is evidenced by the fact that secreted APP could be detected within 20 min of chase in pulse-chase experiments. Consequently, membrane-spanning APP must have a very short half-life. Treatment with mitogenic lectin PHA induced a drastic increase in APP secretion that may be due to increased APP-secretase activity. However, we have not detected a concomitant increase of detectable COOH-terminal APP fragments that are also generated by secretase. On the contrary, we observed a decrease in the amount of detectable COOH-terminal fragments which may suggest that APP secretion is physiologically linked to a mechanism responsible for the degradation of these fragments. This raises the question whether such a secretase-linked degradation pathway also exists in neuronal cells and opens the possibility that differences in stability of COOH-terminal APP fragments may have fundamental consequences for the pathways leading to the release of β/A4 amyloid subunit. Our preliminary experimental data indicate that indeed COOH-terminal fragments of APP are more stable in neurons than in cells of the periphery.

REGULATION OF β/A4 AGGREGATION

Conditioned media of cells expressing APP contain soluble β/A4 which does not *per se* cause amyloid deposition.[6] To study the regulation of the aggregation of β/A4 at physiological concentrations we expressed the β/A4 peptide in the wheat-germ extract.[7] This resulted in a single strong monomeric band at 4 kDa when analyzed by SDS-PAGE. However, the translation of β/A4 mRNA in a cell-free rabbit reticulocyte lysate (RRL) was very inefficient and the translation products were barely detectable. The transformation of non-aggregated β/A4 from the wheat germ extract could be performed by hemoglobin, hemin, or iron in combination with hydrogen peroxide. These factors which promote β/A4 aggregation are radical generation systems which are already present in the RRL and probably responsible for the problems that we encountered with the translation of β/A4 mRNA in this system. To gain further support for the idea that the observed aggregation of β/A4 or of a COOH-terminal fragment, which includes the β/A4 sequence, the transmembrane, and cytoplasmic domains of APP (termed A4CT), is due to radical attack and protein cross-linking we studied the effect of radical scavengers on the aggregation which was induced by oxidative stress (metal-catalyzed oxidation systems).[7] The inhibition of the aggregation by ascorbic acid and trolox, a vitamin E derivative, supports our suggestion that the aggregation involves radical attack and protein cross-linking. Because the addition of amino acids also had an inhibitory effect, the aggregation may be due to oxidation of amino acids. We propose that cross-linking of preformed aggregates of amyloidogenic APP fragments such as β/A4 or A4CT by radical attack may be a prerequisite for the formation of the protease-resistant β/A4 deposits in Alzheimer's disease (FIG. 2). Thus, this aggregation induced by oxidative stress may be the primary event that leads to amyloid formation. After generation of a core of cross-linked amyloidogenic fragments as outlined in FIGURE 2, further APP fragments may extend the deposition without further involvement of metal-catalyzed oxidation systems. Thus AD may represent a specific brain vulnerability to age-related oxidation which together with the age-associated changes in APP mRNA splicing may account for the fact that advancing age is the most prominent risk factor for this disease.

REGULATION OF APP FUNCTION AND THE SITE OF β/A4 AMYLOID DEPOSITION

The function of APP is not yet known in detail but growing evidence exists that APP may mediate cell interactions with cell surface or soluble glycoproteins.[5] Although secreted APP and transmembrane APP belong to the same family, it could be envisaged that they are involved in different cell-cell interaction activities. It seems an intriguing hypothesis that transmembrane APP could function directly as a cell-adhesion molecule, while secreted APP may be involved in indirect cell interactions by generating intracellular signals important for regulation of cell interactions via a yet undefined cell-surface receptor. Since APP expression is not restricted to lymphocytes but expressed in all cells that participate in cell-cell interaction we postulate that APP may be involved in initial, perhaps weak adhesion to target cells and, additionally, in the mediation of signals activating specific and strong cell-cell interactions. The weak adhesion may be due to adhesive interactions of transmembrane APP to extracellular matrix components such as laminin, collagen, and proteoglycans followed by binding of secretory APP to a putative receptor on the target cells. The APP-receptor interaction may trigger a cell-specific adhesion cascade as exemplified by integrins, selectins, and members of the immunoglobulin superfamily, thereby generating a specific intracellular activation signal.

In brain APP serves a synaptic function. We have shown that APP is located in neuronal perikarya and concentrated at axosomatic and other synaptic sites in brain.[12] Accordingly, APP expression and metabolism might be linked to synaptic activity. Recently, a receptor-activated APP release has been demonstrated and has been suggested that a neurotransmitter receptor-controlled APP shedding may be mediated through intracellular activation signals such as phosphorylation by kinases.[17]

The clinical symptomatology of AD is tightly linked to the development of synapse pathology and synapse loss. Therefore synapses which are essential for the maintenance of intellectual brain function would be an early and critical site of amyloid deposition for β/A4 derived from neuronal APP.

REFERENCES

1. GLENNER, G. G. & C. W. WONG. 1984. Alzheimer's disease and Down's syndrome sharing a unique cerebrovascular amyloid fibril protein. Biochem Biophys. Res. Commun. **122**:1131–1135.
2. MASTERS, C. L., G. SIMMS, N. A. WEINMAN, G. MULTHAUP, B. L. MCDONALD & K. BEYREUTHER. 1985. Amyloid plaque core protein in Alzheimer's disease and Down's Syndrome. Proc. Natl. Acad. Sci. USA **82**:4245–4249.
3. KANG, J., H.-G. LEMAIRE, A. UNTERBECK, J. M. SALBAUM, C. L. MASTERS, K. H. GRZESCHIK, G. MULTHAUP, K. BEYREUTHER & B. MÜLLER-HILL. 1987. The precursor of Alzheimer's disease amyloid A4 protein resembles a cell surface receptor. Nature **325**:733–736.
4. KÖNIG, G., U. MÖNNING, R. PRIOR, R. BANATI, U. SCHREITER-GASSER, J. BAUER, C. L. MASTERS & K. BEYREUTHER. 1992. Identification of a novel, leukocyte-derived isoform of the Alzheimer amyloid precursor protein. J. Biol. Chem. **267**:10804-10809.
5. MÖNNING, U., G. KÖNIG, R. B. BANATI, H. MECHLER, C. CZECH, J. GEHRMANN, U. SCHREITER-GASSER, C. L. MASTERS & K. BEYREUTHER. 1992. Alzheimer β/A4 amyloid precursor proteins in immuno-competent cells. J. Biol. Chem. **267**:2390–2396.
6. CITRON, M., T. OLTERSDORF, C. HAAS, L. MCCONLOGUE, A. Y. HUNG, P. SEUBERT, C. VIGO-PELFREY, I. LIEBERBERG, & D. J. SELKOE. 1992. Mutation in the β-amyloid precursor protein in familial Alzheimer's disease increases β-protein production. Nature **360**:672–674.
7. DYRKS, T., E. DYRKS, T. HARTMANN, C. L. MASTERS & K. BEYREUTHER. 1992. Amyloidogenicity of β/A4 and β/A4-bearing APP fragments by metal catalysed oxidation. J. Biol. Chem. **267**:18210–18217.
8. SCHELLENBERG, G. D., T. D. BIRD, E. M. WIJSMAN, H. T. ORR, L. ANDERSON, E. NEMENS, J. A. WHITE, L. BONNYCASTLE, J. L. WEBER, M. E. ALONSO, H. POTTER, L. L. HESTON & G. M. MARTIN. 1992. Genetic linkage evidence for a familial Alzheimer's disease locus on chromosome 14. Science **258**:668–671.
9. RUMBLE, B., R. RETALLAK, C. HILBICH, G. SIMMS, G. MULTHAUP, R. MARTINS, A. HOCKEY, P. MONTGOMERY, K. BEYREUTHER & C. L. MASTERS. 1989. Amyloid A4 protein and its precursor in Down's syndrome and Alzheimer's disease. N. Engl. J. Med. **320**:1446–1452.

10. DAVIES, L., B. WOLSKA, C. HILBICH, G. MULTHAUP, K. MARTINS, G. SIMMS, K. BEYREUTHER & C. L. MASTERS. 1988. A4 amyloid deposition and the diagnosis of Alzheimer's disease: Prevalence in aged brains determined by immunocytochemistry compared with conventional neuropathologic techniques. Neurology **38**:1688–1693.

11. ROBERTS, G. W., S. M. GENTLEMAN, A. LYNCH & D. I. GRAHAM. 1991. β/A4 amyloid protein deposition in brain after head trauma. Lancet **338**:1422–1423.

12. SCHUBERT, W., R. PRIOR, A. WEIDEMANN, H. DIRCKSEN, G. MULTHAUP, C. L. MASTERS & K. BEYREUTHER. 1991. Localization of Alzheimer β/A4 amyloid precursor protein at central and peripheral synaptic sites. Brain Res. **563:** 184–194.

13. POLLWEIN, P., C. L. MASTERS & K. BEYREUTHER. 1992. The expression of the amyloid precursor protein (APP) is regulated by two GC-elements in the promoter. Nucl. Acid Res. **20**:63–68.

14. SALBAUM, J. M., A. WEIDEMANN, H.-G. LEMAIRE, C. L. MASTERS & K. BEYREUTHER. 1988. The promoter of Alzheimer's disease amyloid A4 precursor gene. EMBO J. **7**:2807–2813.

15. POLLWEIN, P. 1993. Overlapping binding sites of two different transcription factors in the promoter of the human gene for the Alzheimer amyloid precursor protein. Biochem. Biophys. Res. Commun. **190**:637–647.

16. KÖNIG, G., C. L. MASTERS & K. BEYREUTHER. 1992. Expression of Alzheimer's amyloid gene in development, aging and Alzheimer's disease. *In* Reihe der Villa Vigoni, Band 1. Biology of Aging. R. Zwilling & C. Baldini, Eds. 82–99. Springer-Verlag. Heidelberg.

17. NITSCH, R., B. E. SLACK, R. J. WURTMAN & J. H. GROWDON. 1992. Release of Alzheimer amyloid precursor derivatives stimulated by activation of muscarinic acetylcholine receptors. Science **258**:302–307.

Production of Amyloid β Protein from Normal Amyloid β-Protein Precursor (βAPP) and the Mutated βAPPS Linked to Familial Alzheimer's Disease[a]

TODD E. GOLDE, XIAO-DAN CAI, MIKIO SHOJI,
AND STEVEN G. YOUNKIN[b]

*Division of Neuropathology, Institute of Pathology, Case Western Reserve
University, Cleveland, Ohio USA 44106*

ABSTRACT: The ~4 kD (39–43 amino acid) polypeptide (amyloid β protein, Aβ) deposited as amyloid in Alzheimer's disease (AD) is derived from a set of 695–770 residue precursor proteins collectively referred to as the amyloid β-protein precursor (βAPP). Using immunoblotting techniques, metabolic labeling, and sequencing we have analyzed βAPP derivatives in medium conditioned by (1) human mononuclear leukemic (K562) cells expressing a model βAP-bearing carboxyl-terminal βAPP derivative (2) human neuroblastoma (M17) cells transfected with constructs expressing full length βAPP and (3) M17 cells expressing only endogenous βAPP. In each case, we observed the release of a ~4 kD βAPP derivative essentially identical to the Aβ found in AD amyloid. A similar, if not identical, βAPP fragment was readily detected in CSF from both Alzheimer's disease patients and controls. These observations indicate that the Aβ is produced and released by normal processing of the βAPP. To determine if the production of Aβ or Aβ-tearing COOH-terminal βAPP derivatives is altered in cells expressing the mutant βAPPs linked to familial AD, we have compared M17 cells expressing wild type βAPP with those expressing mutant βAPPs ($\beta APP_{\Delta I}$ or $\beta APP_{\Delta NL}$). After continuous metabolic labeling for 8 hours, cells expressing the $\beta APP_{\Delta NL}$ mutant showed a 5-fold increase in the relative amount of an ~11.4 kD Aβ-bearing carboxyl-terminal βAPP derivative, and they released 6-fold more 4 kD Aβ into the medium. These observations provide strong evidence that (1) the pathway producing Aβ in cultured cells is highly relevant to AD and (2) the $\beta APP_{\Delta NL}$ mutant causes AD because its processing is altered in a way that releases increased amounts of Aβ.

[a] This work was supported by NIH grant AG06656 and an ADRDA Zenith award.

[b] *Send correspondence to:* Steven G. Younkin, Division of Neuropathology, Institute of Pathology, Case Western Reserve University, Cleveland, OH USA 44106; TEL: (216) 368-3381; FAX: (216) 844-1810.

In each of the 695–770 residue amyloid β protein precursor (βAPP) iso-forms, the 43 residue amyloid β protein (Aβ) is an internal peptide that begins 99 residues from the carboxyl end of the βAPP and extends from the extracellular/intraluminal region of the βAPP into the middle of its hydropho-bic membrane-spanning domain. The βAPP is normally processed in a consti-tutive secretory pathway[1–3] and by alternative processing. In the secretory pathway, the βAPP is cleaved within the Aβ[4,5] to produce a large secreted derivative and a small membrane associated fragment that cannot produce amyloid because neither contains the entire Aβ. Alternative processing, which occurs at least in part in the endosomal/lysosomal system, produces a complex set of carboxyl-terminal derivatives that includes potentially amyloidogenic forms with the entire Aβ at or near their amino terminus.[6–8]

To determine whether Aβ can be produced from Aβ-bearing carboxyl-terminal βAPP derivatives, human mononuclear leukemic (K562) cells were stably transfected with LC_{99}, a construct that begins with the 17 amino acid βAPP signal peptide, continues with the leucine that normally follows the βAPP signal peptide, and ends with the 99 amino acids at the carboxyl end of the βAPP, a sequence that begins with the Aβ. To detect Aβ released from $K562\text{-}LC_{99}$ cells, we used SGY2134, a rabbit antiserum raised to synthetic $A\beta_{1-40}$ that recognizes primarily $A\beta_{1-16}$, to immunoprecipitate the protein in medium conditioned with $K562\text{-}LC_{99}$ cells. The immunoprecipitated protein was separated on 10/16% tris/tricine gels,[6] transferred to immobilon P, and labeled with 4G8, a mouse monoclonal antibody to $A\beta_{17-24}$. As a control, synthetic $A\beta_{1-40}$ was added to culture medium and analyzed identically. Using this approach, a 4 kD protein that comigrated with synthetic $A\beta_{1-40}$ was identified in medium conditioned with $K562\text{-}LC_{99}$ cells but not in me-dium conditioned with K562 cells transfected with vector alone.[9] This 4 kD protein was definitively identified as Aβ by isolating it from a large volume of culture medium and directly sequencing it. Thus cells transfected with a model Aβ-bearing carboxyl-terminal derivative process that derivative to re-lease Aβ into the medium.

The same assay used to detect synthetic $A\beta_{1-40}$ and the Aβ released from $K562\text{-}LC_{99}$ cells was employed to determine whether Aβ is also released into human CSF and by cultured cells expressing full length βAPP. In our initial experiment on CSF, we analyzed 3 ml samples obtained at autopsy from 7 AD patients and 7 controls. Strong signals were obtained in 5 of the 7 autopsy-confirmed AD cases, but considerable Aβ was also present in 3 of the 7 controls. We also examined 3 ml samples of CSF from living patients, 5 from patients with probable AD and 5 from age matched non-AD patients. Again, there was considerable overlap in the amount of Aβ observed in the AD and non-AD group. Thus our initial survey[9] indicates that there is (1) readily detectable Aβ in the CSF of AD and control patients, (2) considerable appar-ent interindividual variation in the amount of Aβ in CSF, and (3) no obvious correlation between AD and the amount of Aβ in CSF. Additional studies are needed, however, to determine whether the measurement of Aβ in CSF will be useful in the diagnosis or management of AD patients and to determine, in particular, if high levels of Aβ are a significant risk factor in the development of AD.

To determine whether Aβ is released by cultured cells expressing full length βAPP, we analyzed medium conditioned with human neuroblastoma (M17) cells stably transfected with a $βAPP_{695}$ expression construct. In our initial experiments,[9] the transfected M17 cells were differentiated for 7 days with retinoic acid to induce the formation of long neurites. These differentiated $M17-βAPP_{695}$ cells released readily detectable levels of 4 kDa Aβ. Subsequent experiments showed the same to be true for undifferentiated M17 cells. Remarkably, some 4 kD Aβ was also detected in the medium of M17 cells expressing only endogenous βAPP. Thus our analysis of human CSF and transfected cells[9] showed that normal cellular processing of the βAPP produces significant amounts of a soluble extracellular 4 kD drivative essentially identical to the Aβ that forms amyloid in AD. Similar results have been reported by others.[10,11]

In rare families, AD is inherited as an autosomal dominant trait. Strong evidence that amyloid deposition plays a critical role in the development of AD has come from the identification of familial AD (FAD) kindreds in which the AD phenotype cosegregates with mutations in the βAPP gene. Three of the FAD-linked βAPP mutations convert the valine located three residues carboxyl to $Aβ_{43}$ (val_{717} in $βAPP_{770}$), to isoleucine (ΔI),[12–15] phenylalanine (ΔF),[16] or glycine (ΔG).[17] A fourth double mutation (ΔNL) alters the lysine-methionine located immediately amino to $Aβ_1$ (lys_{670}-met_{671} in $βAPP_{770}$) to asparagine-leucine.[18] The location of these mutations in close proximity to Aβ immediately suggests that they may cause AD by altering βAPP processing in a way that is amyloidogenic.

To evaluate production of Aβ and Aβ-bearing COOH-terminal derivatives in cells expressing the FAD-linked mutant βAPPs, we compared human neuroblastoma (M17) cells stably transfected with mutant (ΔI, ΔNL) or wild type (WT) $βAPP_{695}$.[19] In our initial experiment, two ΔNL lines, a ΔI line, a WT line, and a line transfected with vector alone (CEP4β) were metabolically labeled with [^{35}S]methionine for 20 min to assess βAPP synthesis, and for 12 hours to analyze the COOH-terminal βAPP derivatives accumulating in cells and the Aβ released into the medium. After 12 hours of continuous labeling, the WT and ΔI lines were similar with respect to the COOH-terminal βAPP derivatives that accumulated and the Aβ that was released. In contrast, the 8–12 kD COOH-terminal derivatives accumulating in the two ΔNL lines were completely different showing a marked increase in the relative amount of the 11.4 kD derivative, a derivative that has Aβ at its amino terminus. In addition, the medium conditioned by the two ΔNL lines contained, on average, 15-fold more 4 kD Aβ than the medium conditioned by the WT and ΔI lines. After pulse labeling for 20 minutes, the two 695 ΔNL lines contained 5-fold more full length βAPP than the WT and ΔI lines, but this increased expression did not account for the 15-fold increase in Aβ.

To pursue this observation, we retransfected M17 cells producing new stably transfected 695WT, 695 ΔI, and 695 ΔNL lines. During pulse labeling for 20 minutes, the three new ΔI and the three new ΔNL lines accumulated comparable amounts of full-length βAPP, but the three new WT lines accumulated 3.3-fold more βAPP indicating that expression was 3.3-fold higher in these lines. Despite βAPP expression less than one third that of the WT lines, the ΔNL lines accumulated considerably more of the 11.4 kD Aβ-bearing COOH-terminal derivative after 8 hours of continuous labeling and medium conditioned with the ΔNL lines contained considerably more 4 kD Aβ. Quantitative analysis of these results using phosphorimaging technology showed that, in cells pulse labeled for 8 hours, the ratio of the 11.4 to 8.7 kD cell-associated derivatives was over 5-fold higher in the ΔNL as compared to the WT or ΔI lines. When the amount of Aβ in medium was normalized to the full-length βAPP present after pulse labeling for 20 minutes, Aβ was over 6 times higher in the ΔNL than in the ΔI or WT lines. Recently, Citron, Oltersdorf and their colleagues have reported that 293 cells expressing βAPP$_{\Delta NL}$ show a similar increase in Aβ release.[20]

The observation that M17 cells expressing βAPP$_{\Delta NL}$ show a marked increase in Aβ-bearing COOH-terminal derivatives and release increased amounts of 4 kD Aβ provides strong evidence that βAPP$_{\Delta NL}$ causes AD because its processing is altered in a way that releases increased amounts of Aβ thereby fostering amyloid deposition. More generally, the linkage of this form of FAD to a βAPP$_{\Delta NL}$ mutation demonstrated to increase Aβ production in cultured cells (1) provides strong evidence that the pathway producing Aβ in cultured cells is highly relevant to AD and (2) greatly strengthens the hypothesis that amyloid deposition plays a central role in the development of all forms of AD.

If amyloid deposition is invariably pivotal in the development of AD, then one would also expect the βAPP$_{717}$ mutations (ΔI, ΔF, and ΔG) to alter βAPP processing in a way that is amyloidogenic. In an extensive series of experiments examining the turnover of full-length βAPP$_{\Delta I}$ and the secretion of its large amino-terminal derivative, we have observed significant differences in the processing of βAPP$_{\Delta I}$ as compared to βAPP$_{WT}$. However, neither these data, which will be published in a separate report, nor the data presented here provide evidence that the processing of βAPP$_{\Delta I}$ in M17 cells is altered in a way that would obviously promote amyloidogenesis. In fact, both our unpublished data and the data presented here suggest that, if anything, M17 cells expressing βAPP$_{\Delta I}$ produce less secreted 4 kD Aβ than those producing wild type βAPP. As discussed more fully elsewhere,[19] it is possible that the aberrant processing of $\beta APP_{\Delta I}$ that produces amyloid in the brain does not occur in transfected M17 cells or that amyloidogenic processing occurring in M17 cells has so far gone undetected. Thus it seems likely, given the positive results obtained with the ΔNL mutation, that continued analysis of the βAPP_{717} mutations will ultimately reveal altered processing that is highly informative with regard to the mechanism through which these mutations produce AD.

REFERENCES

1. WEIDEMANN, A., G. KÖNIG, D. BUNKE, *et al.* 1989. Identification, biogenesis, and localization of precursors of Alzheimer's disease A4 amyloid protein. Cell **57**:115–126.
2. PALMERT, M. R., M. B. PODLISNY, D. S. WITKER, *et al.* 1989. The β-amyloid protein precursor of Alzheimer disease has soluble derivatives found in human brain and cerebrospinal fluid. Proc. Natl. Acad. Sci. USA **86**:6338–6342.
3. SCHUBERT, D., M. LACORBIERE, T. SAITOH & G. COLE. 1989. Characterization of an amyloid β precursor protein that binds heparin and contains tyrosine sulfate. Proc. Natl. Acad. Sci. USA **86**:2066–2069.
4. SISODIA, S. S., E. H. KOO, K. BEYREUTHER, A. UNTERBECK & D. L. PRICE. 1990. Evidence that beta-amyloid protein in Alzheimer's disease is not derived by normal processing. Science **248**:492–495.
5. ESCH, F. S., P. S. KEIM, E. C. BEATTIE, *et al.* 1990. Cleavage of amyloid beta peptide during constitutive processing of its precursor. Science **248**: 1122–1124.
6. ESTUS, S., T. E. GOLDE, T. KUNISHITA, *et al.* 1992. Potentially amyloidogenic carboxyl-terminal derivatives of the amyloid protein precursor. Science **255**: 726–728.
7. GOLDE, T. E., S. ESTUS, L. YOUNKIN, D. J. SELKOE & S. G. YOUNKIN. 1992. Processing of the amyloid protein precursor to potentially amyloidogenic derivatives. Science **255**:728–730.
8. HAASS, C., E. H. KOO, A. MELLON, A. Y. HUNG & D. J. SELKOE. 1992. Targeting of cell surface β-amyloid precursor protein to lysosomes: Alternative processing into amyloid-bearing fragments. Nature **357**:500–503.
9. SHOJI, M., T. E. GOLDE, J. GHISO, *et al.* 1992. Production of the Alzheimer amyloid β protein by normal proteolytic processing. Science **258**:126–129.
10. HAASS, C., M. G. SCHLOSSMACHER, A. Y. HUNG, *et al.* 1992. Amyloid β-peptide is produced by cultured cells during normal metabolism. Nature **359**: 322.
11. SEUBERT, P., C. VIGO-PELFREY, F. ESCH, *et al.* 1992. Isolation and quantitation of soluble Alzheimer's β-peptide from biological fluids. Nature **359**:325.
12. GOATE, A., M.-C. CHARTIER-HARLIN, M. MULLAN, *et al.* 1991. Segregation of a missense mutation in the amyloid precursor protein gene with familial Alzheimer's disease. Nature **349**:704–706.

13. NARUSE, S., S. IGARASHI, K. AOKI, *et al.* 1991. Mis-sense mutation Val-Ile in exon 17 of amyloid precursor protein in Japanese familial Alzheimer's disease. Lancet **337:**978–979.
14. YOSHIOKA, K. 1991. Biochem. Biophys. Res. Commun **178:**1141–1146.
15. HARDY, J. 1991. Lancet **337:**1342.
16. MURRELL, J., M. FARLOW, B. GHETTI & M. D. BENSON. 1991. A mutation in the amyloid precursor protein associated with hereditary Alzheimer's disease. Science **254:**97–99.
17. CHARTIER-HARLIN, M.-C., F. CRAWFORD, H. HOULDEN, *et al.* 1991. Early-onset Alzheimer's Disease caused by mutations at codon 717 of the β-amyloid precursor protein gene. Nature **353:**844–846.
18. MULLAN, M., F. CRAWFORD, K. AXELMAN, *et al.* 1992. A pathogenic mutation for probable Alzheimer's disease in the APP gene at the N-terminus of β-amyloid. Nature Genet. **1:**345–347.
19. CAI, X., T. E. GOLDE & S. G. YOUNKIN. 1993. Release of excess amyloid β protein from a mutant amyloid β protein precursor. Science **259:**514–516.
20. CITRON, M., T. OLTERSDORF, C. HAASS, *et al.* 1992. Mutation of the β-amyloid precursor protein in familial Alzheimer's disease causes increased β-protein production. Nature. **360:**672–674.

Normal Cellular Processing of the β-Amyloid Precursor Protein Results in the Secretion of the Amyloid β Peptide and Related Molecules[a]

CHRISTIAN HAASS,[b,d] ALBERT Y. HUNG,[b]
MICHAEL G. SCHLOSSMACHER,[b,e] TILMAN OLTERSDORF,[c]
DAVID B. TEPLOW,[b] AND DENNIS J. SELKOE[b]

[b] *Department of Neurology and Program in Neuroscience, Harvard Medical School, and Center for Neurologic Diseases, Brigham and Women's Hospital, Boston, Massachusetts 02115 USA*
[c] *Athena Neuroscience Inc., South San Francisco, California 94090 USA*

ABSTRACT: Alzheimer's disease is characterized by the extracellular deposition in the brain and its blood vessels of insoluble aggregates of the amyloid β peptide (Aβ). This peptide is derived from a large integral membrane protein, the β-amyloid precursor protein (βAPP), by proteolytic processing. The Aβ has previously been found only in the brains of patients with Alzheimer's disease or advanced aging. We describe here the finding that Aβ is produced continuously by normal processing in tissue culture cells. Aβ and closely related peptides were identified in the media of cells transfected with cDNAs coding for βAPP in a variety of cell lines and primary tissue cultured cells. The identity of these peptides was confirmed by epitope mapping and radiosequencing. Peptides of a molecular weight of ~3 and ~4 kDa are described. The 4 kDa range contains mostly the Aβ and two related peptides starting N-terminal to the beginning of Aβ. In the 3 kDa range, the majority of peptides start at the secretase site; in addition, two longer peptides were found starting at amino acid $F^{(4)}$ and $E^{(11)}$ of the Aβ sequence. To identify the processing pathways which lead to the secretion of these peptides, we used a variety of drugs known to interfere with certain cell biological pathways. We conclude that lysosomes may not play a predominant role in the formation of 3 and 4 kDa peptides. We show that an acidic environment is necessary to create the N-terminus of the Aβ and postulate that alternative secretory cleavage might result in the formation of the N-terminus of Aβ and related

[a] This work was supported by NIH grants 06173 (LEAD Award) and AG 07911 to D.J.S. and grants from the Deutsche Forschungsgemeinschaft to C.H. and Merck Sharp and Dohme Research Laboratories to A.Y.H.
[d] *Send correspondence to:* Christian Haass, Department of Neurology and Program in Neuroscience, Harvard Medical School; and Center for Neurologic Diseases, Brigham and Women's Hospital, Boston, MA 02115 USA; TEL: 617-732-6454; FAX: 617-732-7787.
[e] *Present address:* Research Unit of Experimental Neuropathology, Austrian Academy of Science, Vienna A 1090 Austria

peptides. This cleavage takes place either in late Golgi, at the cell-surface or in early endosomes, but not in lysosomes. The N-terminus of most of the 3 kDa peptides is created by secretory cleavage on the cell surface or within late Golgi.

INTRODUCTION

During Alzheimer's disease and aging, a 40 amino acid hydrophobic peptide—amyloid β-peptide (Aβ)—accumulates in the brain and its blood vessels.[1] The accumulation results in the formation of vascular deposits and amyloid plaques. Aβ is derived from the large membrane spanning βAPP.[2] The Aβ domain is in part inserted in the membrane making it difficult to understand how this peptide can be formed. To date, two different processing pathways of βAPP have been described. The secretory pathway described by Weidemann *et al.*[3] seems to exclude the formation of Aβ (FIG. 1). Upon

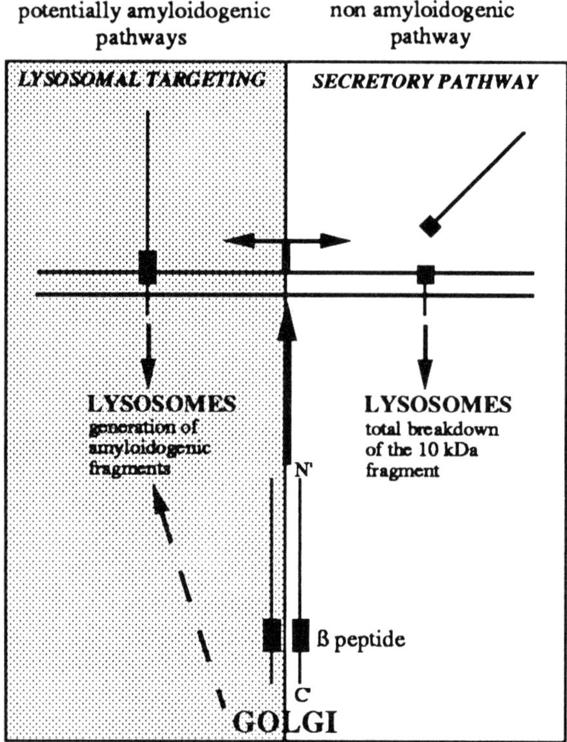

FIGURE 1. Schematic describing the secretory and endosomal/lysosomal pathway of βAPP. Dashed line indicates a potential direct targeting pathway of βAPP from trans Golgi to the lysosome.

maturation within the Golgi, βAPP reaches the cell surface, where it is cleaved[4,5] by an enzyme called secretase. The secretase cleaves βAPP within the Aβ domain thus clearly preventing amyloidogenesis. The soluble form of βAPP (APPs) is released and a 10 kDa C-terminal fragment is retained within the membrane.[6–9]

In addition to the secretory pathway, an endosomal/lysosomal processing pathway of βAPP has been described[4,10,11] which results in the formation of amyloid-bearing C-terminal fragments of βAPP. These fragments as well as the 10 kDa C-terminal fragment and full-length βAPP were detected within isolated lysosomes.[4] Furthermore, cell surface biotinylation demonstrated the reinternalization of full-length βAPP and its targeting to lysosomes (FIG. 1[4]). Full-length βAPP and the 10 kDa C-terminal fragment have also been detected in coated vesicles.[12] So far, it is not clear whether in addition to the reinternalization pathway, a direct transport of βAPP from the trans-Golgi to the lysosome exists (FIG. 1). Since full-length βAPP and a variety of amyloid-bearing fragments are detected within isolated lysosomes, this pathway, in contrast to the constitutive secretory pathway, is potentially amyloidogenic. Although amyloid-bearing fragments were detected within lysosomes, Aβ itself has so far been found only in the brain of patients with Alzheimer's disease and aged individuals. Recently, we[13] and others[14,15] (Yankner, personal communication) have described the identification of soluble Aβ in the media of tissue culture cells. These peptides are released by normal proteolytic processing; no membrane injury or cell death is necessary for the formation of these peptides.

RESULTS AND DISCUSSION

In order to determine whether tissue cultured cells are able to produce Aβ directly via a normal processing pathway, we metabolically labeled human kidney 293 cells stably transfected with βAPP 695 for ~12 hour. Conditioned media were immunoprecipitated with a polyclonal antibody against Aβ 1–40. We detected a 3 and a 4 kDa peptide, the latter comigrating with radio-iodinated Aβ 1–40. These peptides were strongly augmented when we compared their amounts in transfected versus untransfected 293 cells, indicating that they are derived from βAPP. Epitope mapping with a variety of poly-clonal and monoclonal antibodies against different regions of Aβ was consis-tent with the hypothesis that the 4 kDa peptide is indeed the Aβ, and that the 3 kDa peptide starts at the constitutive secretase site (Aβ).[17] These data were confirmed by radiosequencing the isolated 3 and 4 kDa peptides after metabolic labeling with [^{3}H]phenylalanine. In the 4 kDa range, we found three different peptides starting at Asp$^{(1)}$ (Aβ), Val$^{(-3)}$ and Ile$^{(-6)}$ relative

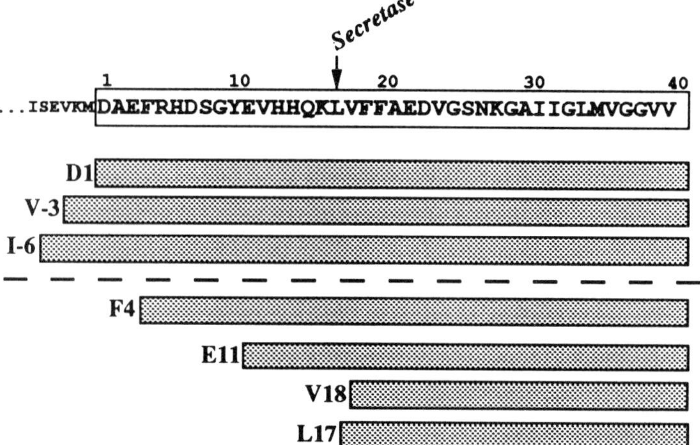

FIGURE 2. Radio-sequencing of the 3 and 4 kDa peptides reveals a variety of peptides starting with different N-termini. The sequence within the white box corresponds to Aβ 1–40. The site of secretase cleavage is indicated. The gray bars represent the different peptides found in the 4 kDa range *(above dashed line)* or the 3 kDa range *(below dashed line)*. The precise C-terminus of these peptides has not been determined.

to the Aβ sequence (FIG. 2). The 3 kDa band was shown to consist of four different peptides starting at Phe[4], Glu[11], Val[18], and Leu[17]. The latter two are close to or at the secretase site (FIG. 2). The relative abundance of these peptides is shown in FIGURE 3. About 62% of the 3 kDa peptides start at Val[18], the second amino acid after the secretase site. About 31% of the

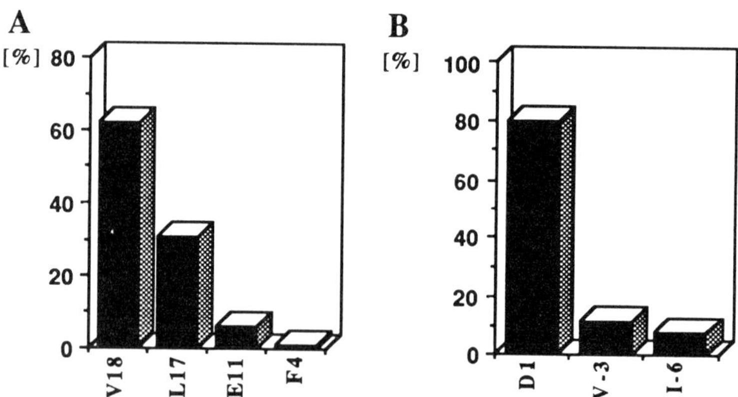

FIGURE 3. Relative ratios of the different peptides found in the 3 kDa range **(a)** and in the 4 kDa range **(b)**.

peptides have a N-terminus at the secretase site [Leu[17]; FIG. 3a]. Two minor species were identified in addition [6% Glu[11]; 1% Phe[4]]. About 80% of the 4 kDa range peptides consists of the Aβ [Asp[1]], followed by the Val[(−3)] species at 12% and the Ile[(−6)] species at 8% (FIG. 3b). These peptide species are found reproducibly after every isolation. Since the isolation protocol is a very rapid one step procedure, the minor peptides are unlikely to be due to proteolytic degradation. Instead, we favor the hypothesis that these peptides are produced by alternative cleavage by one and the same enzyme or by a family of closely related enzymes. Currently, we do not know the precise C-terminus of these peptides. However, preliminary results using mass-spectometry indicate a C-terminus at amino acid 40 for at least some of these peptides (I. Lieberburg, personal communication). The findings in the tissue culture system are consistent with the observation that most Aβ molecules isolated from the brain of Alzheimer's patients end at amino acid 40.[16] Surprisingly, the Aβ peptides were found to be completely soluble. After a $100,000 \times g$ spin for 1 hour, we completely recovered these peptides in the supernatant. The SDS-extracted pellet contained no 3 or 4 kDa peptides. Furthermore, the production of the peptides is independent of the specific spliced form of Aβ. Cells transfected with the three major isoforms, βAPP 695, 751, and 770[1] produced similar amounts of 3 and 4 kDa peptides. Recently, an additional isoform of βAPP has been described in brain microglia and leukocytes which lacks exon 15.[17] Transfection of this cDNA results in generation of amounts of 3 and 4 kDa peptides similar to those from other βAPP isoforms.

On the basis of the data described above, one may ask if the lysosomal pathway is directly involved in the production of these peptides. Immunoprecipitations of extracts from isolated lysosomes purified from metabolically labeled 293 cells did not detect any 3 or 4 kDa peptides. This could indicate that only the precursors are made within the lysosome, and upon their release into the media, Aβ and the related peptides are formed extracellular. In order to determine which cellular compartments are involved in the production of these peptides, we treated 293 cells with a variety of drugs known to interfere with certain cellular processing pathways[18] (TABLE 1). Since it is known that microtubles are necessary for the fusion of late endosomes with lysosomes, we depolymerized microtubules with nocodazole or colchicine. Cells treated with these drugs still produced 3 and 4 kDa peptides. To determine whether lysosomal proteases may be involved in the generation of these peptides, 293 cells were treated with leupeptin. Increasing amounts of leupeptin had no influence on the generation of both peptides, despite the fact that this protease inhibitor causes a substantial accumulation of Aβ-containing C-terminal fragments of βAPP in the lysosomes of these cells.[4] In contrast, increasing amounts of NH_4Cl clearly inhibited the formation of both peptides in a dose dependent manner, indicating that an acidic cellular compartment is involved.

TABLE 1. The Effect of Colchicine, Nocodazole, Leupeptin, NH$_4$Cl, Monensin and Brefeldin A on the Production of 3 kDa Peptides and Aβ in Kidney Cells Stably Transfected with βAPP695

	3 kDa Peptides	Aβ
Control	+ + + +	+ + +
Colchicine	+ + + +	+ + +
Nocodazole	+ + + +	+ + +
Leupeptin	+ + + +	+ + +
NH$_4$Cl	+ +	+
Monensin	+ +	(+)
Brefeldin A	–	–

The monovalent ionophore, monensin, known to inhibit both late Golgi and endo-somal/lysosomal functions, had a strong dose-dependent inhibitory effect on the formation of the 3 and 4 kDa peptides. The possibility of Aβ formation within the ER or early Golgi was excluded by the use of Brefeldin A (BFA), which causes a redistribution of Golgi into ER. Under these conditions, 3 and 4 kDa peptides could not be detected either in the media or inside the cell. These experiments also exclude the possibility that Aβ might be formed within the cytoplasm after incomplete translocation of βAPP into the ER, since such a process would be unaffected by BFA. Interestingly, we could not detect any intracellular Aβ in the extracts of the cells treated with each of the different drugs described above.

Taken together, our data indicate that an acidic environment is necessary for the formation of Aβ. It seems unlikely that end-stage lysosomes are involved in this process since agents which interfere with transport to lysosomes or which inhibit lysosomal proteases have no effect on Aβ or p3 generation. The N-terminus of Aβ might be generated within the acidic environment of early endosomes or within late Golgi or on the cell surface. In either case, we speculate that the N-terminus of Aβ is created by an alternative secretory cleavage. Such a cleavage taking place at the N-terminus of Aβ has been described recently by Seubert *et al.*[19] The N-terminus of most of the 3 kDa peptides is created by a normal secretase cleavage that creates the 10 kDa C-terminal fragment. In both cases, we would like to propose that the C-terminal cleavage takes place on the cell surface by the same enzyme. Upon cleavage, 3 and 4 kDa peptides are than immediately released into the media. This model would explain why we[13] and others[14,15] (Yankner, personal communication) have been unable to detect these peptides within cell lysates.

REFERENCES

1. SELKOE, D. J. 1987. The molecular pathology of Alzheimer's disease. Neuron 6:487–498.

2. KANG, J., H.-G. LEMAIRE, A. UNTERBECK, J. M. SALBAUM, C. L. MASTERS, K.-H. GRZESCHIK, G. MULTHAUP, K. BEYREUTHER & B. MÜLLER-HILL. 1987. The precursor of Alzheimer's disease amyloid A4 protein resembles a cell-surface receptor. Nature **325**:733–736.

3. WEIDEMANN, A., G. KÖNIG, D. BUNKE, P. FISCHER, J. M. SALBAUM, C. L. MASTERS & K. BEYREUTHER. Identification, biogenesis, and localization of precursors of Alzheimer's disease A4 amyloid protein. Cell **57**:115–126.

4. HAASS, C., E. H. KOO, A. MELLON, A. Y. HUNG & D. J. SELKOE. 1992. Targeting of cell surface β-amyloid precursor protein to lysosomes: Alternative processing into amyloid-bearing fragments. Nature **357**:500–503.

5. SISODIA, S. S. 1992. β-amyloid precursor protein cleavage by a membrane-bound protease. Proc. Natl. Acad. Sci. USA **89**:6075–6079.

6. SELKOE, D. J., M. B. PODLISNY, C. L. JOACHIM, E. A. VICKERS, G. LEE & T. OLTERSDORF. 1988. β-Amyloid precursor protein of Alzheimer disease occurs as a 110- to 135- kilodalton membrane-associated proteins in neuronal and nonneuronal tissues. Proc. Natl. Acad. Sci. USA **85**:7341–7345.

7. OLTERSDORF, T., P. J. WARD, T. HENRIKSSON, E. C. BEATTIE, R. NEVE, I. LIEBERBURG & L. C. FRITZ. 1990. The Alzheimer amyloid precursor protein of Alzheimer disease occurs as 100-135-kilodalton membrane-associates proteins in neuronal and nonneuronal issues. J. Biol. Chem. **265**:4492–4497.

8. ESCH, F. S., P. S. KEIM, E. C. BEATTIE, R. W. BLACHER, A. R. CULWELL, T. OLTERSDORF, D. MCCLURE & P. J. WARD. 1990. Cleavage of amyloid β peptide during constitutive processing of its precursor. Science **248**:1122–1124.

9. WANG, R., J. F. MESCHIA, R. J. COTTER & S. S. SISODIA. 1991. Secretion of the β/A4 amyloid precursor protein. J. Biol. Chem. **266**:16960–16964.

10. ESTUS, S., T. E. GOLDE, T. KUNISHITA, D. BLADES, D. LOWERY, M. EISEN, M. USIAK, X. QU, T. TABIRA, B. D. GREENBERG & S. G. YOUNKIN. 1992. Potentially amyloidogenic, carboxyl-terminal derivatives of the amyloid protein precursor. Science **255**:726–728.

11. GOLDE, T. E., S. ESTUS, L. H. YOUNKIN, D. J. SELKOE & S. G. YOUNKIN. 1992. Processing of the amyloid protein precursor to potentially amyloidogenic derivatives. Science **255**:728–730.

12. NORSTEDT, C., G. L. CAPORASO, J. THYBERG, S. E. GANDY & P. GREENGARD. 1993. Identification of the Alzheimer β/A4 amyloid precursor protein in clathrin-coated vesicles purified from PC12 cells. J. Biol. Chem. In press.

13. HAASS, C., M. G. SCHLOSSMACHER, A. Y. HUNG, C. VIGO-PELFREY, A. MELLON, B. L. OSTASZEWSKI, I. LIEBERBURG, E. H. KOO, D. SCHENK, D. B. TEPLOW & D. J. SELKOE. 1992. Amyloid β-peptide is produced by cultured cells during normal metabolism. Nature **359**:322–325.

14. SEUBERT, P., C. VIGO-PELFREY, F. ESCH, M. LEE, H. DOVEY, D. DAVIS, S. SINHA, M. SCHLOSSMACHER, J. WHALEY, C. SWINDELHURST, R. MCCORMACK, R. WOLFERT, D. J. SELKOE, I. LIEBERBURG & D. SCHENK. 1992. Isolation and quantification of soluble Alzheimer's β-peptide from biological fluids. Nature **359**:325–327.

15. SHOJI, M., T. E. GOLDE, T. T. CHEUNG, J. GHISO, S. ESTUS, L. M. SHAFFER, X. D. CAI, D. M. MCKAY, R. TINTNER, B. FRANGIONE & S. G. YOUNKIN.

1992. Production of the Alzheimer amyloid β protein by normal proteolytic processing. Science **258**:126–129.

16. MORI, H., K. TAKIO, M. OGAWARA & D. J. SELKOE. 1992. Mass spectrometry of purified amyloid β protein in Alzheimer's disease. J. Biol. Chem **267**: 17082–17086.

17. KÖNIG, G., U. MÖNNING, C. CZECH, R. PRIOR, R. BANATI, U. SCHREITER-GASSER, J. BAUER, C. L. MASTERS & K. BEYREUTHER. 1992. Identification and differential expression of a novel alternative splice isoform of the βA4 amyloid precursor protein (APP) mRNA in leukocytes and brain microglia cells. J. Biol. Chem. **267**:10804–10809.

18. HAASS, C., A. Y. HUNG, M. G. SCHLOSSMACHER & D. J. SELKOE. 1993. β-amyloid peptide and a 3 kDa fragment are derived by distinct cellular mechanisms. J. Biol. Chem. **268**:3021–3024.

19. SEUBERT, P., T. OLTERSDORF, M. G. LEE, R. BARBOUR, C. BLOMQUIST, D. L. DAVIS, K. BRYANT, L. C. FRITZ, D. GALASKO, L. J. THAL, I. LIEBERBURG & D. B. SCHENK. 199■. β-amyloid precursor protein is cleaved at the amino-terminus of the β-amyloid peptide n an alternative secretory pathway. Nature. **361**:260–263.

Protein Phosphorylation Regulates Relative Utilization of Processing Pathways for Alzheimer β/A4 Amyloid Precursor Protein[a]

SAMUEL E. GANDY,[b] GREGG L. CAPORASO,
JOSEPH D. BUXBAUM, ODETE DA CRUZ E SILVA,
KERSTIN IVERFELDT, CHRISTER NORDSTEDT,
TOSHI SUZUKI, ANDREW J. CZERNIK,
ANGUS C. NAIRN, AND PAUL GREENGARD

*Laboratory of Molecular and Cellular Neuroscience, The Rockefeller University,
New York, New York 10021*
*Department of Neurology and Neuroscience, The New York Hospital-Cornell
Medical Center, New York, New York 10021 USA*

ABSTRACT: The Alzheimer amyloid precursor protein (APP) is a phosphoprotein, and the phosphorylation state of APP at Ser^{655} can be regulated by protein kinase C, calcium/calmodulin-dependent protein kinase II, and okadaic acid-sensitive protein phosphatases. Other enzymes may also play a role at Ser^{655} of APP and, perhaps, at other residues.

Signal transduction via protein phosphorylation regulates APP metabolism. In particular, APP processing via the nonamyloidogenic secretory cleavage pathway is increased following the activation of protein kinase C or the inactivation of okadaic acid-sensitive protein phosphatases.

The mechanism(s) by which protein phosphorylation regulates APP secretory cleavage include (among others): substrate activation, substrate redistribution, protease activation and/or protease redistribution. Current experimental evidence will be discussed, addressing the relative importance of each of these possibilities and the implications for these events in the modulation of β/A4-amyloidogenesis.

In 1986, we noted that the predicted cytoplasmic domain of APP contains amino acid sequences that resemble consensus acceptor sequences for phosphorylation by several serine/threonine-, or tyrosine-protein kinases. We

[a] This work was supported by USPHS AG 09464, AG 10491 and AG 11508.

[b] *Send correspondence to:* Dr. Samuel Gandy, Laboratory of Molecular and Cellular Neuroscience, The Rockefeller University, 1230 York Avenue, New York, NY 10021 USA; TEL: 212-746-6560; FAX: 212-746-8082.

therefore characterized the efficiency of short synthetic peptides corresponding to these APP sequences to serve as substrates for phosphorylation, using either purified protein kinases or endogenous protein kinase activities in homogenates of rat cerebral cortex.[1] After a comparison of kinetic parameters of protein phosphorylation determined for the APP peptides and for peptides corresponding to known physiological substrates, we identified an efficient site for phosphorylation of the APP cytoplasmic tail, located seven amino acid residues from the plasma membrane. Protein kinase C (PKC) rapidly phosphorylates Ser^{655} (numbering for APP_{695}) whereas calcium/calmodulin-dependent protein kinase II rapidly phosphorylates Thr^{654} and Ser^{655}.[1] Recently, PKC-dependent phosphorylation at Ser^{655} has been demonstrated in studies using either a 50-amino acid synthetic peptide corresponding to the entire APP cytoplasmic domain (S. Gandy and P. Greengard, unpublished observations) or APP holoprotein.[2] In addition, the studies of the phosphorylation of APP holoprotein[2] implicate the okadaic acid-sensitive protein phosphatases 1 and/or 2A in catalyzing the dephosphorylation of APP holoprotein. The APP holoprotein has also been demonstrated to be phosphorylated in cultures of intact human cells stably transfected with APP[3] and in intact untransfected PC12 cells (Suzuki *et al.*, unpublished observations); the determination of the site(s) of *in vivo* phosphorylation and the identity of the APP kinase(s) and phosphatase(s) is in progress.

On the basis of precedents from studies of several transmembrane proteins, the physiological effects of the phosphorylation of APP by PKC may be anticipated. The epidermal growth factor receptor (EGFR) and the interleukin-2 receptor (IL-2R) are integral membrane phosphoproteins which are phosphorylated by PKC. The endocytosis of both EGFR and IL-2R is regulated by PKC-dependent phosphorylation. By analogy, we proposed that phosphorylation of APP by PKC might stimulate its intracellular trafficking, and that such accelerated trafficking might regulate the catabolism of APP and hence the process of amyloidogenesis. More recently, PKC has been demonstrated to be an important regulator of the proteolytic processing of other integral membrane molecules, including the precursor of transforming growth factor-α and the receptor for colony stimulating factor-1. The mechanism for regulating of these processing events by PKC is currently unknown, but possibilities include intracellular redistribution and enhanced co-compartmentation of enzyme and/or substrate, direct phosphorylation of substrate ("substrate activation"), direct phosphorylation of protease(s) such as APP secretase ("enzyme activation"), or some combination of these.

To examine the effects of protein phosphorylation on APP metabolism directly, the biology of endogenous APP was studied in PC12 cells, an immortalized neuroendocrine cell line derived from a rat pheochromocytoma. These cells were chosen because of their neuronal lineage and their high levels of APP expression. Since the primary sequence of APP is highly conserved among many mammalian species, data obtained from studies of PC12 cells should be relevant to our understanding of the biology of APP in human neurons.

Using [^{35}S]methionine labeling in a pulse-chase protocol, we discovered that agents which regulate protein phosphorylation have dramatic effects on the proteolytic processing of APP.[4] Phorbol ester, which stimulates PKC, rapidly accelerates APP processing, increasing the level of a low molecular mass (*ca.* 15 kDa) carboxyl-terminal fragment of APP.[4] Okadaic acid, a compound structurally unrelated to phorbols, increases the state of protein phosphorylation by inhibiting protein phosphatases 1 and 2A, and was observed to increase the level of the identical fragment.[4] Thus, the enzymes that can regulate the state of APP phosphorylation in studies performed *in vitro*[1,2] are implicated in the regulation of APP metabolism in intact cells.[4] Furthermore, in some experiments where both phorbol ester and okadaic acid have been used in combination to produce a supraphysiological elevation of the state of protein phosphorylation, no further increase in production of the 15 kDa fragment is observed (as compared with either agent alone). However, a slightly larger fragment is recovered in addition to the 15 kDa species.[4] In order to completely understand how these phenomena relate to the process of amyloidogenesis, substantially more information on cellular APP processing routes is required. In an effort to dissect this process at the cellular level, we have extended our studies and discovered that two alternative trafficking and processing routes exist for APP molecules.

In one study,[5] we have obtained evidence that in PC12 cells only a minor population of molecules is targeted to the standard pathway for proteolytic cleavage within the β/A4-amyloid domain. Since this cleavage pathway is coupled to secretion of a large amino-terminal fragment, we have termed it the "standard secretory cleavage pathway." We have observed that the targeting of APP molecules to this standard pathway is regulated by protein phosphorylation, since compounds that either activate PKC or inhibit protein phosphatases 1 and 2A can independently stimulate the activity of the pathway. In the course of analyzing the products of the standard secretory cleavage pathway for APP in PC12 cells, we discovered that the majority of the newly synthesized APP molecules were apparently degraded via a different route. Inhibitors of organelle function were used to investigate the subcellular localization of APP degradation.[6] Treatment of PC12 cells with brefeldin A, a compound that causes retention of newly synthesized proteins in the endoplasmic reticulum (ER), totally inhibited secretion and revealed that APP secretory cleavage probably did not occur within the ER or early Golgi. Similar results were obtained with monensin, an ionophore which inhibits distal Golgi function.

Additional studies along this line provided evidence for degradation of APP within an intracellular acidic organelle.[6] The weak base chloroquine, which acts to neutralize acidic intracellular compartments, was particularly useful. Chloroquine treatment results in the inhibition of acid-dependent intravesicular proteolysis, as might occur in either the endocytic pathway (*i.e.,* early and late endosomes, lysosomes) or within the trans-Golgi network. Chloroquine had no effect on APP synthesis, maturation, or secretion under conditions in which vesicular neutralization could be observed.[6] This demonstrated that the drug did not exert a generalized toxicity for the cells and that the standard secretory cleavage pathway was relatively insensitive to changes in the acidification of intravesicular compartments. However, chloroquine dramatically diminished the intracellular degradation of mature APP holoprotein. Furthermore, chloroquine inhibited the degradation of the small carboxyl-terminal fragment generated by cleavage of APP holoprotein in the standard secretory cleavage pathway.

This series of experiments has allowed us to develop a scheme for the trafficking of APP molecules within PC12 cells. In this scheme, some mature APP molecules are targeted directly to a chloroquine-sensitive compartment for degradation, whereas others are targeted for intra-β/A4-amyloid cleavage and secretion in a pathway regulated by PKC and protein phosphatases 1 and 2A. Following secretory cleavage of mature APP, the carboxyl-terminal fragment thus generated is targeted to a chloroquine-sensitive compartment for degradation. Determination of the precise cellular locations where the APP standard secretory cleavage and chloroquine-sensitive degradation occur awaits further study. Definitive identification of which (if either) of these intracellular trafficking routes can be a source for potentially amyloidogenic carboxyl-terminal APP fragments has not yet been conclusively determined.

The identification of the subcellular site(s) which participate in APP cleavage is one step toward identification and isolation of the enzymes that catalyze the processing of APP, and the characterization of the regulation (perhaps by protein phosphorylation) of these enzymes. It seems likely that signal transduction via protein phosphorylation regulates the balance of the activities of these various pathways, some of which are nonamyloidogenic and others of which are likely to be amyloidogenic. In addition to defining the cleavage sites that generate amyloidogenic fragments, and identifying the proteases and protease inhibitors which regulate APP cleavage, it will be of great interest to elucidate the signal transduction components that modulate the relative activities of the various pathways. It seems likely that disturbance of these signals may be relevant to the pathogenesis of Alzheimer's disease, and particularly to the complex biochemical events that lead to the final common pathway of amyloidogenesis. Many of the components of these proteolytic and signal transduction systems (*e.g.,* proteases cleaving APP, protein kinases and protein phosphatases acting on APP or APP proteases, neurotransmitters/receptors which are linked to the relevant signaling pathways[7]) may eventually serve as targets for rational drug therapy by antiamyloidogenic agents.[8]

ACKNOWLEDGMENT

The authors thank Jodi Pliml for technical and secretarial support.

REFERENCES

1. GANDY, S. E., A. J. CZERNIK & P. GREENGARD. 1988. Phosphorylation of Alzheimer disease amyloid precursor peptide by protein kinase C and calcium/calmodulin-dependent protein kinase II. Proc. Natl. Acad. Sci. USA **85:** 6218–6221.
2. SUZUKI, T., A. NAIRN, S. GANDY & P. GREENGARD. 1992. Phosphorylation of Alzheimer amyloid precursor protein by protein kinase C. Neuroscience **48:** 755–761.
3. OLTERSDORF, T. L., P. J. WARD, T. HENRIKSSON, E. C. BEATTIE, R. L. NEVE, I. L. LIEBERBURG & L. C. FRITZ. 1990. The Alzheimer amyloid precursor protein: Identification of a stable intermediate in the biosynthetic/degradative pathway. J. Biol. Chem. **265:**4492–4497.
4. BUXBAUM, J. D., S. E. GANDY, P. CICCHETTI, M. E. EHRLICH, A. J. CZERNIK, R. P. FRACASSO, T. V. RAMABHADRAN, A. J. UNTERBECK & P. GREENGARD. 1990. Processing of Alzheimer β/A4 amyloid precursor protein: Modulation by agents that regulate protein phosphorylation. Proc. Natl. Acad. Sci. USA **87:** 6003–6006.
5. CAPORASO, G. L., S. E. GANDY, J. D. BUXBAUM, T. V. RAMABHADRAN & P. GREENGARD. 1992. Protein phosphorylation regulates secretion of Alzheimer β/A4 amyloid precursor protein. Proc. Natl. Acad. Sci. USA **89:**3055–3059.
6. CAPORASO, G. L., S. E. GANDY, J. D. BUXBAUM & P. GREENGARD. 1992. Chloroquine inhibits intracellular degradation but not secretion of Alzheimer β/A4 amyloid precursor protein. Proc. Natl. Acad. Sci. USA **89:**2252–2256.
7. BUXBAUM, J. D., M. OISHI, H. I. CHEN, R. PINKAS-KRAMARSKI, E. A. JAFFE, S. E. GANDY & P. GREENGARD. 1992. Cholinergic agonists and interleukin 1 regulate processing and secretion of Alzheimer β/A4 amyloid protein precursor. Proc. Natl. Acad. Sci. USA **89:**10075–10078.
8. GANDY, S. & P. GREENGARD. 1992. Amyloidogenesis in Alzheimer's disease: Some possible therapeutic opportunities. Trends Pharmacol. Sci. **13:**108–113.

Receptor-coupled Amyloid Precursor Protein Processing[a]

ROGER M. NITSCH,[b,c,e] BARBARA E. SLACK,[b]
STEVEN A. FARBER,[b] PAUL R. BORGHESANI,[b]
JOACHIM G. SCHULZ,[b] CINDY KIM,[b] CHRISTIAN C. FELDER,[d]
JOHN H. GROWDON,[c] AND RICHARD J. WURTMAN[b]

[b] *Department of Brain and Cognitive Sciences, Massachusetts Institute of
Technology, Cambridge, Massachusetts 02139 USA*

[c] *Department of Neurology, Massachusetts General Hospital,
Boston, Massachusetts 02114 USA*

[d] *Laboratory of Cell Biology, National Institutes of Mental Health,
Bethesda, Maryland 20892 USA*

ABSTRACT: The family of β-amyloid protein precursors (APP) can be processed via several alternative proteolytic pathways. Some generate potentially amyloidogenic APP derivatives, whereas others preclude the formation of such fragments. The cellular mechanisms regulating the relative activities of these pathways are thus important in determining the factors contributing to the formation of amyloidogenic APP derivatives. In order to investigate whether cell-surface receptor activity can regulate APP processing, HEK 293 cell lines stably expressing human muscarinic acetylcholine receptors (mAChR; subtypes m1, m2, m3, m4) were stimulated with the muscarinic agonist carbachol, and the release of APP derivatives was measured. Carbachol increased the release of large amino-terminal APP-fragments 4- to 6-fold in cell lines expressing the m1 or m3 receptors but not in those expressing m2 or m4 subtypes. This increase was blocked by various protein kinase inhibitors and mimicked by phorbol esters, indicating that it is mediated by protein kinase activation, presumably by protein kinase C (PKC). To determine whether additional cell-surface receptor types linked to this signal transduction pathway could also regulate APP processing, we stimulated differentiated PC-12 cells with bradykinin and found that this neuropeptide also increased the secretion of amino-terminal APP derivatives. We next investigated the possibility that neuronal depolarization might affect APP processing in mammalian brain. Electrically stimulated rat hippocampal slices released two times more amino-terminal APP derivatives than unstimulated control slices. This release increased with increasing stimulation frequencies in the physiological firing range of hippocampal pyramidal cells, and was blocked by tetrodotoxin. These results suggest that, in brain, APP processing is regulated by neuronal activity.

[a] This work was funded by NIA, NIMH, CBSMCT, and the Hoffman Fellowship for Alzheimer's Disease at MGH.

[e] *Send correspondence to:* Dr. R. M. Nitsch, Department of Brain and Cognitive Sciences, E25-604/M.I.T., Cambridge, MA 02139 USA, TEL: 617-253-6733; FAX: 617-253-6882.

INTRODUCTION

Amyloid deposits in the brains of Alzheimer's disease patients are primarily constituted of aggregates of 39–43 amino-acid peptides termed βA4 or Aβ. These peptides are derivatives of APP, a larger family of integral membrane glycoproteins. After maturation, full-length mature APP molecules can be cleaved within the βA4 domain[1] by a membrane-bound endoprotease[2] to generate two non-amyloidogenic breakdown products: a large amino-terminal derivative which is released and a remaining 10 kDa carboxyl-terminal fragment. This pathway has been referred to as "d-secretase processing." Alternatively, APP can be processed intracellularly in an endosomal-lysosomal compartment which generates multiple APP derivatives of various sizes. Some of these fragments are potentially amyloidogenic.[3] A further alternative processing pathway results in the direct secretion of soluble $\beta A4_{1-40}$ peptides.[4,5] In unstimulated cell cultures, approximately one fifth of full-length, mature APP molecules are processed via the constitutive secretory pathway[6] and the rest largely by the internal processing pathways. Only a small proportion of total cellular APP is processed to yield secreted soluble $\beta A4_{1-40}$ (1–5%, estimated from ref. 4).

It has previously been shown that activation of protein kinase C by phorbol esters accelerates the rate of APP turnover and promotes the release of amino-terminal APP derivatives.[7,8] Physiologically, PKC is activated in response to stimulation of cell-surface receptors which are coupled, via G proteins, to phospholipases generating diacylglycerol from membrane phospholipids.[9] Neurotransmitter receptors coupled to this signal transduction pathway include the muscarinic acetylcholine receptor (mAChR) subtypes m1 and m3, as well as bradykinin receptors.

MUSCARINIC ACETYLCHOLINE RECEPTORS REGULATE APP PROCESSING

To investigate the role of mAChR in regulating APP processing, we used human 293 cell lines which express endogenous human APP at high levels, and which release large amino-terminal APP derivatives indicative of constitutive APP secretion in this cell line. These cells were stably transfected with cDNA's encoding for human mAChR subtypes m1, m2, m3, or m4.[10] Stimulation of the transfected mAChR subtypes m1 and m3 increased the release of large amino-terminal APP derivatives by 4- to 6-fold.[11] The released amino-terminal APP derivatives lacked the carboxyl terminus suggesting that they are similar to the products generated by normal secretory cleavage. The increase in release occurred within minutes of the onset of receptor stimulation (maximum release was reached at 30 minutes) and was not blocked by cycloheximide. In contrast, the levels of full-length APP, basal and elevated secretion of amino-terminal APP derivatives were decreased by cycloheximide after treatment for more than 1 hour. These results indicate that derivatives of preexisting APP molecules are released in response to receptor activation. In parallel with the increase in secretion of amino-terminal APP derivatives, cell-associated full-length APP decreased in response to receptor activation. The receptor-coupled increase in release of amino-terminal APP derivatives was not blockable by colchicine, suggesting that the mechanism of the acceleration in APP cleavage and release does not require colchicine-sensitive vesicular transport. Together, these data indicate that stimulation of mAChRs rapidly induce proteolytic cleavage of preexisting full-length APP molecules which could be located at the plasma membrane or in colchicine-insensitive secretory vesicles.

A ROLE OF OTHER CELL-SURFACE RECEPTORS IN APP PROCESSING

Wild-type PC-12 cells, which can be differentiated into a neuronal phenotype with nerve growth factor, express endogenous bradykinin receptors which generate inositol trisphosphate and diacylglycerol in response to agonist binding. Inositol phosphate formation was increased 7-fold by bradykinin in differentiated PC-12 cells verifying the existence of functionally intact bradykinin receptors, coupled to phospholipase C, in the cell clones used. Concomitantly, bradykinin caused a 2-fold increase in the release of amino-terminal APP derivatives lacking the APP carboxyl-terminus, similar to the derivatives released by carbachol-stimulated cells expressing m1 or m3 receptors. Bradykinin-induced acceleration of APP processing was blocked by a bradykinin receptor antagonist, indicating a specific interaction of the peptide with the receptor. These data indicate that endogenous levels of neurotransmitter receptors are sufficient to accelerate APP processing in response to agonist binding. Recently, our initial finding that muscarinic m1 receptors accelerate APP processing has been confirmed;[12] moreover, it has been reported that interleukin 1 receptors also stimulate the release of these APP derivatives. Together, these data support the possibility that other cell-surface receptors coupled to PKC activation can also affect APP processing.

SIGNAL TRANSDUCTION

Muscarinic acetylcholine receptor subtypes m1 and m3 are coupled to multiple distinct signal transduction pathways.[9] Those include activation of several phospholipase C subtypes via G-proteins and the subsequent formation of diacylglycerol with or without concomitant formation of inositol trisphosphates. In addition, both m1 and m3 receptors activate phospholipases D and A_2, tyrosine kinases, receptor-operated calcium channels,[14] and a proton exchange pump; and stimulate cAMP formation.

To investigate signal transduction pathways involved in receptor-coupled APP processing, we measured the receptor-mediated increase in release of amino-terminal APP derivatives in the presence of the protein kinase inhibitors staurosporine, chelerythrine chloride, and calphostin C. All three inhibitors blocked the increase in APP release and chelerythrine chloride also inhibited basal release of the amino-terminal APP derivatives. Additionally, activation of PKC with phorbol esters mimicked the receptor-induced release of those fragments. These data suggest that receptor-coupled acceleration of APP processing is mediated by protein kinases, possibly PKC.[13]

Stimulation with carbachol in the absence of Ca^{++} also increased the release of amino-terminal APP derivatives, the magnitude of the effect, however, was somewhat reduced. This implies that, while Ca^{++} is not necessary for mediating the release, it potentiates the effect of m1 or m3 receptors when present. This assumption is compatible with the findings that Ca^{++} mobilization and PKC activation act synergistically on a variety of cellular responses.[9] The ionophore A23187 did not affect the release of APP derivatives, indicating that increased cellular Ca^{++} alone is not sufficient for mediating the release.

Activation of phospholipase A_2 with mellitin did not mimic the effect of m1 or m3 activation on the release of amino-terminal APP derivatives, suggesting that generation of arachidonic acid alone does not mediate this effect. Similarly, cAMP does not seem to be involved in regulating APP processing, inasmuch as receptor-mediated inhibition of adenylyl cyclase activity by m2 or m4 mAChR activation with carbachol failed to affect release. Increasing the formation of cAMP with forskolin also failed to affect APP processing.

In concert, these findings suggest that receptor-coupled acceleration of the release of amino-terminal APP derivatives is mediated by diacylglycerol-induced activation of PKC, possibly potentiated by a concomitant transient increase in intracellular Ca^{++}.

APP PROCESSING IN BRAIN CAN BE REGULATED BY NEURONAL ACTIVITY

To investigate whether APP processing in mammalian brain might also be controlled by neurotransmitters released with neuronal activity, we induced the synchronous electrical depolarization of rat hippocampal slices using field stimulation in a superfusion chamber system. Physiological depolarization frequencies (5 to 30 Hz) increased the release of endogenous neurotransmitters (*e.g.*, acetylcholine and glutamate) manyfold. This increase was inhibited by tetrodotoxin, which blocks voltage-sensitive sodium channels.

Electrical field stimulation of the hippocampal slices increased by 2-fold the release of amino-terminal APP derivatives lacking the APP carboxyl terminus. Release of these derivatives increased linearly with increasing stimulation frequency, over a range from 8 to 18 Hz; this range corresponds to the physiological firing frequencies of hippocampal pyramidal cells.[15] This suggests that, in rat hippocampus, the physiological regulation of APP processing depends on neuronal firing rates. The increase in the release of these derivatives was blocked by tetrodotoxin, demonstrating that action potentials regulate brain APP processing. To control for unspecific protein release and to verify the structural integrity of the slices during electrical stimulation, we determined whether stimulation also elicited the release of lactate dehydrogenase, or proteins separated by SDS-PAGE. Both were unaffected by electrical stimulation.

FUTURE DIRECTIONS

The functional significance of the coupling of APP processing to neurotransmission clearly awaits discovery. Perhaps this coupling relates to a hypothesized function of APP as an adhesive molecule. This mechanism may be involved in the pathophysiology of Alzheimer's disease, which is characterized by both alterations in neurotransmission and APP processing to amyloid. These initial findings suggest the use of receptor-active drugs to suppress the formation of amyloidogenic fragments from APP.

ACKNOWLEDGMENT

We thank Dr. Julius Axelrod for his advice.

REFERENCES

1. SISODIA, S. S., E. H. KOO, K. BEYREUTHER, A. UNTERBECK & D. L. PRICE. 1990. Evidence that β-amyloid protein in Alzheimer's disease is not derived by normal processing. Science **248:**492–495.
2. SISODIA, S. S. 1992. β-Amyloid precursor protein cleavage by a membrane-bound protease. Proc. Natl. Acad. Sci. USA **89:**6075–6079.
3. GOLDE, T. E., S. ESTUS, L. H. YOUNKIN, D. J. SELKOE & S. G. YOUNKIN. 1992. Processing of the amyloid protein precursor to potentially amyloidogenic derivatives. Science **255:**728–730.

4. HAASS, C., M. G. SCHLOSSMACHER, A. HUNG, C. VIGO-PELFREY, A. MELLON, B. OSTASZEWSKY, I. LIEBERBURG, E. KOO, D. SCHENK, D. TEPLOW & D. J. SELKOE. 1992. Amyloid β-peptide is produced by cultured cells during normal processing. Nature **359**:322–325.

5. SHOJI, M., T. E. GOLDE, J. GHISO, T. T. CHEUNG, S. ESTUS, L. M. SHAFFER, X-D. CAI, D. M. MCKAY, R. TINTNER, B. FRANGIONE, & S. G. YOUNKIN. 1992. Production of the Alzheimer amyloid β protein by normal proteolytic processing. Science **258**:126–129.

6. WEIDEMANN, A., G. KÖNIG, D. BUNKE, P. FISCHER, J. M. SALBAUM, C. L. MASTERS & K. BEYREUTHER. 1989. Identification, biogenesis, and localization of precursors of Alzheimer's disease A4 amyloid protein. Cell **57**:115–126.

7. BUXBAUM, J. D., S. E. GANDY, P. CICCHETTI, M. E. EHRLICH, A. J. CZERNIK, R. P. FRACASSO, T. V. RAMABHADRAN, A. J. UNTERBECK & P. GREENGARD. 1990. Processing of Alzheimer βA4 amyloid precursor protein: Modulation by agents that regulate protein phosphorylation. Proc. Natl. Acad. Sci. USA **87**: 6003–6006.

8. CAPORASO, G. L., S. E. GANDY, J. D. BUXBAUM, T. V. RAMABHADRAN & P. GREENGARD. 1992. Protein phosphorylation regulates secretion of Alzheimer βA4 amyloid precursor protein. Proc. Natl. Acad. Sci. USA **89**:3055–3059.

9. NISHIZUKA, Y. 1992. Intracellular signalling by hydrolysis of phospholipids and activation of protein kinase C. Science **258**:607–614.

10. PERALTA, E. G., A. ASHKENAZI, J. W. WINSLOW, J. RAMACHANDRAN & D. J. CAPON. 1988. Differential regulation of PI hydrolysis and adenylyl cyclase by muscarinic receptor subtypes. Nature **334**:434–437.

11. NITSCH, R. M., B. E. SLACK, R. J. WURTMAN, & J. H. GROWDON. 1992. Release of Alzheimer amyloid precursor derivatives stimulated by activation of muscarinic acetylcholine receptors. Science **258**:304–307.

12. BUXBAUM, J. D., M. OISHI, H. I. CHEN, P. PINKAS-KRAMARSKI, E. A. JAFFE, S. E. GANDY & P. GREENGARD. 1992. Cholinergic agonists and interleukin 1 regulate processing and secretion of the Alzheimer β/A4 amyloid protein precursor. Proc. Natl. Acad. Sci. USA **89**:10075–10078.

13. SLACK, B. E., R. M. NITSCH, E. LIVNEH, G. M. KUNZ, JR., H. ELDAR & R. J. WURTMAN. 1993. Regulation of amyloid precursor protein release by protein kinase C in Swiss 3T3 fibroblasts. Ann. N.Y. Acad. Sci. **695**:128–131. This volume.

14. FELDER, C. C., M. O. POULTER & J. WESS. 1992. Muscarinic receptor-operated Ca^{2+} influx in transfected fibroblast cells is independent of inositol phosphates and release of intracellular Ca^{2+}. Proc. Natl. Acad. Sci. USA **89**:509–513.

15. NITSCH, R. M., S. A. FARBER, J. H. GROWDON & R. J. WURTMAN. 1993. Release of amyloid β-protein precursor derivative by electrical depolarization of rat hippocampal slices. Proc. Natl. Acad. Sci. USA **90**:5191–5193.

Regulation of Amyloid Precursor Protein Release By Protein Kinase C in Swiss 3T3 Fibroblasts[a]

BARBARA E. SLACK,[b,e] ROGER M. NITSCH[b,c] ETTA LIVNEH,[d]
GEORGE M. KUNZ, JR.,[b] HAGIT ELDAR,[d]
AND RICHARD J. WURTMAN[b]

[b] *Department of Brain and Cognitive Sciences, Massachusetts Institute of
Technology, Cambridge, Massachusetts 02139*
[c] *Department of Neurology, Massachusetts General Hospital and Harvard Medical
School ACC 830, Fruit Street, Boston, Massachusetts 02114 USA*
[d] *Department of Chemical Immunology, The Weizmann Institute of Science,
Rehovot 76100 Israel*

ABSTRACT: Release of the amyloid precursor protein (APP) of Alzheimer's disease from Swiss 3T3 fibroblasts was stimulated in a concentration-dependent manner by phorbol 12-myristate 13-acetate. In fibroblasts overexpressing protein kinase Cα (PKCα), the EC_{50} for this response was 7 nM, while in control cells the EC_{50} was 63 nM. The effect of PMA was inhibited by the PKC antagonist H-7 in control cells, but not in cells that overexpressed PKCα. Basal release of APP was higher in cells that overexpressed PKCα, and was not affected by the phosphatase inhibitor okadaic acid, although this compound doubled APP release from control cells. The results suggest that PKCα regulates APP processing in mammalian cells. Alterations in the activity of PKC have been reported to occur in Alzheimer's disease and might potentially contribute to abnormalities of APP metabolism characteristic of this disorder.

INTRODUCTION

The amyloid precursor proteins (APP) of Alzheimer's disease (AD) make up a family of integral membrane proteins found in a variety of cell types. The extracellular N-terminal portion of mature APP is released from the cell following cleavage at a site located approximately 11 amino acids external to

[a] This work was supported in part by a grant from the National Institute of Mental Health (MH 28783).
[e] *Send correspondence to:* Dr. Barbara Slack, Department of Brain and Cognitive Sciences, E25-604/M.I.T., Cambridge, MA 02139 USA; TEL: (617) 253-6732, -8371; FAX: (617) 253-6882.

the cell membrane, leaving behind a small C-terminal fragment.[1–4] This process is stimulated by activation of receptors linked to membrane phosphatidylinositol (PtdIns) turnover, and appears to be mediated by protein kinase C (PKC).[5,6] The involvement of PKC in the release of soluble derivatives of APP is further suggested by the observation that the release of APP N-terminal derivatives into the medium of cultured cells[7] and the formation of a cell-associated C-terminal fragment[8] are both increased by treatment of cells with phorbol esters, which directly activate PKC, or with okadaic acid, a phosphatase inhibitor. At least 10 different subtypes of PKC have been identified, which vary in their sensitivity to lipid activators.[9] The alpha subtype of PKC (PKCα) is found in all tissues, and is activated by diacylglycerol and by fatty acids.[9] In order to determine whether PKCα is involved in the regulation of APP processing, APP release from fibroblasts overexpressing this PKC subtype and from control cells was determined both under basal conditions and in response to the PKC activator PMA (phorbol 12-myristate 13-acetate).

METHODS

Swiss 3T3 fibroblasts were infected with virus particles containing the full-length PKCα gene and a neomycin resistance gene, or with the neomycin resistance gene alone.[10] Two of the resulting PKCα-overexpressing clones (designated SF 1.4 and SF 3.2) and one control (neomycin-resistant) clone (SC1) were examined. The cells were maintained in Dulbecco's Modified Eagle Medium (D-MEM) containing 10% calf serum (GIBCO, Grand Island, NY) in an atmosphere of 5% CO_2. Prior to experiments, cells were subcultured onto 35 or 60 mm dishes and grown to confluency. To measure APP release, the cells were incubated at 37°C in serum-free D-MEM. Various concentrations of PMA or vehicle (dimethylsulfoxide) were added to the medium, and at the end of the incubation period (usually 1 hour in duration), media and cells were collected, and APP content in both was assayed by Western blot using anti-PreA4 (Mab clone 22C11; Boehringer Mannheim, Indianapolis, IN) according to the method of Nitsch *et al.*[5] The bands were quantitated by scanning densitometry (LKB, Bromma, Sweden). Quantitative comparisons were made between samples processed simultaneously on one blot.

RESULTS AND DISCUSSION

Both control and PKCα-overexpressing cell lines released APP consitutively into the medium. The released protein appeared as one major band on Western blots with an approximate molecular weight of 108 kDa. PMA increased APP release from both control and PKCα overexpressing cell lines in a concentration-dependent manner over a concentration range of 1 nM to 1 μM. The amount of APP released by 1 μM PMA after one hour was similar in control (SC1) and in PKCα-overexpressing (SF 1.4) cells, but the EC_{50} of the response was significantly lower in SF 1.4 cells (7 nM) than in control cells (63 nM). The increased sensitivity of the response to PMA observed in SF 1.4 cells suggests that PKCα regulates APP release. The PKC antagonist H-7 inhibited PMA-induced APP release from control cells, but not from SF 1.4 cells. The high levels of PKCα in the latter could account for the ineffectiveness of the inhibitor in these cells. The phosphatase inhibitor okadaic acid increased release from control cells, but not from SF 1.4 cells, which, however, exhibited elevations in basal APP release relative to controls. An increase in the basal phosphorylation state of APP could explain these observations, but has not yet been directly demonstrated. The levels of cell-associated APP in the SC1 cell line were not different from those in SF 1.4 cells. Preliminary experiments in a second clone that overexpresses PKCα (SF 3.2) again revealed a shift of approximately 5-fold in the EC_{50} to PMA with respect to control cells, with no change in the absolute amount of APP released by 1 μM PMA. Although it has been shown that PMA increases synthesis of APP mRNA,[11] the effects of PMA described here were not sensitive to cycloheximide, and hence can be attributed to processing of pre-existing APP via activation of PKC.

These results implicate PKCα in the regulation of APP release. This conclusion is supported by a recent report that co-infection with PKCα increased the phosphorylation and processing of APP introduced into cultured Sf9 insect cells via a recombinant baculovirus vector.[12] The observation that levels of membrane-associated PKCα and PKCβ are depressed in some brain regions in AD patients[13] suggests that alterations in one or more subtypes of PKC may participate in the abnormalities of APP processing that characterize this disease.

ACKNOWLEDGMENTS

The authors would like to thank Mr. Jeffrey Breu for expert technical assistance, and Boehringer Mannheim for the generous gift of anti-PreA4 antibody.

REFERENCES

1. WEIDEMANN, A., G. KÖNIG, D. BUNKE, P. FISCHER, J. M. SALBAUM, C. L. MASTERS, & K. BEYREUTHER. 1989. Identification, biogenesis, and localization of precursors of Alzheimer's disease A4 amyloid protein. Cell **57:**115–126.

2. OLTERSDORF, T., P. J. WARD, T. HENRIKSSON, E. C. BEATTIE, R. NEVE, I. LIEBERBURG & L. C. FRITZ. 1990. The Alzheimer amyloid precursor protein. Identification of a stable intermediate in the biosynthetic/degradative pathway. J. Biol. Chem. **265:**4492–4497.

3. ESCH, F. S., P. S. KEIM, E. C. BEATTIE, R. W. BLACHER, A. R. CULWELL, T. OLTERSDORF, D. MCCLURE & P. J. WARD. 1990. Cleavage of amyloid β peptide during constitutive processing of its precursor. Science **248:**1122–1124.

4. SISODIA, S. S., E. H. KOO, K. BEYREUTHER, A. UNTERBECK & D. L. PRICE. 1990. Evidence that β-amyloid protein in Alzheimer's disease is not derived by normal processing. Science **248:**492–495.

5. NITSCH, R. N., B. E. SLACK, R. J. WURTMAN, & J. H. GROWDON. 1992. Release of Alzheimer amyloid precursor derivatives stimulated by activation of muscarinic acetylcholine receptors. Science **258:**304–307.

6. BUXBAUM, J. D., M. OISHI, H. I. CHEN, R. PINKAS-KRAMARSKI, E. A. JAFFE, S. E. GANDY & P. GREENGARD. 1992. Cholinergic agonists and interleukin 1 regulate processing and secretion of the Alzheimer β/A4 amyloid protein precursor. Proc. Natl. Acad. Sci. USA **89:**10075–10078.

7. CAPORASO, G. L., S. E. GANDY, J. D. BUXBAUM, T. V. RAMABHADRAN, & P. GREENGARD. 1992. Protein phosphorylation regulates secretion of Alzheimer β/A4 amyloid precursor protein. Proc. Natl. Acad. Sci. USA **89:**3055–3059.

8. BUXBAUM, J. D., S. E. GANDY, P. CICCHETTI, M. E. EHRLICH, A. J. CZERNIK, R. P. FRACASSO, T. V. RAMABHADRAN, A. J. UNTERBECK, & P. GREENGARD. 1990. Processing of Alzheimer β/A4 amyloid precursor protein: modulation by agents that regulate protein phosphorylation. Proc. Natl. Acad. Sci. USA **87:** 6003–6006.

9. NISHIZUKA, Y. 1992. Intracellular signaling by hydrolysis of phospholipids and activation of protein kinase C. Science **258:**607–614.

10. ELDAR, H., Y. ZISMAN, A. ULLRICH & E. LIVNEH. 1990. Overexpression of protein kinase C α-subtype in Swiss/3T3 fibroblasts causes loss of both high and low affinity receptor numbers for epidermal growth factor. J. Biol. Chem. **265:**13290–13296.

11. GOLDGABER, D., H. W. HARRIS, T. HLA, T. MACIAG, R. J. DONNELLY, J. S. JACOBSEN, M. P. VITEK & D. C. GAJDUSEK. 1989. Interleukin 1 regulates synthesis of amyloid β-protein precursor mRNA in human endothelial cells. Proc. Natl. Acad. Sci. USA **86:**7606–7610.

12. SHAPIRO, I. P., L. MCCONOLOGUE, K. E. EIDMAN & T. R. SODERLING. 1992. Phosphorylation of β/A4 amyloid precursor protein (APP) in vivo. Soc. Neuroscience Abstracts **18:**1442.

13. MASLIAH, E., G. COLE, S. SHIMOHAMA, L. HANSEN, R. DETERESA, R. D. TERRY & T. SAITOH. 1990. Differential involvement of protein kinase C isozymes in Alzheimer's disease. J. Neurosci. **10:**2113–2124.

Cellular Processing and Proteoglycan Nature of Amyloid Precursor Proteins[a]

NIKOLAOS K. ROBAKIS,[b] DIDO VASSILACOPOULOU,
SPIROS EFTHIMIOPOULOS, KUMAR SAMBAMURTI,
LAWRENCE M. REFOLO, AND JUNICHI SHIOI

*Department of Psychiatry and Fishberg Research Center for Neurobiology,
Mount Sinai School of Medicine, New York, New York 10029 USA*

ABSTRACT: Amyloid β protein (β/A_4 or $A\beta$), the main proteinaceous component of the amyloid depositions of the Alzheimer's brain, derives from the proteolytic processing of the amyloid precursor protein (APP). Cleavage of the amyloid precursor by at least two distinct secretase activities produces soluble secreted APP. The major secretase cleavage (site I) takes place between $A\beta$ 16 and 17, while the minor cleavage (site II) takes place after $A\beta$ Lys 28 and may produce potentially amyloidogenic secreted APP. Full-length cellular APP is cleaved by secretase intracellularly in the Trans-Golgi Network (TGN) or in post-Golgi vesicles. The resultant soluble APP is transported to the plasma membrane and exocytosed.

The biological activity of the APP is still not completely understood, although it seems to act as a cell adhesion molecule. Recent studies have shown that in glioma cells, most of the soluble secreted APP occurs as a chondroitin sulfate proteoglycan (CSPG). In addition, full length APP CSPG has been detected in neuroblastoma and fibroblast cells as well as on the surface of glioma cells, and in human brain. These results suggest that the proteoglycan nature of the APP proteins may be important for their biological function.

INTRODUCTION

The amyloid fibrils of Alzheimer's disease (AD) accumulate in the neuritic plaque cores and cerebral blood vessels. The major component of these amyloid depositions is a small peptide 28 to 42 residues long ($\beta/A4$ or $A\beta$), derived from a larger amyloid precursor protein (APP). Molecular cloning of the gene encoding APP[1–4] led to the discovery of at least three APP isoforms—APP_{695}, APP_{751}, APP_{770}—two of which contain a region homologous to the Kunitz-type serine protease inhibitor (KPI).[5] Full-length APP's are membrane-bound proteins comprising a large extracytoplasmic section, a transmembrane region, and a small cytoplasmic domain. The longest $A\beta$

[a] This work was supported by National Institute on Aging Grants AGO8200 and AGO5138.
[b] *Send correspondence to:* Dr. Nikolaos K. Robakis, Mount Sinai School of Medicine, Department of Psychiatry and Fishberg Research Center for Neurobiology, One Gustave Levy Place, Box 1229, New York, NY 10029 USA; TEL: (212) 241-9380; FAX: (212) 831-1947.

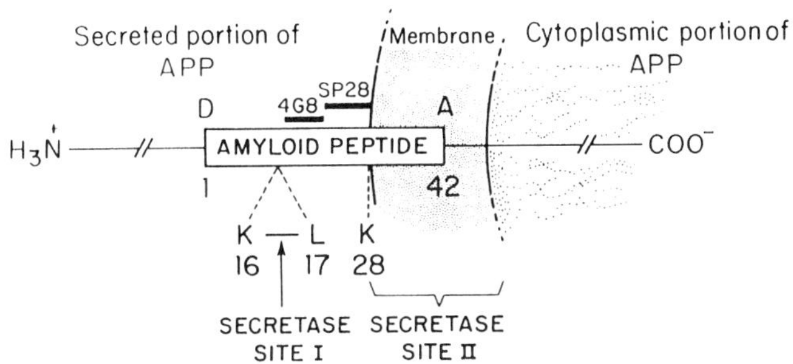

FIGURE 1. A diagram illustrating the APP sequence recognized by monoclonal antibody 4G8 and polyclonal antiserum SP28, and the location of two secretase cleavage sites. For more details about the antibodies see ref. 14. Secretase site II is located after Lys 28. Asp 1 (D1) is the N-terminus of the amyloid peptide and corresponds to $APP_{770}672$. Ala 42 is the C-terminus of the plaque amyloid. Vascular amyloid may contain 28 to 39 residues. See also text.

sequence includes the last 28 amino acids of the extracytoplasmic region of APP and about 14 amino acids of the transmembrane domain (FIG. 1). In addition to the membrane-associated full length forms, constitutively secreted APP, lacking the transmembrane and cytoplasmic sequences have been detected in the conditioned media of cell cultures and in human plasma and cerebrospinal fluid. Sequencing studies showed that secreted APP is produced after full length molecules are cleaved by an unidentified enzyme (APP secretase) between amino acids Lys 16 and Leu 17 (secretase cleavage I) of the Aβ sequence (FIG. 1).[6] Thus, this cleavage event is incompatible with production of the intact amyloid peptide. Based on this observation, it was suggested that cellular inability to process all APP's through the secretase pathway may result in altered APP catabolism that leads to the production of Aβ.[7,8] In this context, it is interesting to note that treatment of cell cultures by several agents, including NGF,[9] phorbol esters,[10] and cholinergic agonists[11] increased the secretory cleavage of APP. Soluble extracellular Aβ containing 40 residues was recently detected as a product of the normal cellular metabolism,[12,13] but it is still not clear whether this Aβ species are produced intracellularly or extracellularly from secreted precursors. In addition, although the detected Aβ is a potential precursor of the vascular amyloid, it may not serve as a precursor of the 42-residue plaque amyloid, since it lacks the last two residues of the Aβ. Our group has been working on the proteolytic processing and post-translational modifications of APP. In the next paragraphs, we discuss our most recent results on the post-translational processing of these proteins.

DETECTION OF AN ALTERNATIVE SECRETASE CLEAVAGE OF APP

Rat PC12 cell cultures grown on collagen coated plates were induced to differentiate in a neuronal phenotype by nerve growth factor (NGF). Recently, we have shown that this treatment increases the secretion of the KPI-containing APP[9] and that most of the secreted APP is cleaved between Aβ Lys[16] and Leu[17].[6] However, when purified secreted APP was probed on immunoblots with monoclonal antibody 4G8 directed against Aβ Leu[17]-Val[24] (FIG. 1), a small portion of the secreted APP reacted.[14] These results suggest that a fraction of the secreted APP molecules are cleaved further downstream of Aβ Lys[16]. The 4G8-reactive APP was affinity purified by an immobilized 4G8 antibody. The purified protein was recognized by several antibodies directed against the extracytoplasmic region of APP. In addition, this protein reacted with antiserum SP28 directed against Aβ[21–28], which corresponds to APP$_{751}$ sequence 673–680 (FIG. 1). Similar results were obtained from secreted APP isolated from a human embryonic kidney cell line transfected with APP$_{751}$.[14] These results indicate that a portion of the secreted APP is produced after the full-length protein is cleaved at a site further downstream of Aβ Lys[16]. Although the exact cleavage site of the 4G8-reactive secreted APP (secretase cleavage II) is not yet determined, our results suggest it is located either at Aβ Lys[28], which is the last residue of the extracytoplasmic domain of APP, or within the transmembrane region (FIG. 1). The secreted molecules did not react with several antisera directed against the cytoplasmic portion of APP, nor where they precipitated at $100,000 \times g$. These results exclude the possibility that our preparations were contaminated with full-length APP or with membrane fragments that may contain full-length protein. Therefore, our data indicate the presence of an alternative APP secretase cleavage activity. Cleavage by secretase II within the transmembrane sequence would imply that this region of APP may not always be inserted into a membrane. Presently it is not clear whether both secretase I and secretase II activities reside in the same or two distinct polypeptides. Depending on the exact cleavage site of the 4G8-reactive APP, the secreted isoform could serve as an extracellular precursor of the soluble amyloid detected in culture media.[12,13] Further studies should determine what factors modulate cleavage at secretase sites I and II. This is important because it would determine the potential amyloidogenicity of the secreted APP. The amyloid precursors undergo extensive post-translational modifications, including phosphorylation[15] and addition of glycosaminoglycan chains, which could influence the secretory cleavage site of APP (see below).

APP IS CLEAVED BY SECRETASE INTRACELLULARLY

Production of the Aβ protein is the result of the proteolytic processing of APP. Therefore, an important aspect of the work on AD amyloidosis is the elucidation of the metabolism and post-translational modification of these proteins. The subcellular organelle in which APP is cleaved by secretases is not known, although one hypothesis is that full-length APP is cleaved by secretase on the plasma membrane and the produced soluble APP is then directly released to the medium. However, we detected soluble nexin II in cell extracts suggesting an intracellular secretory cleavage.[16] In addition, in extracts prepared in the absence of detergent, a fraction of the cellular nexin II was associated with membranes. Treatment of these membranes with low concentration of digitonin, a mild detergent used to solubilize lumen proteins while leaving intact the integral membrane proteins, solubilized the membrane associated nexin II. Similar results were obtained after sodium carbonate treatment.[16] These data suggested that nexin II, the secreted form of the KPI-containing APP, is contained in the lumen of vesicles. Pulse chase experiments also showed that cellular nexin II was detected before culture medium nexin II, suggesting an intracellular secretory cleavage. Pulse-labeling experiments using ^{35}S-sulfate, showed that the secretory cleavage of APP takes place immediately after tyrosine sulfation which occurs exclusively in the trans-Golgi compartment.[16] Cell surface labeling revealed very little surface APP in PC12 cells which secrete high levels of nexin II. These results strongly indicate an intracellular cleavage of APP probably at the TGN or in post-TGN transport vesicles (FIG. 2).

Cell surface APP has been detected in several cell lines including C6 glioma cells, indicating that a fraction of the cellular full length APP may reach the cell surface intact. This fraction may increase when the cells synthesize high levels of APP as in the case of transfected cell lines. Inhibition of endocytosis in C6 cells inhibited the secretory cleavage of cell surface-full length APP,

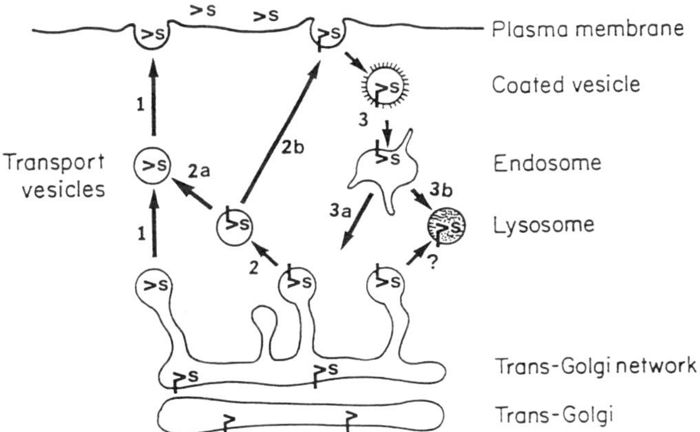

FIGURE 2. Model showing the proposed site(s) of APP cleavage by secretases. Full-length APP is cleaved in the TGN (pathway 1) or in post-Golgi transport vesicles (pathway 2a) and then secreted into the medium.[16] A fraction of full-length APP may reach the cell-surface (pathway 2b). Cell-surface APP is endocytosed (pathway 3) and then transported either to the TNG (pathway 3a) where it is cleaved by APP secretase or to the lysosomes (pathway 3b) where it is degraded (L. M. Refolo and N. K. Robakis, in preparation). It is presently not clear whether some intracellular full-length APP is transported to the lysosomes directly from the TGN (see text for further explanation).

suggesting that cell surface APP is internalized before it is cleaved by secretases. It seems reasonable that internalized APP is transported to the TGN where it is cleaved by secretases and then released to the medium. Treatment of the C6 cultures with chloroquine, an inhibitor of the endosomal/lysosomal system, increased the levels of both cell surface full length APP and cell surface-derived secreted APP, suggesting that a fraction of the cell surface APP may be transported to the lysosomes where it is degraded[17] to smaller fragments. Therefore, after endocytosis cell surface APP may be routed either to the TGN where it is cleaved by secretases or to the endosomal/lysosomal system (L. M. Refolo and N. K. Robakis, in preparation). From these observations, we propose the model showing in FIGURE 2 for the intracellular trafficking, secretory cleavage, and degradation of the full-length APP.

THE CHONDROITIN SULFATE PROTEOGLYCAN FORM OF APP

Recently, we showed that in C6 cells, most of the secreted soluble nexin II occurs as the core protein of a chondroitin sulfate proteoglycan.[18] These molecules consist of a core protein to which one or more chondroitin sulfate (CS) glycosaminoglycan (GAG) chains are covalently attached. Secreted, membrane-bound, and intracellular granule CSPG have been detected. They are involved in a variety of cellular functions including cell adhesion and migration, cell-cell communication, inhibition of axonal growth, and modulation of growth factor activities. Proteoglycans have been shown to play a critical role in several basement membrane-related diseases including atherosclerosis[19] and metastasis.[20] Cell surface labeling experiments in our laboratory indicate that in C6 cells at least 50% of the cell surface full-length APP occurs in the proteoglycan form.[21] Cell surface CSPG promote cell adhesion by interacting with components of the Extracellular Matrix (ECM) while secreted proteoglycan may inhibit cell adhesion by interfering with the binding of cell membrane-associated proteoglycans to the ECM. These observations raise the possibility that the cell surface and secreted AP CSPG modulate cell adhesion by competing for binding sites on the ECM. This hypothesis is supported by recent data suggesting that cell surface APP promotes neural cell adhesion and binds to collagen.[22] Presently, it is not known where the GAG chains are attached on the APP sequence; however, these proteins have only three consensus Ser-Gly sequence that could serve as the attachment sites for the GAG chains, at positions 57, 656, and 679 (numbering according to ref. 5). The last Ser-Gly dipeptide is preceded and followed by acidic residues, making it an excellent consensus sequence for the attachment of a GAG chain. The last 2 consensus GAG attachment sites closely flank Asp-672, the N terminus of Aβ peptide; indeed, Ser-679 is part of the Aβ sequence, corresponding to Aβ amino acid 8, and is also located only 9 residues upstream of the major APP secretase cleavage site.[6] Inhibition of cleavage at this site has been implicated in the production of the Aβ.[8] Given the large charge and size of the GAG chains, attachment of GAG on serine 656 or 679 could affect the proteolytic cleavage(s) that produce the Aβ by, for example, hindering access of the protease that produces the N-terminus of Aβ to the Asp 672. The proteoglycan form of APP was also detected in other cell lines including N2a mouse neuroblastoma and COS monkey fibroblast cells. In addition, this proteoglycan was detected in both fetal and adult human brain tissue. These results suggest that the APP proteoglycan is widely distributed and may perform an essential function in many tissues including the brain. Further research will reveal the biological function of this novel APP form and its role in the development of AD.

ACKNOWLEDGMENT

We thank Ms. N. Maderic for excellent secretarial assistance.

REFERENCES

1. GOLDGABER, D., M. I. LERMAN, W. O. MCBRIDE, U. SAFFIOTTI & D. C. GAJDUSEK. 1987. Characterization anc chromosomal localization of a DNA encoding brain amyloid of Alzheimer's disease. Science **235:**887–880.
2. KANG, J., H. G. LEMAIRE, A. UNTERBECK, J. M. SALBAUM, C. L. MASTERS, K. H. GRZESCHIK, G. MULTHAUP, K. BEYREUTHER & B. MULLER-HILL. 1987. The precursor of Alzheimer's disease amyloid A4 protein resembles a cell-surface receptor. Nature **325:**733–736.
3. ROBAKIS, N. K., N. RAMAKRISHNA, G. WOLFE & H. M. WISNIEWSKI. 1987. Molecular cloning and characterization of a cDNA encoding the cerebrovascular and the neuritic plaque core amyloid peptides. Proc. Natl. Acad. Sci. USA **84:** 4190–4194.
4. TANZI, R. E., J. F. GUSELLA, P. C. WATKINS, G. A. P. BRUNS, P. ST. GEORGE-HYSLOP, M. L. VAN KEUVEN, D. PATTERSON, S. PAGAN, D. M. KURNIT & R. L. NEVE. 1987. Amyloid β protein gene: cDNA mRNA distribution, and genetic linkage near the Alzheimer's locus. Science **235:**880–884.
5. KITAGUCHI, N., Y. TAKAHASHI, Y. TOKUSHIMA, S. SHIORJIRI & H. ITO. 1988. Novel precursor of Alzheimer's disease amyloid protein shows protease inhibitory activity. Nature **331:**530–532.
6. ANDERSON, J. P., F. S. ESCH, P. S. KEIM, K. SAMBAMURTI, I. LIEBERBURG & N. K. ROBAKIS. 1991. Exact cleavage site of Alzheimer amyloid precursor in neuronal PC-12 cells. Neurosci. Lett. **128:**126–128.
7. SISSODIA, S. S., E. H. KOO, K. BEYREUTHER, A. UNTERBECK & D. L. PRICE. 1990. Evidence that β-amyloid protein in Alzheimer's disease is not derived by normal processing. Science **248:**492–495.
8. ROBAKIS, N. K., K. SAMBAMURTI, J. P. ANDERSON, P. MEHTA & L. M. REFOLO. 1991. *In* Effects of neurotrophic factors on the secretion and metabolism of the Alzheimer's amyloid precursor, growth factors and Alzheimer's disease. H. Bracket & W. Christen, Eds.: 208–215. Heidelberg: Springer-Verlag.

9. REFOLO, L. M., S. R. J. SALTON, J. P. ANDERSON, P. MEHTA & N. K. ROBAKIS. 1989. Nerve and epidermal growth factors induce the release of the Alzheimer amyloid precursor from PC-12 cell cultures. Biochem. Biophys. Res. Commun. 164:664–670.

10. CAPORASO, G. L., S. E. GANDY, J. D. BUXBAUM, T. V. RAMABHADRAN & P. GREENGARD. 1992. Protein phosphorylation regulates secretion of Alzheimer β/A4 amyloid precursor protein. Proc. Natl. Acad. Sci. USA 89:3055–3059.

11. NITSCH, R. M., B. E. SLACK, R. J. WURTMAN & J. H. GROWDON. 1992. Release of Alzheimer amyloid precursor derivatives stimulated by activation of muscarinic acetylcholine receptors. Science 258:304–307.

12. HAASS, C., M. G. SCHLOSSMACHER, A. Y. HUNG, C. VIGO-PELFREY, A. MELLON, B. L. OSTASZEWSKI, I. LIEBERBURG, E. H. KOO, D. SCHENK, B. D. TEPLOW & D. J. SELKOE. 1992. Amyloid β-peptide is produced by cultured cells during normal metabolism. Nature 359:322–325.

13. SHOJI, M., T. E. GOLDE, J. GHISO, T. T. CHEUNG, S. ESTUS, L. M. SHAFFER, X. D. CAI, D. M. McKAY, R. TINTER, B. FRANGIONE & S. G. YOUNKIN. 1992. Production of the Alzheimer amyloid β protein by normal proteolytic processing. Science 258:126–129.

14. ANDERSON, J. P., Y. CHEN, K. S. KIM & N. K. ROBAKIS. 1992. An alternative secretase cleavage produces soluble Alzheimer Amyloid Precursor Protein containing a potentially amyloidogenic sequence. J. Neurochem. 59:2328–2331.

15. OLTERSDORF, T., P. J. WARD, T. HENRIKSSON, E. C. BEATTIE, R. NEVE, I. LIEBERBURG & L. C. FRITZ. 1990. The Alzheimer's amyloid protein identification of a stable intermediate in the biosynthetic/degradation pathway. J. Biol. Chem. 263:4492–4497.

16. SAMBAMURTI, K., J. SHIOI, J. P. ANDERSON, M. A. PAPPOLLA & N. K. ROBAKIS. 1992. Evidence for intracellular cleavage of the Alzheimer's amyloid precursor in PC12 cells. J. Neurosci. Res. 33:319–329.

17. HAAS, C., E. H. KOO, A. MELLON, A. Y. HUNG & D. J. SELKOE. 1992. Targeting of cell-surface β-amyloid precursor protein to lysosomes: Alternative processing into amyloid-bearing fragments. Nature 357:500–503.

18. SHIOI, J., J. P. ANDERSON, J. A. RIPELLINO & N. K. ROBAKIS. 1992. Chondroitin sulfate proteoglycan form of the Alzheimer's β-amyloid precursor. J. Biol. Chem. 267:13819–13822.

19. WAGNER, W. D., B. G. J. SALISBURY & H. A. ROWE. 1986. A proposed structure of chondroitin 6-sulfate proteoglycan of human normal and adjacent atherosclerotic plaque. Arteriosclerosis 6:407–417.

20. NEWMAN, S. A., D. A. FRENZ, E. HASEGAWA & S. K. AKIYAMA. 1987. Matrix-driven translation: Dependence on interaction of amino-terminal domain of fibronectin with heparin-like surface components of cells or particles. Proc. Natl. Acad. Sci. USA 84:4791–4795.

21. SHOI, J., L. M. REFOLO, S. EFTHIMIOPOULOS & N. K. ROBAKIS. 1993. Chondroitin sulfate proteoglycan form of cellular and cell-surface Alzheimer amyloid precursor. Neurosci. Lett. 154:121–124.

22. BREEN, K. C. 1992. APP-collagen interaction is mediated by heparin bridge mechanism. Mol. Chem. Neuropathol. 16:109–121.

Sequestration of Amyloid β-Peptide[a]

D. GOLDGABER,[b,d] A. I. SCHWARZMAN,[b] R. BHASIN,[b]
L. GREGORI,[b] D. SCHMECHEL,[c] A. M. SAUNDERS,[c]
A. D. ROSES,[c] AND W. J. STRITTMATTER[c]

[b] *Department of Psychiatry and Behavioral Science, State University of New York,
Stony Brook, New York 11794-8101 USA*

[c] *Department of Medicine (Neurology), Joseph and Kathleen Bryan Alzheimer's
Disease Research Center, Duke University Medical Center,
Durham, North Carolina 27710 USA*

ABSTRACT: Amyloid β-protein, or β/A4, is a 4-kilodalton peptide that forms poorly soluble extracellular depositions of amyloid in brains and leptomeninges of patients with Alzheimer's disease (AD), Down's syndrome (DS), and hereditary cerebral hemorrhage with amyloidosis-Dutch type (HCHWA-D). β/A4 peptide is a derivative of a large transmembrane glycoprotein (APP) and is found in the extracellular space, *i.e.*, in the cerebrospinal fluid and serum of individuals with and without AD and in the conditioned media of many different cells grown in culture.[1] The mechanism by which normally produced amyloid β peptide forms extracellular aggregates in patients is unknown. One possible explanation is a failure of a mechanism for removal of the β/A4 peptide that prevents this highly aggregating peptide from forming extracellular amyloid depositions.

In order to identify molecules that interact with β/A4 and could thus either prevent or facilitate its aggregation, a solid phase assay employing synthetic β/A4 peptide was developed. Synthetic β/A4 peptide or two control peptides were covalently linked to nylon membranes. One control peptide had the same amino acids as β/A4, but the sequence was scrambled and predicted a hydrophobic profile without significant hydrophobicity or hydrophylicity (peptide E.H.). The other peptide had a hydropathy profile very similar to that of β/A4 but was composed of different amino acids (peptide H.M.). Cerebrospinal fluid (CSF) was incubated with immobilized β/A4 or control peptides, and membranes were washed with different solutions. Proteins that were retained by the immobilized peptides after the most stringent washes were analyzed by SDS PAGE followed by silver staining or Western blotting.

[a] This work was supported by Alzheimer's Association grants IIRG-90-193 and Zenith Award ZEN-91-017 to D. Goldgaber; NIA LEAD Award AG-07922, NIA Alzheimer's Disease Center AG-05128 to A. D. Roses; NIGMS Clinical Research Center grant RR-30 to Duke University.

[d] *Send correspondence to:* D. Goldgaber, Department of Psychiatry and Behavioral Science, State University of New York, Stony Brook, NY 11794-8101 USA; TEL: (516) 444-1369; FAX: (516) 444-7534.

A number of proteins were retained by both β/A4 and H.M. but not E.H. peptides after 5% SDS or 6M guanidine hydrochloride washes. Two CSF proteins that strongly bind to the immobilized β/A4 peptides were identified. These are apolipoprotein E (Apo E) and APP.[2,3]

To determine if ApoE will bind β/A4 peptide in solution, purified ApoE and synthetic β/A4 peptide were mixed together, incubated and analyzed by SDS PAGE and Western blotting. We found that ApoE binds to β/A4 peptide directly. ApoE formed a very stable complex with β/A4 peptide that was not destroyed by boiling for 5 minutes in a sample buffer with 2% SDS. However, this complex was destroyed if β-mercaptoethanol was present in a sample buffer during boiling. The binding appears to be specific, *i.e.*, denaturation of ApoE by boiling prior to incubation abolished ApoE binding to β/A4 peptide. The binding is dose dependent with saturation at 10^{-4}M at neutral pH. The binding is also pH dependent with a maximum at neutral pH and a decrease at lower pH. No binding was observed below pH3.5. ApoE3 and ApoE4 bind to β/A4$_{(1-28)}$ peptide as efficiently as to β/A4$_{(1-40)}$ peptide. The rates of binding to β/A4 peptide are different for ApoE3 and ApoE4. The binding of ApoE4 to β/A4 peptide was detected in five minutes, while the binding of ApoE3 was first detected after two hours incubation at 37°C.[4]

To ascertain whether β/A4 peptide binds to ApoE in CSF, samples of human CSF (non-AD) were incubated with radioiodinated β/A4$_{(1-28)}$ peptide and then subjected to ultracentrifugation in potassium bromide gradient to separate lipoprotein particles from free proteins. Gradient fractions were subjected to SDS PAGE under nonreducing conditions. Radiolabeled β/A4 peptide was detected by autoradiography, and ApoE was detected by Western blotting using an anti-ApoE antibody. In CSF radioactive β/A4 peptide rapidly formed SDS resistant complexes with several electrophoretically distinct proteins. Complex formation was specific and was competed out by two hundred times excess of unlabeled peptide. Western blot analysis identified ApoE as a band that was electrophoretically distinct from β/A4 complexes. After ultracentrifugation, lipid-free ApoE as well as radioactive β/A4 peptide bound to at least two proteins were found at a density of 1.27 g/cm^3. Unbound radioactive β/A4 peptide was found throughout the gradient with a major peak near the bottom at a density of 1.30 g/cm^3. As expected the major peak of ApoE immunoreactivity was detected at the top of the gradient at density less than 1.10 g/cm^3 indicating an association of ApoE with lipoproteins. Only free unbound β/A4 peptide was found in this region of the gradient. In human CSF, the molar ratio of total ApoE (concentration 3 μg/ ml, reference 5) to β/A4 peptide (concentration 5 ng/ml, ref. 6) is approximately 100 to 1, and the molar ratio of free ApoE to β/A4 peptide is approximately 10 to 1. However, neither lipid-free ApoE nor ApoE in lipoprotein particles bind β/A4 peptide. Rapid binding of other CSF proteins to β/A4 peptide at nanomolar concentrations and formation of SDS resistant complexes suggest another high affinity interaction. We observed similar binding of serum proteins to β/A4 peptide.

Because β/A4 is a highly aggregating peptide, could be toxic for cells, and readily binds to a number of extracellular proteins, the following hypothesis of amyloid formation in AD and related disorders is proposed. We postulate the existence of a mechanism for sequestration and clearance of β/A4 peptide from the extracellular space. Failure of this mechanism in patients leads to the formation of amyloid. Our experiments unequivocally show that several CSF proteins bind β/A4 peptide to form very tight SDS resistant complexes. β/A4 peptide complexes are probably removed by one or more scavenger systems. Evidence supporting the existence of such a system was provided by recently reported internalization of β/A4 peptide by human fibroblast cells[7] from media with fetal calf serum that contains proteins binding β/A4 peptide.

The inefficient removal of β/A4 peptide, its aggregation and formation of amyloid could be due to 1) overproduction of β/A4 peptide, 2) disbalance in the level of sequestering proteins, 3) impairment or inability of sequestering proteins to form complexes with β/A4 peptide, 4) defects in the clearance mechanism, or 5) combination of the above. In AD, both ApoE and APP genes are overexpressed.[8] Local overproduction of β/A4 peptide and ApoE could lead to the formation of ApoE-β/A4 complexes due to the successful competition of the overproduced ApoE with proteins that normally sequester β/A4. Failure of the scavenger system to remove these complexes would result in amyloid depositions. The highly significant association of the ApoE-ε4 allele with late onset AD,[9] massive cerebrovascular amyloid depositions in ApoE-ε4 homozygotes with AD,[10] greater ability of ApoE4 isoform to bind β/A4 peptide, and presence of ApoE immunoreactivity in plaques, tangles and cerebrovascular amyloid[9–12] strongly support the direct involvement of ApoE in AD amyloidosis of the brain and cerebral blood vessels.

The binding of ApoE to the β/A4 peptide is a new and unexpected finding, but interaction of ApoE with other proteins is not unprecedented. ApoE is a lipid transporter molecule that is a constituent of all but LDL lipoprotein particles.[13] Unlike other apolipoproteins ApoE is expressed in many tissues and is the only apolipoprotein prominent in the brain and CSF. ApoE is also found as a free protein not associated with lipids. ApoE interacts with several receptors. At least two of these are also expressed in the brain. ApoE3 forms homodimers and complexes with ApoA-II. ApoE forms tetramers. It was proposed that activation of hepatic lipase by ApoE is the result of protein-protein interaction.[14] Very little is known about ApoE functions other than its role in lipid metabolism. Several receptors described modification of cellular responses by free ApoE. ApoE inhibited adherence and modulated outgrowth of neuronal processes of dorsal root ganglion cells, induction of ovarian androgen production, and mitogen stimulated lymphocyte activation.[15–17] Collectively, this suggests that free ApoE may interact with other proteins.

On the basis of our experimental data we propose a new role for ApoE: sequestration of peptides. There are two main domains in ApoE: the receptor-binding aminoterminal domain and the lipid-binding carboxyterminal domain. The interaction of ApoE with β/A4 peptide could be similar in nature to the interaction of ApoE with lipids and involve the lipid-binding carboxy-terminal amphipathic helices of ApoE. Such interaction would allow ApoE to interact with receptors via its receptor-binding domain. Overexpression of ApoE in response to tissue damage,[18] detection of ApoE in amyloid depositions in the brains of patients with AD,[10–12] and demonstration of direct interaction and complex formation of ApoE and β/A4 peptide presented in this report provide support for our hypothesis.

REFERENCES

1. SELKOE, D. J. 1987. The molecular pathology of Alzheimer's disease. Neuron **6:**487–498.
2. STRITTMATTER, W. J., A. M. SAUNDERS, D. SCHMECHEL, M. PERICAK-VANCE, J. ENGHILD, G. S. SALVESEN & A. D. ROSES. 1993. Apolipoprotein E: High avidity binding to β-amyloid and increased frequency of type 4 allele in familial Alzheimer's disease. Proc. Natl. Acad. Sci. USA. In press.
3. STRITTMATTER, W. J., D. Y. HUANG, R. BHASIN, A. D. ROSES & D. GOLD-GABER. 1993. Selective binding of βA amyloid to its own precursor. J. Exp. Neurol. Submitted.
4. ROSES, A. D., M. A. PERICAK-VANCE, A. M. SAUNDERS, D. SCHMECHEL, D. GOLDGABER & W. J. STRITTMATTER. 1993. Complex genetic disease: Can genetic strategies in Alzheimer's disease and new genetic mechanisms be applied to epilepsy? Epilepsy. In press.
5. PITAS, R. E., J. K. BOYLES, S. H. LEE, D. HUI, K. H. WEISGRABER. 1987. Lipoproteins and their receptors in the central nervous system. J. Biol. Chem. **262:**14352–14360.
6. FRANGIONE, B. Personal communication.
7. KNAUER, M. F., B. SOREGHAN, D. BURDICK, J. KOSMOSKI & C. G. GLABE. 1992. Intracellular accumulation and resistance to degradation of the Alzheimer amyloid A4/β protein. Proc. Natl. Acad. Sci. USA **89:**7437–7441.
8. DEDRICH, J. F., H. MINNIGAN, R. I. CARP, J. N. WHITAKER, R. RACE, W. FREY II & A. T. HAASE. 1991. Neuropathological changes in scrapie and Alzheimer's disease are associated with increase expression of apolipoprotein E and catepsin D in astrocytes. J. Virol. **65:**4759–4768.
9. SAUNDERS, A. M., W. J. STRITTMATTER, P. H. ST GEORGE-HYSLOP, M. A. PERICAK-VANCE, S. H. JOO, B. L. ROSI, D. SCHEMECHEL, M. J. ALBERTS, C. HULETTE, B. CRAIN, D. CRAPPER-MCLACHLAN, D. GOLDGABER & A. D.

ROSES. 1993. Association of apolipoprotein E type 4 allele with late-onset familial and sporadic Alzheimer's disease. Neurology. Submitted.

10. SCHMECHEL, D. Personal communication.

11. NAMBA, Y., M. TOMONAGA, H. KAWASAKI, E. OTOMO & K. IKEDA. 1991. Apolipoprotein E immunoreactivity in cerebral amyloid deposits and neurofibrillary tangles in Alzheimer's disease and kuru plaque amyloid in Creutzfeldt-Jakob disease. Brain Res. **541:**163–166.

12. WISNIEWSKI, T. & B. FRANGIONE. 1992. Apolipoprotein E: A pathological chaperone protein in patients with cerebral and systemic amyloid. Neurosci. Lett. **135:**235–238.

13. MAHLEY, R. W. 1988. Apolipoprotein E: Cholesterol transport protein with expanding role in cell biology. Science **240:**662–630.

14. THUREN T., K. H. WEISGRABER, P. SISSON & M. WAITE. 1992. Role of apolipoprotein in hepatic lipase catalyzed hydrolysis of phospholipid in high-density lipoproteins. Biochemistry **31:**2332–2338.

15. HANDELMAN, G. E., J. K. BOYLES, K. H. WEISGRABER, R. W. MAHLEY & R. E. PITAS. 1992. Effects of apolipoprotein E, β-very low density lipoproteins, and cholesterol on the extension of neurites by rabbit dorsal root ganglion neurons in vitro. J. Lipid Res. **33:**1677–1688.

16. DYER, C. A. & L. K. CURTIS. 1988. Apoprotein E-rich high density lipoproteins inhibit ovarian androgen synthesis. J. Biol. Chem. **263:**10965–10973.

17. PEPE, M. C. & L. K. CURTIS. 1986. Apolipoprotein E is a biologically active constituent of the normal immunoregulatory lipoprotein, LDL-In. J. Immun. **136:**3716–3723.

18. DAWSON, P. A., N. SCHECHTER & D. WILLIAMS. 1986. Induction of rat E and chicken A-I apolipoproteins and mRNAs during optic nerve degeneration. J. Biol. Chem. **261:**5681–5684.

The C-Terminus of the β Protein is Critical in Amyloidogenesis[a]

JOSEPH T. JARRETT, ELIZABETH P. BERGER,
AND PETER T. LANSBURY, JR.[b]

*Department of Chemistry, Massachusetts Institute of Technology,
Cambridge, Massachusetts 02139 USA*

ABSTRACT: The β amyloid protein found in extracellular deposits in Alzheimer's disease (AD) is heterogeneous at its C-terminus; proteins ending at residues 40, 42, and 43 have been identified in neuritic deposits, while protein in vascular amyloid appears to end at residue 39 or 40. Studies of synthetic β proteins (β1-39, β1-40, β1-42), and model peptides (β26-39, β26-40, β26-42, β26-43) demonstrate that amyloid formation is a nucleation-dependent phenomenon. Peptides ending at residues 39 or 40 were kinetically soluble for hours to days, while peptides ending at residues 42 or 43 aggregated immediately; all eventually reached similar thermodynamic solubility. The kinetically soluble variants could be seeded with the kinetically insoluble variants. The secondary structure of β26-39 fibrils was different from that of β26-42 fibrils, however, seeding β26-39 with β26-42 produces mixed fibrils with structure similar to β26-42. These results suggest that neuritic plaques may be seeded by their minor component; this may determine the structure and properties of amyloid in AD.

INTRODUCTION

The neuritic plaques characteristic of AD are composed of the ca. 4 kD β proteins; however, there is debate as to the precise N- and C-termini of the proteins found in various deposits. Original reports identified β1-42 as the primary component of neuritic plaque cores.[1,2] A recent report found that neuritic plaques are primarily composed of β1-40, while β1-43 is a minor component.[3] Another study reports that neuritic plaques contain β1-42,

[a] We thank the National Institutes of Health (AG08470-01), the Camille and Henry Dreyfus Foundation, the Sloan Foundation and the National Science Foundation (Presidential Young Investigator Award; contributions from Parke-Davis, Monsanto, and Hoechst-Celanese) for support of this work. P. T. L. is the Firmenich Assistant Professor of Chemistry. E. B. thanks Eli Lilly for support in the form of a graduate fellowship. J. T. J. is an NIH predoctoral trainee (1T32GM08318-01).

[b] *Send correspondence to:* Dr. Peter T. Lansbury, Jr., Department of Chemistry, 18-498/Massachusetts Institute of Technology, Cambridge, MA 02139 USA; TEL: (617) 253-5787; FAX: (617) 258-7500.

while vascular plaques contain β1-40.[4] Reports have indicated that the apparent solubility of synthetic β proteins is affected by the C-terminus.[5,6] Using synthetic peptides, we have studied the effect of the C-terminus on the formation and structure of amyloid fibrils.

AMYLOID FORMATION IS A NUCLEATION-DEPENDENT ASSEMBLY PROCESS

The aggregation of synthetic β peptides (β1-39, β1-40, β1-42) and model peptides (β26-39, β26-40, β26-42, β26-43) was followed by measuring the turbidity of buffered solutions (20-200 µM). The typical aggregation profile is shown for β26-40 (FIG. 1A). Aggregation is characterized by an initial phase during which the peptide is kinetically soluble, lasting for seconds (β1-42, β26-42, β26-43), hours (β26-40), or days (β1-39, β1-40, β26-39). Aggregation eventually occurs, leading to a growth phase, which reaches an apparent equilibrium within a few hours to several days. After equilibrium is reached, the solubility of these peptides was similar (2-10 µM). The aggregation of those variants with long lag times could be seeded with preformed fibrils from any of the variants; for example, β26-40 could be seeded with itself or with β26-43 (FIG. 1B). This kinetic behavior is characteristic of nucleation-dependent processes; well understood examples include tubulin polymerization[7] and protein crystallization.[8]

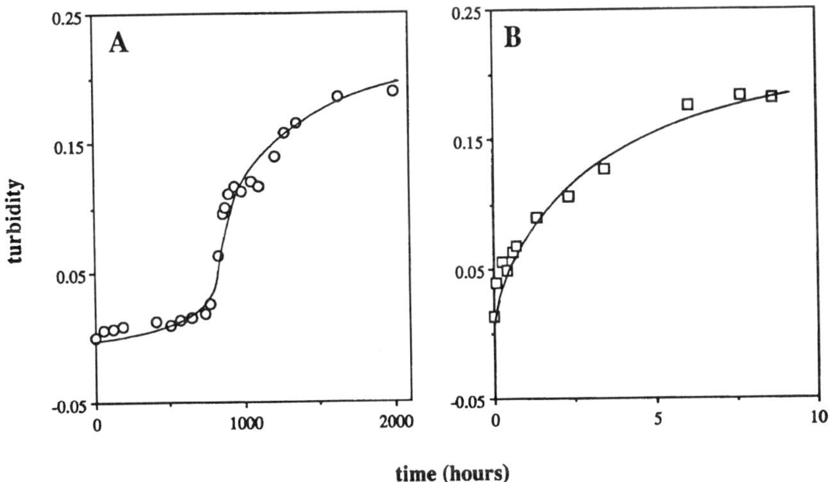

FIGURE 1. Aggregation profile for β26-40. **A:** Unseeded aggregation; **B:** Seeded with β26–43 (<10% by moles).

AMYLOID FIBRIL STRUCTURE VARIES AND DEPENDS ON THE SEED PROTEIN

The model peptides (β26-39, β26-40, β26-42, β26-43) formed amyloid fibrils which were indistinguishable by electron microscopy. However, infrared spectroscopy indicates differences at the secondary structure level. Spectra of each peptide show a strong band at ~1630 cm^{-1} (FIG. 2), possibly indicative of the presence of antiparallel β-sheet.[9] However, spectra of β26-39 and β26-40 also contain bands at ~1665 cm^{-1}, indicating some disordered, non β-sheet structures. If β26-39 aggregation is seeded with β26-42 (5 mol %), this disordered structure disappears. The spectrum obtained from these seeded fibrils (2:1 β26-39/β26-42 by mass spec.) was similar to the spectrum of β26-42. Similar results are obtained if β26-40 is seeded with β26-43. This suggests that a conformational change is induced upon binding of β26-39/40 to β26-42/43 nuclei, and that this structure may be continued throughout the growing fibril.

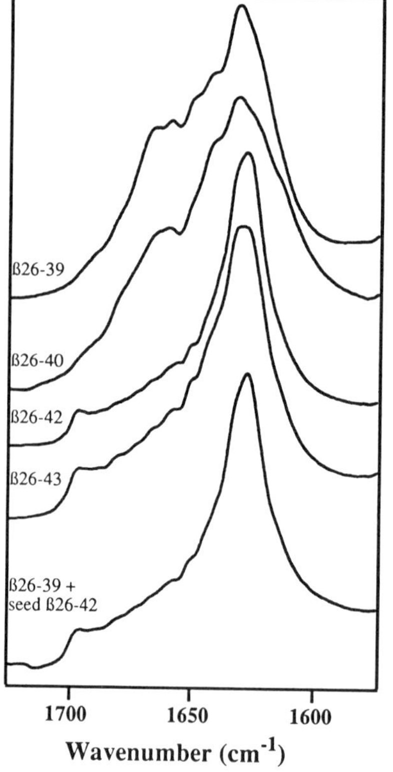

FIGURE 2. Spectra of model peptides (see text).

CONSEQUENCES FOR AMYLOID DEPOSITION IN ALZHEIMER'S DISEASE

These findings have important consequences for amyloid formation in AD. Nucleation-dependent mechanisms are characterized by the high concentration dependence of nucleus formation, which must precede aggregation. A slight elevation in *in vivo* β protein concentration could result in a dramatic increase in the rate of deposition. In addition, the kinetically soluble variant β1-40 may be seeded by the kinetically insoluble β1-43. Thus, the normal cleavage which produces extracellular β1-40 may become defective in AD, producing small amounts of β1-43, which initiates amyloid deposition. The mutations at codon 717 of APP may alter the binding of the protease responsible for normal cleavage at residue 40, resulting in production of β1-43; this variant deposits rapidly, possibly explaining the early onset of these cases of familial AD. The structure of β1-40 and β1-43 may be different; as suggested by model peptides. β1-43 and seeded β1-40 deposits may be more ordered than unseeded β1-40 deposits, resulting in plaques which are difficult to solubilize *in vitro* and difficult to clear *in vivo*.

REFERENCES

1. GLENNER, G. G. & C. W. WONG. 1984. Alzheimer's disease: Initial report of the purification and characterization of a novel cerebrovascular amyloid protein. Biochem. Biophys. Res. Commun. **120**:885–890.
2. KANG, J., H. G. LEMAIRE, A. UNTERBECK, J. M. SALBAUM, C. L. MASTERS, K. H. GRZESCHIK, G. MULTHAUP, K. BEYREUTHER & B. MULLER-HILL. 1987. The precursor of Alzheimer's disease amyloid A4 protein resembles a cell-surface receptor. Nature **325**:733–736.
3. MORI, H., K. TAKIO, M. OGAWARA & D. J. SELKOE. 1992. Mass spectrometry of purified amyloid β protein in Alzheimer's disease. J. Biol. Chem. **267**: 17082–17086.
4. MILLER, D. L., I. A. PAPAYANNOPOULOS, J. STYLES, S. A. BOBIN, Y. Y. LIN, K. BIEMANN & K. IQBAL. 1993. Peptides compositions of the cerebrovascular and senile plaque core amyloid deposits of Alzheimer's disease. Arch. Biochem. Biophys. In press.
5. BURDICK, D., B. SOREGHAN, M. KWON, J. KOSMOSKI, M. KNAUER, A. HENSCHEN, J. YATES, C. COTMAN & C. GLABE. 1992. Assembly and aggregation properties of synthetic Alzheimer's A4/β amyloid peptide analogs. J. Biol. Chem. **267**:546–554.
6. BARROW, C. J. & M. G. ZAGORSKI. 1991. Solution structure of the β peptide and its constituent fragments: Relation to amyloid deposition. Science **253**: 179–182.
7. KIRSCHNER, M. & T. MITCHISON. 1986. Beyond self-assembly: From microtubules to morphogenesis. Cell **45**:329–342.

8. FEHER, G. & Z. KAM. 1985. Nucleation and growth of protein crystals: General principles and assays. Meth Enzymology **114:**77–112.

9. LANSBURY, P. T. 1992. In pursuit of the molecular structure of amyloid plaque: New technology provides unexpected and critical information. Biochemistry **31:**6865–6870.

10. SPENCER, R. G. S., K. J. HALVERSON, M. AUGER, A. E. McDERMOTT, R. G. GRIFFIN & P. T. LANSBURY. 1991. An unusual peptide conformation may precipitate amyloid formation in Alzheimer's disease: Application of solid-state NMR to the determination of protein secondary structure. Biochemistry **30:**10382–10387.

Biologically Active Domain of the Secreted Form of the Amyloid β/A4 Protein Precursor[a]

JEAN-MARC ROCH,[b,d] LEE-WAY JIN,[b] HARUAKI NINOMIYA,[b] DAVID SCHUBERT,[c] AND TSUNAO SAITOH[b]

[b] Department of Neurosciences, University of California San Diego,
La Jolla, California USA
[c] Salk Institute for Biological Studies, San Diego, California USA

ABSTRACT: The amyloid β/A4 protein precursor (APP), a large transmembrane protein, is expressed ubiquitously in many organisms, as well as in a variety of cultured cells. Studies of the synthesis and processing of APP have revealed several intricate metabolic pathways for this protein. One of these pathways involves the cleavage of APP in the middle of the β/A4 domain and results in the secretion of the large amino-terminal portion of the protein. The biological function of this secreted form of APP has been the subject of intense investigation by several groups and various activities have been described for the different domains of APP studied. Our initial approach was to create a fibroblast cell line in which APP expression is dramatically reduced. These fibroblasts, called A-1, have a very slow growth rate. Addition of exogenous APP in the medium of A-1 cells restores their growth to the level of normal parent fibroblasts, demonstrating a growth factor-like activity for the secreted form of APP. Using APP fragments made in bacteria as well as synthetic peptides, we have been able to locate the active site of APP within a domain of 17 amino-acids (Ala319-Met335). This domain of APP can stimulate neurite extension of cultured neuroblastoma cells and it is proposed that APP mediates this effect through binding to a cell surface receptor, triggering intracellular transduction mechanisms. Thus, the secreted form of APP can function as a growth and/or differentiation factor and the site involved in these activities is within a 17-mer domain in the middle of the molecule. Our current lines of research seek to further characterize the mechanisms of APP function as well as its activity *in vivo*.

INTRODUCTION

The amyloid β/A4 protein is a peptide of approximately 4.2 kDa found in cerebrovascular amyloid deposits as well as in the core of the neuritic

[a] This work was supported by grants from Swiss National Science Foundation (# 823A-028366), and NIH (AG 05131, NS07078, and TW04602).
[d] *Send correspondence to:* Jean-Marc Roch, Department of Neurosciences 0624, UC San Diego, La Jolla, CA 92093 USA; TEL: 619/534-2545; FAX: 619/534-5569.

149

plaques[1] in the brain tissue of Alzheimer's disease (AD) patients. The molecular cloning of a cDNA coding for the amyloid β/A4 protein revealed that it is synthesized as a large precursor molecule, the amyloid β/A4 protein precursor (APP). Because the production of amyloid β/A4 protein requires the cleavage of its precursor, the biogenesis and metabolism of APP have been studied in depth by several groups.[1-3] It is also of primary importance to understand the biological activities of APP and this has been under intense investigation. Because the β/A4 protein is found in the core of the neuritic plaques, many of these studies have focused on the biological effects of this region of APP (reviewed in refs. 1–3). Both neurotrophic and neurotoxic activities have been reported for the β/A4 peptide, depending on various factors such as the type of cells used (PC12, neuroblastoma, primary hippocampal or cortical neurons, *etc.*), the domain of the β/A4 sequence, and the concentration of the active peptide in the culture medium. The activity of the secreted form of APP has also been the subject of intense investigation. The secreted forms of APP-770 and APP-751 (identical to protease Nexin II) have been implicated in the regulation of extracellular protease activity.[1-3] This activity has been shown to regulate neurite extension.[4] However, the non–KPI-containing form of APP (APP-695) has also been shown to stimulate neurite extension.[5,6] APP may also play a role in the regulation of blood coagulation, as suggested by the finding that APP is released by stimulated platelets and inhibits the coagulation factor XIa.[1-3] APP has also been shown to be involved in cell adhesion[1] and growth.[7-9]

APP IS A GROWTH FACTOR

In the investigation of the biological function of APP, our initial approach was to dramatically reduce the expression of APP in cultured cells.[7] This was achieved by transfection of a human lung fibroblast cell line (AG2804) with a plasmid vector (pNCA) driving the expression of an antisense APP RNA (FIG. 1). These cells grew very poorly unless we added medium that had previously been conditioned by the parent fibroblasts. The effect of this conditioned medium (CM) was dose-dependent with an optimal concentration of about 30%. Among the several clones isolated, we chose to analyze the clone A-1 because it showed the greatest dependence on conditioned medium for a normal growth rate. We thought that the factor present in the conditioned medium which was capable of restoring the growth of A-1 cells could be APP itself. Indeed, we found that the growth-restoring activity of the CM was abolished by passing it through an anti-APP affinity column, indicating that APP was the growth-stimulating factor. Another piece of evidence came from the following experiment: the kidney cell line 293 was transfected with

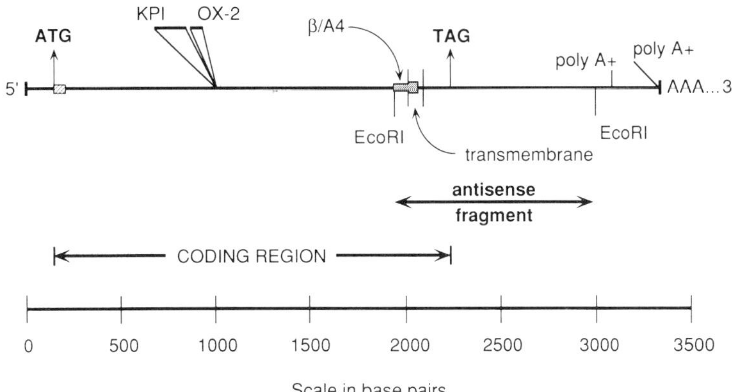

FIGURE 1. Creation of a low APP-producing cell line. This map of APP cDNA shows the 1.1 kb EcoR I fragment that was ligated in the expression vector pMSG to create the plasmid pNCA.[7] This new construct was used to transfect the human lung fibroblast cell line AG2804. Stable transfectants were selected for HAT resistance (conferred by the vector) and several clones were isolated. The cells transfected with pNCA express extremely low levels of APP mRNA and translation products as compared to the parent fibroblasts. The level of APP secreted into the medium of the transfected cells is also dramatically reduced.

vectors driving the over-expression of two isoforms of APP. The cells over-expressing APP-695 were called Amy-695 and those over-expressing APP-751 were called Amy-751. The medium conditioned by these transfected cells contained approximately 10 times more APP than the medium conditioned by the non-transfected 293 cells. Whereas we needed about 30% of CM from the 293 cells to restore the growth of A-1 fibroblasts, we needed only 3% of CM from either Amy-695 or Amy-751. This again suggested that the secreted form of APP is capable of stimulating the growth of fibroblasts. Furthermore, this activity is present in both the 695 and 751 isoforms. Finally, we showed that APP purified from brain stimulated the growth of A-1 cells in a dose-dependent way, with an optimal concentration between 1 and 10 ng/ml which corresponds to 10 to 100 picomolar. In summary, we demonstrated that the secreted forms of both APP-695 and APP-751 are growth factor-like molecules that can stimulate the growth of fibroblasts. Because the 751 isoform contains a KPI domain, it can stimulate cell growth through inhibition of extracellular protease activity. However, another mechanism must be postulated for the secreted form of APP-695 which lacks the KPI. We considered two possibilities: APP-695 may stimulate cell growth via cell adhesion or alternatively by stimulation of transduction mechanisms probably through binding to a cell-surface receptor. Recently, we have shown that the adhesion properties of A-1 cells are reduced compared to parent cells. However, addition of APP in the medium did not change A-1 cells adhesion although their growth was stimulated (unpublished results). Thus, we think that APP-695 acts through binding to a receptor on the surface of fibroblasts, although the presence of this receptor is yet to be established.

FUNCTIONAL MAPPING OF APP

To further characterize the biological activity of APP, we carried out a functional mapping of the molecule.[8] For that purpose, we decided to synthesize in bacteria APP fragments which spanned different regions of the secreted form of APP-695 (FIG. 2A). These fragments were then tested for the ability to stimulate the growth of A-1 cells. This strategy allowed us to narrow down the active site within a domain of 40 amino acids, from Thr296 to Met335. Confirming these results, we showed that a chemically synthesized 40-mer peptide corresponding to this region of APP was also active. The precise active site was then further defined using smaller and smaller peptides spanning different regions of the 40-mer[9,10] (FIG. 2B). We found that a 17-mer peptide (Ala319-Met335), an 11-mer peptide (Ala325-Met335), and finally a pentameric peptide (Arg-Glu-Arg-Met-Ser) were all active in stimulating the growth of A-1 cells. The activity of these peptides was sequence-specific because a peptide having the reverse sequence of that of the 17-mer (called rs-17-mer) was not active. Furthermore, KB75δ, a variant of KB75 in which the domain Thr306-Met335 (including the active 17-mer peptide) is deleted, was not active in the A-1 cells growth assay, which showed that the active site RERMS is unique in the APP molecule. Some of the small peptides we used were not able to stimulate the growth of A-1 cells (FIG. 2B). This was the case for the 5-mer N-terminal portion and the 7-mer C-terminal portion of the 11-mer peptide, among others. These peptides were added in a 1000-fold excess (10 nanomolar) into the medium of A-1 cells, along with either the 17-mer or KB75 (at 10 picomolar). We found that three peptides, partially overlapping the RERMS sequence, totally abolished the growth stimulating activity of the 17-mer and KB75. These peptides were the 7-mer and 6-mer C-terminal portions of the 11-mer, and the tetramer RMSQ. These data suggested that these peptides might be antagonists of APP-695, and confirmed the uniqueness of the active RERMS site in APP.

THE 17-MER DOMAIN OF APP HAS NEUROTROPHIC PROPERTIES

To study the activity of APP on cells of neuronal origin, we chose the rat neuroblastoma cell line B103 which expresses several neuronal markers, but no detectable APP (at both mRNA and protein levels). Addition of several APP fragments, either bacterially made or synthetic peptides, stimulated the

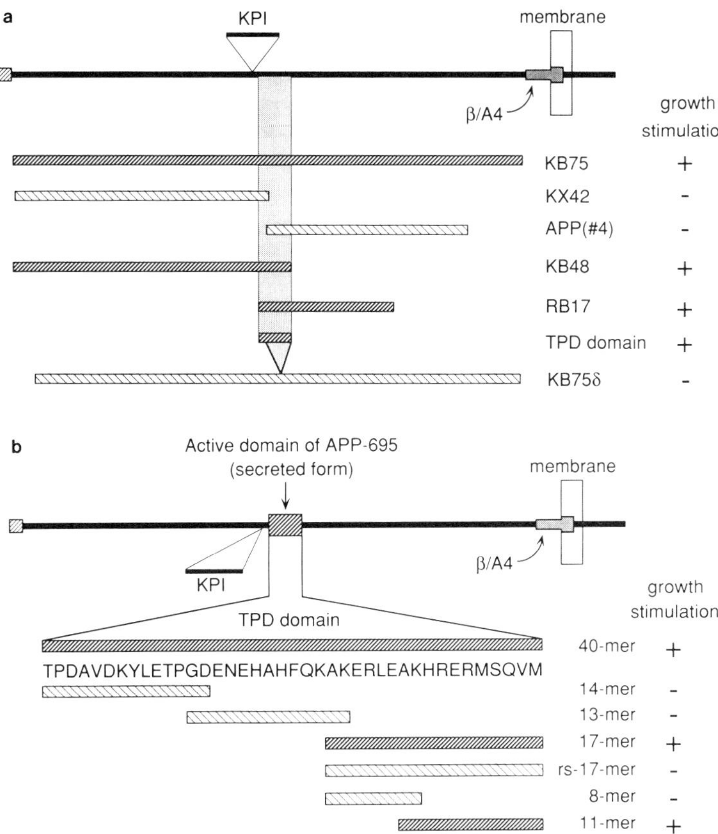

FIGURE 2. Functional mapping of APP. **a.** Fragments spanning different regions of APP were produced in a bacterial expression system and used in the A-1 cells growth assay. None of these fragments contains the KPI domain (represented here only for locating its insertion point). The fragment KB75, corresponding to the secreted form of APP-695, was active at the concentration of 10 picomolar. We then synthesized the fragments KX42, KB48 and RB17. The fragment APP(#4) was given to us by Dr. D. B. Schenk from Athena Neuroscience. Their pattern of activity suggested that the active site was within a domain of 40 residues from Thr296 to Met335. Thus, we chemically synthesized and purified this 40-mer peptide and showed that it was active. Finally, using PCR technology, we produced in our bacterial expression system, a variant of KB75 deleted for the amino acids Thr306 and Met335. This fragment, called KB75δ, was not active in the A-1 cells growth assay. **b.** Peptides of smaller and smaller sizes covering the sequence of the 40-mer in different ways were chemically synthesized and tested for their ability to support the growth of A-1 cells. The 17-mer, 11-mer, and the pentamer RERMS were found to be active. The concentration needed by the pentameric peptide RERMS for full activity was about 10-fold higher than that of the 17-mer, 11-mer, KB75, or APP-695. The fragment APP(#4), (see **a**) was not active, although it contained the complete sequence of the 17-mer. This fragment was made as a fusion protein with the first 99 amino acids of the MS2 polymerase.[8] It appears that the presence of this MS2 polymerase moiety was deleterious to the activity of fragment APP(#4).

neurite extension of B103 cells.[6] Both the number of neurites per cell and the average neurite length were significantly increased in the presence of APP. The active fragments were KB75, the 17-mer, and the 11-mer peptides (FIG. 3, columns A and B). The effect of these fragments was concentration-dependent, with an optimal concentration between 10 and 100 nanomolar (which is approximately a thousand-fold higher than the concentration needed for growth stimulation of fibroblasts). At the same concentration, both the rs-17-mer peptide and KB75δ had no significant activity, thus showing the sequence-specificity of our assay and the uniqueness of this active site in the APP molecule. Interestingly, the small peptides that could antagonize the effect of KB75 and the 17-mer on A-1 fibroblasts, as described above, were also able to antagonize the activity of KB75 and the 17-mer on B103 cells. We had previously hypothesized that one possible mechanism of action of

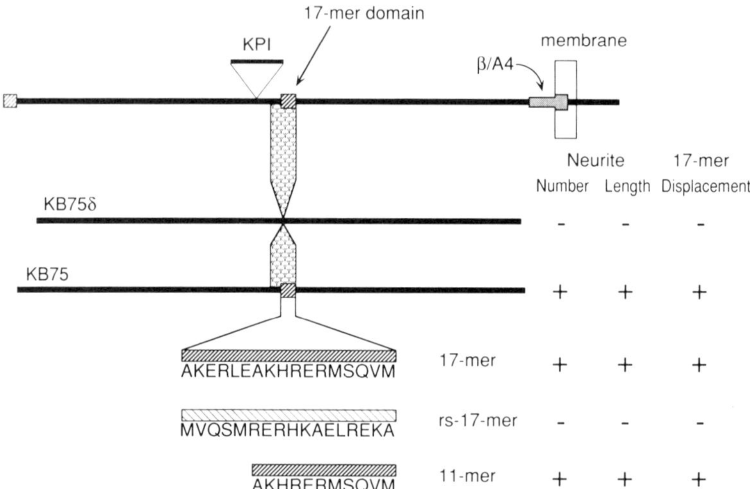

FIGURE 3. Effect of KB75 and derivative peptides on B103 cells. The KB75 peptide, representing the secreted form of APP-695, its deletion variant KB75δ, and chemically synthesized peptides were added to the culture medium of B103 neuroblastoma at various concentrations, and tested for biological activity. We report here the presence or absence of activity at the optimal peptide concentration, 40 nanomolar. The sign + indicates an effect significantly different from the control medium, and the sign − indicates the absence of effect, or an effect non-significantly different from the control medium. *Number of neurites per cell:* this number was significantly increased in presence of KB75, the 17-mer and the 11-mer, at 40 nanomolar, while the 17-mer of reverse sequence and KB75δ were not active. *Neurite length:* the pattern of activity of the different peptides was identical to the number of neurites. *Displacement of 17-mer binding:* the 17-mer peptide was labeled with ^{125}I and used as a radioligand in binding experiments with B103 monolayer. The + sign indicates a total displacement of the labeled peptide by a 1000-fold excess of cold peptide, and the − sign indicates no displacement at all. The binding of ^{125}I-17-mer was completely displaced by addition of 1000-fold excess of cold KB75, 17-mer and 11-mer, but not at all by KB75δ or the reverse-sequence 17-mer.

APP could be the binding of APP to a cell surface receptor and the stimulation of an intracellular cascade (see above). The data of the antagonist peptides support this notion. As a first step in the search for this receptor, we performed binding assays to intact B103 cells, using the 17-mer peptide radiolabeled with [125]I.[11] Our results (Fig. 3, column C) showed that the 17-mer binds to the surface of B103 cells, that this binding is saturable, and can be displaced by KB75, the 17-mer itself, and the 11-mer. In brief, we have demonstrated that the secreted form of APP-695 has neurotrophic activity, as shown by the stimulation of neurite extension of B103 neuroblastoma cells. The site of APP responsible for this activity is within the 17-mer domain, which binds to B103 cells in a saturable and displaceable way. The activity of both KB75 and the 17-mer can be antagonized by small peptides partially overlapping the C-terminal portion of the RERMS sequence.

CONCLUSION

We have presented evidence that the secreted form of APP-695 can function as a growth factor and/or a differentiation (neurotrophic) factor, depending on the type of cells studied. The active site responsible for these effects is entirely included within a domain of 17 residues from Ala319 to Met335. Interestingly, the sequence of this domain is very well conserved through evolution: the 17-mer sequence is conserved with 100% homology in rat, mouse, monkey and human. The Drosophila APP-like protein contains the sequence REKVT[12] which, considering the similarity of the side chains of the amino acids, is very close to the human RERMS motif.[9] This high degree of conservation suggests that this domain of APP is responsible for a fundamental biological function. Because the 17-mer domain is present in all APP isoforms, it potentially represents the active site of them all. Indeed, the secreted form APP-751 (identical to Nexin II) can also stimulate the growth of fibroblasts.[7] However, as the 17-mer domain is very close to the site of insertion of the KPI domain, it is possible that this KPI domain conceals the 17-mer domain in the KPI-containing isoforms of APP. Even if the KPI domain per se does not hinder the activity of the 17-mer, the binding of proteases such as chymotrypsin to the KPI might do so. If this hypothesis is true, it implies that the mechanisms of action of APP-695 and the KPI-containing forms of APP would be mutually exclusive. Considering that APP-695 is expressed almost exclusively in the brain, it is tempting to speculate that the 17-mer domain is the key molecule to a brain-specific mechanism. We are currently studying the biological activity of the different isoforms of APP, in order to determine whether or not the 17-mer domain is actually used by the KPI-containing forms of APP. In any case, it is clear that Nexin II regulates the level of extracellular protease activity. Since the secreted form of APP-695 lacks the KPI domain, we think that it acts through binding to a cell surface receptor, and activation of intracellular transduction mechanisms. In support of this idea, we have found binding sites for APP-695 and its 17-mer domain on the surface of B103 neuroblastoma cells. In addition, the secreted form of APP has recently been shown to reduce the intracellular levels of calcium in primary cultures of hippocampal and cortical neurons,[13,14] which could represent one reaction in the cascade of events triggered by the binding of APP to its receptor. The same study demonstrated that APP had a protective effect against glucose deprivation.[14] In addition, the 17-mer of APP could reduce neurological damage in ischemia.[15] Moreover, because APP induces a reduction of the intracellular calcium concentration, it is also possible that it confers a relative protection against glutamate-induced toxicity.[14] Combining the possible secretion of APP in the hippocampus[16] with the finding that APP undergoes fast anterograde axonal transport,[1] one might thus consider APP as an important factor involved in neuronal cell homeostasis and in the maintenance or stability of synaptic structures and functions. The search for the APP receptor and the elucidation of the molecular events triggered by APP are necessary steps toward a better understanding of the function of this protein.

REFERENCES

1. SELKOE, D. J. 1991. The molecular pathology of Alzheimer's disease. Neuron **6:**487–498.
2. KOSIK, K. S. 1992. Alzheimer's disease: A cell biological perspective. Science **256:**780–783.
3. SELKOE, D. J. 1991. Amyloid protein and Alzheimer's disease. Sci. Am. **265(5):** 68–78.
4. ROBAKIS, N. K., L. D. ALTSTIEL, L. M. REFOLO & J. P. ANDERSON. 1990. Function and metabolism of the protease inhibitor-containing Alzheimer amyloid precursors. *In* T. Miyatake, D. J. Selkoe & Y. Ihara, Eds. 179–188. Molecular Biology of Alzheimer's Disease. Elsevier Science Publishers B. V. Amsterdam. 1992.
5. MILWARD, E. A., R. PAPADOPOULOS, S. J. FULLER, R. D. MOIR, D. SMALL, K. BEYREUTHER & C. L. MASTERS. 1992. The amyloid protein precursor of Alzheimer's disease is a mediator of the effects of nerve growh factor on neurite outgrowth. Neuron **9:**129–137.
6. JIN, L.-W., E. MASLIAH, H. NINOMIYA, J.-M. ROCH, D. A. C. OTERO, D. SCHUBERT, & T. SAITOH. 1992. Biological activity of amyloid β/A4 protein precursor. II. Neurotrophic effect of an APP peptide on a rat brain neuroblastoma cell line. Soc. Neurosci. Abstr. **18:**1466.
7. SAITOH, T., M. P. SUNDSMO, J.-M. ROCH, N. KIMURA, G. M. COLE, D. SCHUBERT, T. OLTERSDORF & D. B. SCHENK. 1989. Secreted form of amyloid β

protein precursor is involved in the growth regulation of fibroblasts. Cell **58:** 615–622.

8. ROCH, J.-M., I. P. SHAPIRO, M. P. SUNDSMO, D. A. C. OTERO, L. M. REFOLO, N. K. ROBAKIS & T. SAITOH. 1992. Bacterial expression, purification, and functional mapping of the amyloid β/A4 protein precursor. J. Biol. Chem. **276:** 2214–2221.

9. NINOMIYA, H., J.-M. ROCH, M. P. SUNDSMO, D. A. C. OTERO & T. SAITOH. 1993. Amino acid sequence RERMS represents the active domain of amyloid β/A4 protein precursor that promotes fibroblast growth. J. Cell Biol. **121:** 879–886.

10. ROCH, J.-M., H. NINOMIYA, D. A. C. OTERO, & T. SAITOH. 1992. Biological activity of the amyloid β/A4 protein precursor. I. Functional mapping of growth promoting activity. Soc. Neurosci. Abstr. **18:**1465.

11. NINOMIYA H., L.-W. JIN, J.-M. ROCH, D. A. C. OTERO & T. SAITOH. 1992. Biological activity of the amyloid β/A4 protein precursor. III. Binding of iodinated 17-mer peptide (Ala319-Met335 of APP695) to rat neuroblastoma (B103) cell monolayer. Soc. Neurosci. Abstr. **18:**1466.

12. ROSEN, D. R., L. MARTIN-MORRIS, L. LUO & K. WHITE. 1992. A Drosophila gene encoding a protein resembling the human β-amyloid protein precursor. Proc. Natl. Acad. Sci. USA **86:**2478–2482.

13. MATTSON, M. P., I. LIEBERBURG & R. E. RYDEL. 1992. Secreted form of amyloid precursor protein regulates intraneuronal calcium levels: role for APPs in neuronal plasticity. Soc. Neurosci. Abstr. **18:**1438.

14. MATTSON , M. P., B. CHENG, A. R. CULWELL, F. S. ESCH, I. LIEBERBURG & R. E. RYDEL. 1993. Evidence for excitoprotective and intraneuronal calcium regulating roles for the secreted forms of the β-amyloid precursor protein. Neuron **10:**243–254.

15. BOWES, M. P., T. SAITOH, J. A. ZIVIN, J.-M.ROCH & K. UÉDA. 1992. A 17-mer peptide segment of the amyloid β/A4 protein (APP) reduces neurologic damage in rabbit spinal cord ischemia model. Soc. Neurosci. Abstr. **18:**1437.

16. FARBER, S. A., R. M. NITSCH & R. J. WURTMAN. 1992. Alzheimer amyloid precursor protein can be released from hippocampal slices in vitro. Soc. Neurosci. Abstr. **18:**765.

β-Amyloid Precursor Protein Mismetabolism and Loss of Calcium Homeostasis in Alzheimer's Disease[a]

S. W. BARGER,[b] V. L. SMITH-SWINTOSKY,[b] R. E. RYDEL,[c] AND
M. P. MATTSON[b,d]

[b] Sanders-Brown Center on Aging and Department of Anatomy & Neurobiology,
University of Kentucky Medical Center, Lexington, Kentucky 40536-0230 USA
[c] Athena Neurosciences, Inc., 800 F. Gateway Boulevard,
South San Francisco, California 94080 USA

ABSTRACT: The suspected involvement of the β-amyloid precursor protein (βAPP) in the etiology of Alzheimer's disease (AD) has been strengthened by recent genetic evidence, but pursuit of the mechanisms involved will initially require basic cell biology approaches. Several studies have concentrated on toxic activities of β-amyloid peptide (βAP) itself, illuminating its contributions to excitotoxicity and calcium-mediated degeneration in general. We now know that generation of βAP from βAPP also compromises the production of an important set of trophic factors: the secreted forms of βAPP (APP^S), which may act—ironically—by conferring protection from calcium-mediated insults. Therefore, conditions which contribute to the formation of βAP (possibly including ischemia) not only produce an agent which exacerbates calcium-mediated cell death, but also reduce the levels of one of the few factors able to rescue calcium homeostasis. The implications of these postulates and their relationship to the process of aging are discussed.

INTRODUCTION

Definitive diagnosis of Alzheimer's disease (AD) still relies on the identification of characteristic neuropathologies at autopsy, including abnormally high numbers of the amyloid plaques present at lower densities in the normally aging brain. From the time it was identified as the principal component of these plaques, the β-amyloid peptide (βAP) has been incorporated into many theories of AD etiology.[1] Although the tide of opinion has repeatedly shifted between views of βAP as a cause or result of AD, several lines of evidence are beginning to support at least a permissive involvement of βAP

[a] The original research described herein was supported by grants to M.P.M. from the NIH and the Alzheimer's Association, and by Athena Neurosciences, Inc. and Eli Lilly & Co.
[d] Send correspondence to: Dr. Mark P. Mattson, 211 Sanders-Brown Bldg., University of Kentucky, Lexington, KY 40536-0230 USA; TEL: (606) 257-6040; FAX: (606) 258-2866.

and its parent molecule—amyloid precursor protein (βAPP)—in neurode-generative mechanisms. The most convincing data concern recent genetic linkage of mutations in the βAPP gene to a limited number of the lineages in which familial AD (FAD) occurs. Although the number of FAD lineages which lack these mutations refutes their causation of all cases of FAD, cosegregation of the mutations and disease among affected individuals strongly argues that βAPP does play a role in the etiology of AD.

βAPP is a transmembrane glycoprotein that exists in different forms that either lack (βAPP$_{695}$ and βAPP$_{714}$) or contain (βAPP$_{751}$ and βAPP$_{770}$) a protease inhibitor domain near the aminoterminus. β-amyloid peptide is a fragment derived from a region of βAPP that spans extracellular and transmembrane sequences. Two alternative pathways of βAPP metabolism have been identified (FIG. 1). One pathway involves an enzymatic cleavage at the cell surface (within the βAP sequence) that results in liberation of secreted forms of βAPP (APP^S) into the extracellular milieu, thereby precluding the generation of βAP. The alternative pathway apparently involves processing of βAPP in an acidic (possibly lysosomal) compartment; this pathway can result in liberation of intact βAP from cells. Because βAP is the product of

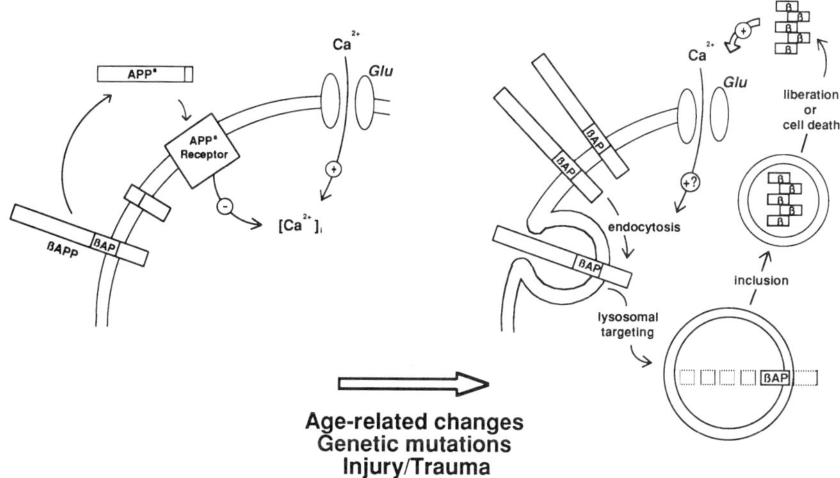

FIGURE 1. Alternative processing of βAPP's. The βAPP's are transmembrane proteins, similar to the precursors for other peptide growth factors. Proteolytic cleavage within the βAP region *(left)* generates the APP^{S}s, which have stabilizing effects on [Ca^{2+}]$_i$ otherwise elevated by glutamate receptor activation, *etc.* The actions of APP^{S}s are consistent with mediation through a cell surface receptor. In Alzheimer's disease, mutations, overexpression, or age-related changes in metabolism may favor endocytosis, lysosomal degradation, and accumulation of βAPP into cell-associated inclusion bodies and/or extracellular deposits *(right)*. As discussed in the text, the latter condition would tend to rob the tissue of the protective APP^S's and generate βAP aggregates which themselves destabilize [Ca^{2+}]$_i$.

a normal metabolic pathway[2] but only accumulates excessively during aging and more dramatically in AD, it seems likely that in AD there is either an increased generation of βAP from βAPP or decreased degradation of βAP. The events which control segregation into these alternate pathways are still poorly understood: activation of protein kinase C, which results in phosphorylation of the βAPPs, has been reported to increase the generation of both βAP-containing fragments and βAP-exclusive APP[S]'s.[3,4]

To understand how such alterations in βAPP metabolism contribute to neuronal degeneration, we and others have been studying the biological activities and mechanisms of action of βAPs. Previous data have suggested that neuronal degeneration could result from toxic activities of βAP, elevated by overexpression of βAPP, or changes in its processing. Here, we consider the neurotoxicity of βAP, especially in relation to excitatory amino acids, calcium homeostasis, and energy availability/utilization. In addition, we discuss our recent demonstration of trophic effects of the secreted forms of βAPP and advance the hypothesis that loss of trophic functions due to alternative processing of βAPP's may be equally as important as the acquisition of toxic ones.

βAPs AND THE LOSS OF CALCIUM HOMEOSTASIS

βAPs can be directly neurotoxic at micromolar concentrations.[5] Perhaps more consistent is the ability of βAPs to increase neuronal vulnerability to other toxic insults (below). Any toxic effects of βAPs are likely to depend on the formation of insoluble peptide aggregates.[6] These aggregates may represent the β-sheet conformation characteristic of amyloid fibrils from AD brain; the generation of these fibrils *in vitro* is pH-dependent,[7] consistent with their hypothetical formation in lysosomes. The mechanism of βAP neurotoxicity seems to involve a destabilization of cellular calcium homeostasis resulting in elevation of intracellular free calcium levels ($[Ca^{2+}]_i$).[8]

The involvement of calcium in βAP toxicity suggests that the peptide could impact upon other calcium-related systems, particularly glutamate and its receptors. Glutamate is the major excitatory transmitter in the brain, evoking an increase in $[Ca^{2+}]_i$ through several different receptors. Overactivation of glutamate receptors or moderate activation during energy depletion can cause calcium-dependent neuronal death, a process termed excitotoxicity. Glutamate and related excitatory amino acids are implicated in an array of neurodegenerative conditions,[9] and a number of studies suggest that excitotoxicity is involved in the dendritic pruning and cell death that occurs in AD. Glutamate can elicit antigenic and ultrastructural changes in culture similar to those seen in the neurofibrillary tangles of AD;[10] similar neurofibrillary tangle-like changes have been induced by excitotoxins *in vivo*.[11] As predicted by its effects on $[Ca^{2+}]_i$, βAP increases the susceptibility of neurons to excitotoxins.[8] Although the mechanism of this increase in vulnerability is unknown, the available data suggest that the neurodegeneration associated with AD involves enhanced vulnerability to calcium due in part to altered metabolism of βAPP or the accumulation of βAP during aging.

NORMAL FUNCTION OF β-APP

Recent findings concerning the normal function of APP[S]s are providing additional clues to the role of altered βAPP metabolism in the pathogenesis of AD. Endogenous APP[S]s are necessary for the normal growth rate of fibroblastic cells, and exogenous APP[S]s can stimulate proliferation in these cells.[12] βAPP is regulated in a way that suggests a cellular signaling function of APP[S]s in brain as well. For example, βAPPs are axonally transported, and neuronal activity causes the release of APP[S]s. Additionally, the production of βAPPs is increased by ischemia.[13]

These kinds of data suggest trophic roles for βAPPs. In this regard, we have found that APP[S]s protect cultured neurons from both hypoglycemia and excitotoxicity.[14] Both APP^S_{695} and APP^S_{751} exhibited these effects, which were attenuated by antibodies to a region shared by both molecules. The APP[S]s effected neuroprotection on rat septal and hippocampal and human cortical neurons, at concentrations as low as 10^{-7} M. The APP[S]s also rapidly elicited an appreciable decrease in resting $[Ca^{2+}]_i$ and, more importantly, prevented the rise in $[Ca^{2+}]_i$ responsible for hypoglycemic damage. These results clearly demonstrate an important trophic activity which may be compromised by events which favor alternative processing of βAPPs.

RELATIONSHIPS TO OTHER RISKS FOR PATHOGENESIS/PROGRESSION OF AD

Age is the major known risk factor for AD. A number of age-associated changes that occur in the brain (*e.g.*, atherosclerosis, accumulation of mitochondrial DNA mutations) would be expected to result in reduced availability of energy to neurons. In addition, deficits in glucose transport systems in cells of the blood-brain barrier and the brain parenchyma have been reported to be a common alteration in AD victims.[15] In addition to reducing availability of the energy that neurons with high metabolic rates require, ischemia or mitochondrial dysfunction may contribute to the deposition of βAP. For instance, Abe *et al.* reported that ischemia causes increased synthesis of βAPP. More importantly, head trauma (which results in brain ischemia and is a probable risk factor for AD) can cause rapid and quite massive deposition of amyloid in humans,[16] suggesting that ischemia or some other aspect of injury can shift the metabolism of βAPP in favor of increased βAP production and/or aggregation.

The mechanism of ischemic injury to neurons involves a destabilization of calcium homeostasis and oxidative damage to proteins and membranes. In light of our earlier data suggesting that glutamate and calcium influx can induce neurofibrillary tangle-like changes, we carried out a study to examine the effects of hypoglycemic conditions on neuronal injury and markers of neurofibrillary tangles.[17] We found that glucose deprivation elicits antigenic changes similar to those seen in Alzheimer's neurofibrillary tangles, and that these alterations and subsequent neuronal death are attenuated by removal of extracellular calcium or application of growth factors which stabilize $[Ca^{2+}]_i$ (bFGF, IGFs, and NGF). Together with the induction of amyloid deposition by head trauma and ischemia (above), the available data suggest that destabilization of $[Ca^{2+}]_i$ itself may be involved in generation or aggregation of βAP.

Our initial observation that bFGF can protect cultured rat hippocampal neurons against glutamate neurotoxicity has led to an explosion of studies examining the roles of growth factors in protecting neurons against excitotoxic/ischemic insults. Many studies have now confirmed the excitoprotective action of bFGF in cultured neurons from several brain regions, and have extended the in vitro findings to animal models of ischemic brain damage.[18] In addition, several other growth factors have been shown to protect neurons against various insults.[17,19] One general mechanism of action of growth factors seems to be prevention of the elevation of $[Ca^{2+}]_i$ that presages neuronal injury; as mentioned above, APP[S]'s actually cause an immediate decrease in $[Ca^{2+}]_i$, an effect unique among neurotrophic factors.

CONCLUSION

Considering the neurotrophic effects of APP[S]s, a two-pronged model of neurodegeneration is suggested whereby aberrant processing of βAPPs—leading to simultaneous diminution of trophic molecules and accumulation of toxic ones—would create a degenerative feedback loop involving excitotoxicity and loss of calcium homeostasis. It seems likely that several age-associated changes that occur in the brain lead to an excitotoxic form of neuronal damage and death, and it may be difficult to decipher whether dysregulation of calcium leads to liberation of βAP or changes in processing of βAPP lead to enhanced calcium vulnerability. Indeed, both events may occur simultaneously, creating an amplification that accelerates neurodegeneration with time and, therefore, aging. Because βAP is toxic and shows uncommon resistance to lysosomal degradation,[20] and because decreases in APP[S] remove a potentially important protective factor, any stimulus which results in alternative metabolism of βAPP (such as excitotoxin-mediated membrane damage or activation of kinases) is likely to result in further accumulation of βAP and amplify itself over time. The multiplicity of insults which could result in these effects (perhaps all involving increases in $[Ca^{2+}]_i$ as a common mediator) is consistent with the apparent heterogeneity in AD etiology.

REFERENCES

1. KOSIK, K. S. 1992. Alzheimer's disease: A cell biological perspective. Science **256**:780–783.
2. SEUBERT, P., C. VIGO-PELFREY, F. ESCH, M. LEE, H. DOVEY, D. DAVIS, S. SINHA, M. SCHLOSSMACHER, J. WHALEY, C. SWINDLEHURST, R. McCORMACK, R. WOLFERT, D. J. SELKOE, I. LIEBERBURG & D. SCHENK. 1992. Isolation and quantitation of soluble Alzheimer's β-peptide from biological fluids. Nature **359**:325–327.
3. BUXBAUM, J. D., S. E. GANDY, P. CICCHETTI, M. E. EHRLICH, A. J. CZERNIK, R. P. FRACASSO, T. V. RAMABHADRAN, A. J. UNTERBECK & P. GREENGARD. 1990. Processing of Alzheimer β/A4 amyloid precursor protein: Modulation by agents that regulate protein phosphorylation. Proc. Natl. Acad. Sci. USA **87**:6003–6006.
4. GILLESPIE, S. L., T. E. GOLDE & S. G. YOUNKIN. 1992. Secretory processing of the Alzheimer amyloid β/A4 protein precursor is increased by protein phosphorylation. Biochem. Biophys. Res. Commun. **187**:1285–1290.
5. YANKNER, B. A., L. R. DAWES, S. FISHER, L. VILLA-KOMAROFF, M. L. OSTER-GRANITE & R. L. NEVE. 1989. Neurotoxicity of a fragment of the amyloid precursor associated with Alzheimer's disease. Science **245**:417–420.
6. PIKE, C. J., A. J. WALENCEWICZ, C. G. GLABE & C. W. COTMAN. 1991. In vitro aging of β-amyloid protein causes peptide aggregation and neurotoxicity. Brain Res. **563**:311–314.
7. BARROW, C. J. & M. G. ZAGORSKI. 1991. Solution structures of beta peptide and its constituent fragments: Relation to amyloid deposition. Science **253**:179–182.
8. MATTSON, M. P., B. CHENG, D. DAVIS, K. BRYANT, I. LIEBERBURG & R. E. RYDEL. 1992. β-amyloid peptides destabilize calcium homeostasis and render human cortical neurons vulnerable to excitotoxicity. J. Neurosci. **12**:376–389.
9. GREENAMYRE, J. T. & A. B. YOUNG. 1989. Excitatory amino acids and Alzheimer's disease. Neurobiol. Aging **10**:593–602.
10. MATTSON, M. P. 1990. Antigenic changes similar to those seen in neurofibrillary tangles are elicited by glutamate and calcium influx in cultured hippocampal neurons. Neuron **4**:105–117.
11. ELLIOT, E., M. P. MATTSON, P. VANDERKLISH, G. LYNCH, I. CHANG & R. M. SAPOLSKY. 1993. Corticosterone exacerbates kainate-induced alterations in hippocampal tau immunoreactivity and spectrin breakdown in vivo. J. Neurochem. In press.

12. SAITOH, T., M. SUNDSMO, J. M. ROCH, M. XIMURA, G. COLE, D. SCHUBERT, T. OLTERSDORF & D. B. SCHENK. 1989. Secreted form of amyloid β protein precursor is involved in the growth regulation of fibroblasts. Cell **58:**615–622.

13. ABE, K., R. E. TANZI & K. KOGURE. 1991. Selective induction of Kunitz-type protease inhibitor domain-containing amyloid precursor protein mRNA after persistent focal ischemia in rat cerebral cortx. Neurosci. Lett. **125:**172–174.

14. MATTSON, M. P., B. CHENG, A. R. CULWELL, F. S. ESCH, I. LIEBERBURG & R. E. RYDEL. 1993. Evidence for excitoprotective and intraneuronal calcium-regulating roles for secreted forms of the β-amyloid precursor protein. Neuron **10:**243–254.

15. JAGUST, W. J., J. P. SEAB, R. H. HUESMAN, P. E. VALK, C. A. MATHIS, B. R. REED, P. G. COXSON & T. F. BUDINGER. 1991. Diminished glucose transport in Alzheimer's disease: Dynamic PET studies. J. Cereb. Blood Flow Metab. **11:**323–330.

16. ROBERTS, G. W., S. M. GENTLEMAN, A. LYNCH & D. I. GRAHAM. 1991. βA4 amyloid protein deposition in brain after head injury. Lancet **338:**1422–1423.

17. MATTSON, M. P. 1992. Calcium as sculptor and destroyer of neural circuitry. Exp. Gerontol. **27:**29–49.

18. NOZAKI, K., S. P. FINKLESTEIN & M. F. BEAL. 1993. Basic fibroblast growth factor protects against hypoxia/ischemia and NMDA neurotoxicity in neonatal rats. J. Cereb. Blood Flow Metab. **13:**221–228.

19. ZHANG, Y., T. TATSUNO, J. M. CARNEY & M. P. MATTSON. 1993. Basic FGF, NGF, and IGF-II protect hippocampal and cortical neurons against iron-induced degeneration. J. Cereb. Blood Flow Metab. **13:**378–388.

20. KNAUER, M. F., B. SOREGHAN, D. BURDICK, J. KOSMOSKI & C. G. GLABE. 1992. Intracellular accumulation and resistance to degradation of the Alzheimer amyloid A4/beta protein. Proc. Natl. Acad. Sci. USA **89:**7437–7441.

A New Hypothesis for the Mechanism of Amyloid Toxicity, Based on the Calcium Channel Activity of Amyloid β Protein (AβP) in Phospholipid Bilayer Membranes

HARVEY B. POLLARD[a], EDUARDO ROJAS,
AND NELSON ARISPE

*Laboratory of Cell Biology and Genetics, National Institute of Diabetes, Digestive,
and Kidney Diseases, Bethesda, Maryland USA*

ABSTRACT: Amyloid β protein (AβP) is the 40-42 residue polypeptide implicated in the pathogenesis of Alzheimer's disease (AD). We have reconstituted this peptide into phosphatidylserine liposomes and then fused the liposomes with a planar lipid bilayer. When incorporated into this bilayer, the AβP forms cation selective channels capable of transporting calcium and some monovalent cations including cesium, lithium, potassium, and sodium. The channels behave in an ohmic fashion and single channels can be shown to exhibit multiple subconductance states. Hitherto, AβP has been presumed to be neurotoxic, although direct demonstration of toxicity has proved elusive. On the basis of the present data we suggest that the ion channel activity of the polypeptide may be the basis of its neurotoxic effects.

INTRODUCTION

Alzheimer's disease (AD) is a chronic dementia affecting increasingly large numbers of the aging population, and is pathologically characterized by extracellular amyloid plaques, intraneuronal neurofibrillary tangles, and by vascular and neuronal damage.[1-6] The major component of brain amyloid is a 38-42 residue peptide, termed amyloid β protein (AβP),[7-11] which is a proteolytic product of amyloid precursor protein (APP). AβP has been circumstantially linked to the toxic principle causing cell damage in the disease, although the mechanism has, until only recently, remained obscure.

[a] *Send correspondence to:* Harvey B. Pollard, MD, Ph.D., Chief, Laboratory of Cell Biology and Genetics, Bldg. 8, Rm. 401, Bethesda, MD 20892; TEL: 301-496-3435; FAX: 301-402-3298; BITNET: HBP@NIHCU.

ION CHANNEL ACTIVITY OF AβP

We have recently reported that amyloid-β-protein (AβP, 1-40; BACHEM, Torrance; CA) forms cation selective channels in planar lipid bilayers.[12] Liposomes containing AβP were allowed to fuse with a planar lipid bilayer separating various symmetric and bi-ionic solutions. We initially picked Cs^+ for our first analysis because many calcium channels efficiently conduct this ion. We immediately observed discrete conductance changes characteristic of typical ion channel activity. Conductance was observed at different voltages and we noted the reversal potential to be at 0 V. The character of the activity indicated that several conductance levels could be delineated at any given voltage. However, since there were complete closures from any one conductance, and there were many examples of interconversion between different conductances, we concluded that only one channel was active in the bilayer (see refs. 13 and 14 for detailed description of subconductance states).

We found that the AβP channels could also conduct other monovalent cations, including lithium, potassium and sodium. Furthermore, the channels also conducted calcium. Interestingly, calcium also blocked the conduction of the monovalent cations. This result is reminiscent of other calcium channels, such as the voltage-gated L-type calcium channel[15] and the calcium release channel of the sarcoplasmic reticulum.[16] However, unlike these conventional calcium channels, the AβP channel is much less sensitive to the blocking activity of calcium and, in addition, is 5- to 10-fold higher in conductance, as estimated from I-V plots.

BLOCKADE OF AβP ION CHANNEL

The AβP channel is also blocked by relatively low concentrations of aluminum. For example, as little as 10 μM $(Al)_2(SO_4)_3$ can block the channel completely. The channel can occasionally escape the block if the voltage is increased to ca. 100 mV. The drug tromethamine (TRIS), in the range of 1−10 mM, can also block the AβP channel. Tromethamine has been employed clinically to treat metabolic and respiratory acidosis since the early 1960s.[17]

CONCLUSION

On the basis of our data published recently[12] and further described here briefly, we suggest that the channel activity of AβP may be responsible for some aspect of its neurotoxic effects. Calcium accumulation in cells is a common mechanism for both pathologic and programmed cell death, and the cell destruction attending AD may well ensue from such a mechanism. A calcium homeostasis defect has been suspected in AD for some time,[18] although clearly many toxic mechanisms can be active and none are excluded by our experiment. However, the experiments with the purified lipid membrane show unambiguously that AβP can have intrinsic toxic effects and that AβP need not necessarily be thought of as only potentiating the action of other factors. Furthermore, if AβP channel activity is indeed responsible for cell death in AD, then the detailed search for inhibitors at the level of the bilayer may be a useful and inexpensive strategy for screening drugs for eventual testing on more complex systems.

REFERENCES

1. NEVE, R. L., L. R. DAWES, B. A. YANKNER, L. I. BENOWITZ, W. RODRIQUEZ & G. A. HIGGINS. 1990. Genetics and biology of the Alzheimer amyloid precursor. *In* Progress in Brain Research, Vol. 86. P. Coleman, C. Higgins & C. Phelps, Eds. :257–267.
2. KATZMAN, R. & T. SAITOH. 1991. Advances in Alzheimer's disease. FASEB J. **5:**278–286.
3. SELKOE, D. J. 1991. The molecular pathology of Alzheimer's disease. Neuron **8:**487–496.
4. McKEE, A. C., K. S. KOSIK & N. W. KOWALL. 1991. Neuritic pathology and dementia in Alzheimer's disease. Ann. Neurol. **30:**156–165.
5. HARDY, J. A. & G. A. HIGGINS. 1992. Alzheimer's Disease: "The amyloid cascade hypothesis." Science **156:**184–185.
6. KOSIK, K. S. 1992. Alzheimer's disease: A cell biological perspective. Science **256:**780–783.
7. ROTH, M., B. E. TOMLINSON & G. BLESSED. 1966. Correlation between scores for dementia and counts of "senile plaques" in cerebral gray matter of elderly subjects. Nature **209:**109–110.
8. TERRY, R. D., A. PECK, R. DeTERESA, R. SCHECHTER & D. S. HOROUPIAN. 1981. Some morphometric aspects of the brain in senile dementia of the Alzheimer's type. Ann. Neurol. **10:**184–192.
9. GLENNER, G. G. & C. W. WONG. 1964. Alzheimer's Disease: Initial report of the purification and characterization of a novel cerebrovascular amyloid protein. Biochem. Biophys. Res. Commun. **120:**885–890.
10. MASTERS, C. L., G. SIMMS, N. A. WEINMAN, G. MULTHAUP, B. L. McDONALD & K. BEYREUTHER. 1985. Amyloid plaque core protein in Alzheimer's disease and Down syndrome. Proc. Natl. Acad. Sci. USA **82:**4245–4249.
11. JOACHIM, C. L., L. K. DUFFY & D. SELKOE. 1988. Protein chemical and immunochemical studies of meningovascular B-amyloid protein in Alzheimer's Disease and normal aging. Brain Res. **474:**100–111.
12. ARISPE, N., E. ROJAS & H. B. POLLARD. 1993. Alzheimer Disease amyloid β protein forms calcium channels in bilayer membranes: Blockade by tromethamine and aluminum. Proc. Natl. Acad. Sci. USA **90:**567–571.

13. Fox, J. A. 1987. Ion channel subconductance states. J. Membr. Biol. **97:**1–8.
14. Meves, H. & K. Nagy. 1989. Multiple conductance states of the sodium channel and other ion channels. Biochim. Biophys. Acta **988:**99–105.
15. Tsien, R. W., P. Hess, E. W. McCleskey & R. L. Rosenberg. 1987. Calcium channels: Mechanisms of selectivity, permeation and block. Ann. Rev. Biophys. Chem. **16:**265–290.
16. Suarez-Isla, B. A., C. Alcayaga, J. J. Marengo & R. Bull. 1990. Calcium channel in sarcoplasmic reticulum membranes isolated from skeletal muscle. *In* Transduction in Biological Systems C. Hidalgo, J. Bacigalupo, E. Jaimovich & J. Vergara. Eds. Plenum Press. New York and London.
17. Nahas, G. G. 1962. The pharmacology of tris (hydroxymethyl)aminomethane (THAM) Pharmacol. Rev. **14:**447–472.
18. Mattson, M. P., B. Cheng, D. Davis, K. Bryant, I. Lieberburg & R. E. Rydel. 1992. β amyloid peptides destabilize calcium homeostasis and render human cortical neurons vulnerable to excitotoxicity. J. Neurosci. **376:**38.

The Role of Extracellular Matrix in the Processing of the Amyloid Protein Precursor of Alzheimer's Disease[a]

DAVID H. SMALL,[b,e] VICTOR NURCOMBE,[c] HEIDI CLARRIS,[b]
KONRAD BEYREUTHER,[d] AND COLIN L. MASTERS[b]

[b] *Department of Pathology and* [c] *Department of Anatomy, University of Melbourne,*
The Mental Health Research Institute of Victoria, Parkville, Victoria 3052
Australia
[d] *Laboratory of Molecular Biology, University of Heidelberg, Heidelberg Germany*

ABSTRACT: Alzheimer's disease (AD) is characterized by the presence of extra-cellular amyloid plaques, which contain a protein referred to as the amyloid or βA4 protein. The βA4 protein is derived from a larger precursor protein (APP). Studies of autosomal-dominant forms of AD have established the central role of APP in the pathogenesis of the disease. Despite considerable research, the function of APP is unknown. APP can be processed by at least two separate routes. The first route involves a protease known as "APP secretase," which cleaves within the amyloid sequence, thereby mitigating amyloid formation. The second route may result in the production of potentially amyloidogenic fragments. Our studies suggest that following release from the cell membrane, APP interacts with components of the extracellular matrix (ECM) such as the heparan sulfate proteoglycans (HSPG's). The interaction of APP with HSPG's may be important for the function of APP. Substratum-bound APP was found to dramatically increase neurite outgrowth and survival of chick sympathetic neurons in vitro. This effect was dependent upon the presence of substratum-bound HSPG. The results suggest that normally, when bound to the ECM, APP functions to promote neurite outgrowth and/or cell survival. Loss of this normal trophic function might occur in AD, when APP is proteolytically processed via the amyloidogenic pathway.

A major neuropathologic feature of Alzheimer's disease (AD) is the deposition of amyloid in extracellular compartments of the cerebral cortex. The major protein component (βA4) of these amyloid plaques is derived from a

[a] This work was supported by grants from the National Health and Medical Research Council of Australia, the Victorian Health Promotion Foundation and the Aluminium Development Council. K.B. is supported by the Deutsche Forschungsgemeinschaft and the Bundesministerium für Forschung und Technologie.

[e] *Send correspondence to:* Dr. David H. Small, Department of Pathology, University of Melbourne, Parkville, Victoria 3052, Australia; TEL: 61-3-344-4205; FAX: 61-3-344-4004.

precursor referred to as the amyloid protein precursor (APP), which has features of a transmembrane cell surface receptor.[1] The βA4 sequence spans a region of 43 amino acid residues, which includes part of the extracellular and transmembrane domains of APP. Studies linking autosomal-dominant forms of AD to mutations in codon 717 of the APP gene have helped to establish the role of APP in the pathogenesis of AD.[2]

AMYLOIDOGENIC PROCESSING OF APP

Cole *et al.*[3] first provided evidence for processing of APP in the lysosomal system. Studies by Younkin and coworkers[4] have shown that processing of APP through the endosomal-lysosomal system may result in the production of a complex set of carboxyl-terminal derivatives, some of which may be amyloidogenic. Studies by Haass *et al.*[5] suggest that intracellular processing of APP is a major pathway in microglia and astrocytes. The possibility that amyloidogenic processing occurs as a result of internalization of the cell surface protein is supported by the presence of a consensus sequence (NPXY) for coated pit-mediated internalization.[6] Despite the intensive research on the mechanism by which amyloid is formed from APP, the role of amyloid in the pathogenesis of AD is unclear. Experiments using isolated neurons in culture suggest that amyloid may be neurotoxic.[7]

NORMAL PROCESSING OF APP

A major route of APP processing involves an enzyme referred to as the "APP secretase." In isolated cultured cells, a proportion of the membrane-bound APP is released into the medium as a C-terminally truncated fragment.[8] The released protein contains a large portion of the extracellular domain. Secreted forms of APP which contain a Kunitz protease inhibitor (KPI) domain have been shown to be identical to protease nexin II,[9] which was described previously as a protease inhibitor.[10] Studies by Sisodia *et al.*[11] and Palmert *et al.*[12] demonstrated that APP is secreted by a proteolytic cleavage within the βA4 sequence. The "APP secretase" cleaves APP adjacent to lysine-16 of βA4, producing a C-terminally truncated form of APP, which is released from the cell membrane.[13]

Our own work[14] has shown that a protease activity associated with the enzyme acetylcholinesterase (AChE) can cleave peptides homologous to the APP secretase site. The AChE-associated protease can also release a form of APP from membranes that is indistinguishable from the secreted form. The AChE-protease activity is not an intrinsic property of AChE, but rather is associated with a specific protease which co-purifies with the enzyme (Michaelson and Small, in press). However, studies using mutagenesis techniques[15] have demonstrated that in some cells, the APP secretase is non-specific in its peptide bond cleavage, unlike the AChE-associated protease. Mutagenesis studies also indicate that the cleavage site for the APP secretase is defined by distance from the cell membrane rather than by primary or secondary protein structure.

Secreted forms of APP may interact with components of the extracellular matrix (ECM).[16] APP possesses a heparin-binding site and can bind tightly to a basement membrane heparan sulfate proteoglycan (HSPG).[17] Thus, HSPG's may be important for the interaction of APP with ECM. Indeed, agents which disrupt the incorporation of HSPG's into ECM significantly decrease the number of APP binding sites on ECM.[16]

THE ROLE OF APP IN NEURITE OUTGROWTH AND CELL SURVIVAL

In the developing chick brain, APP expression is increased during the period in which neurite outgrowth is maximal,[16] suggesting that APP could have a function in neurite outgrowth. Therefore we examined the possibility that APP could be important for regulating cell adhesion or neurite outgrowth. Plastic tissue culture plates were pre-treated by coating them with various proteins. Chick sympathetic neurons were then cultured on the plates for 2–3 days. Cell survival and neurite outgrowth were quantitated by computer-assisted image capture analysis. Using this approach, we found that in the presence of HSPG, APP dramatically promoted both neurite outgrowth (Small *et al.*, manuscript submitted) and cell survival (FIG. 1). Not all forms

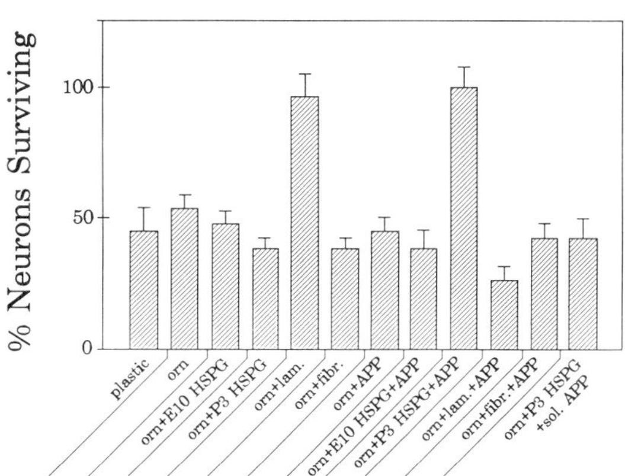

FIGURE 1. Effect of pre-coating tissue culture plates with various protein substrates (10 mg/ml) on the survival of E12 chick sympathetic neurons after 2 days in culture. **Abbreviations:** Polyornithine, orn.; laminin, lam.; fibronectin, fibr.; heparan sulfate proteoglycan, HSPG; amyloid protein precursor, APP.

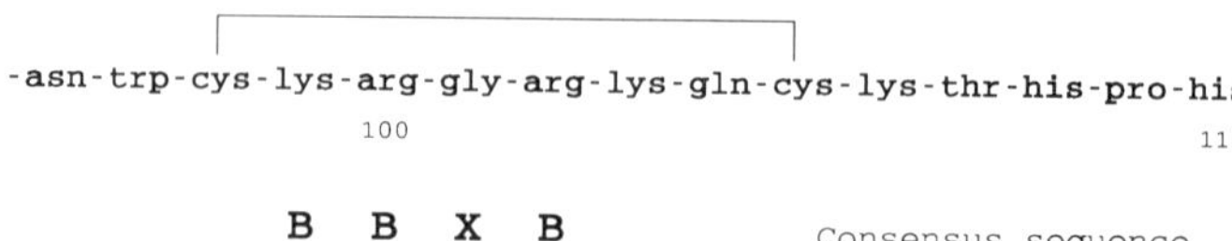

FIGURE 2. Predicted heparin-binding domain in APP. The region between residues 99 and 102 possesses the consequence for heparin binding proposed by Cardin and Weintraub.[18] A peptide homologous to this region of APP (residues 96–110) was found to block the neurite-outgrowth- and cell survival-promoting activity of APP.

of HSPG promoted the effects of APP on cell survival. HSPG purified from P3 mouse brain promoted cell survival, whereas HSPG purified from E10 embryonic mouse brain did not. Thus, specific developmentally regulated HSPG's may be required to promote the effects of APP on cell survival.

We have identified a domain on APP between residues 96 and 110 which is involved in the neurite outgrowth-promoting effects of APP. This domain contains a consensus sequence for heparin binding,[18] and may therefore form part of a heparin-binding site. Computer-assisted algorithms designed to assess secondary structure predict that this domain could form a flexible loop on the surface of APP stabilized by a disulfide bond between two cysteine residues (FIG. 2). A peptide homologous to the region between residues 96 and 110 was found to have a similar affinity for heparin as APP itself. This peptide also potently inhibited the neurite-outgrowth-promoting effects of APP (Small *et al.,* manuscript submitted). Thus, the APP (96–110) peptide may inhibit the binding of APP to the glycan component of HSPG.

THE ROLE OF APP-ECM INTERACTIONS IN ALZHEIMER'S DISEASE

The observation that APP and HSPG promote neurite outgrowth and cell survival has implications for understanding the pathogenesis of AD. The presence of dystrophic neurites surrounding amyloid plaques may result more from the loss of normal APP function rather than from the toxic effects of amyloid. As APP may also interact with cell surface forms of HSPG, it is possible that a defective interaction with such a component may result in abnormal proteolytic processing of the APP, and the eventual formation of amyloid.

REFERENCES

1. KANG, J., H. G. LEMAIRE, A. UNTERBECK, J. M. SALBAUM, C. L. MASTERS, K. H. GRZESCHIK, G. MULTHAUP, K. BEYREUTHER & B. MULLER-HILL.

1987. The precursor of Alzheimer's disease amyloid A4 protein resembles a cell-surface receptor. Nature **325:**733–736.

2. GOATE, A., M. C. CHARTIER-HARLIN, M. MULLAN, J. BROWN, F. CRAWFORD, L. FIDANI, L. GIUFFRA, A. HAYNES, N. IRVING, L. JAMES, R. MANT, P. NEWTON, K. ROOKE, P. ROQUES, C. TALBOT, M. PERICAK-VANCE, A. ROSES, R. WILLIAMSON, M. ROSSOR, M. OWEN & J. HARDY. 1991. Segregation of a missense mutation in the amyloid precursor protein gene with familial Alzheimer's disease. Nature **349:**704–706.

3. COLE, G. M., T. V. HUYNH & T. SAITOH. 1989. Evidence for lysosomal processing of amyloid beta-protein precursor in cultured cells. Neurochem. Res. **14:**933–939.

4. ESTUS, S., T. E. GOLDE, T. KUNISHITA, D. BLADES, D. LOWERY, M. EISEN, M. USIAK, X. M. QU, T. TABIRA, B. D. GREENBERG & S. YOUNKIN. 1992. Potentially amyloidogenic, carboxyl-terminal derivatives of the amyloid protein precursor. Science **255:**726–728.

5. HAASS, C., E. H. KOO, A. MELLON, A. T. HUNG & D. J. SELKOE. 1992. Targeting of cell-surface beta-amyloid precursor protein to lysosomes: Alternative processing into amyloid-bearing fragments. Nature **357:**500–503.

6. CHEN, W. J., J. L. GOLDSTEIN & M. S. BROWN. 1990. NPXY, a sequence often found in cytoplasmic tails, is required for coated pit-mediated internalization of the low density lipoprotein receptor. J. Biol. Chem. **265:**3116–3123.

7. YANKNER, B. A., L. R. DAWES, S. FISHER, L. VILLA-KOMAROFF, M. L. OSTER-GRANITE & R. L. NEVE. 1989. Neurotoxicity of a fragment of the amyloid precursor associated with Alzheimer's disease. Science **245:**417–420.

8. WEIDEMANN, A., G. KÖNIG, D. BUNKE, P. FISCHER, J. M. SALBAUM, C. L. MASTERS & K. BEYREUTHER. 1989. Identification, biogenesis and localization of precursors of Alzheimer's disease A4 amyloid protein. Cell **57:**115–126.

9. OLTERSDORF, T., L. C. FRITZ, D. B. SCHENK, I. LIEBERBURG, K. L. JOHNSON-WOOD, E. C. BEATTIE, P. J. WARD, R. W. BLACHER, H. F. DOVEY & S. SINHA. 1989. The secreted form of the Alzheimer's amyloid precursor protein with the Kunitz domain is protease nexin-II. Nature **341:**144–147.

10. VAN NOSTRAND, W. E. & D. D. CUNNINGHAM. 1987. Purification of protease nexin II from human fibroblasts. J. Biol. Chem. **262:**8508–8514.

11. SISODIA, S. S., E. H. KOO, K. BEYREUTHER, A. UNTERBECK & D. L. PRICE. 1990. Evidence that beta-amyloid protein in Alzheimer's disease is not derived by normal processing. Science **248:**492–495.

12. PALMERT, M. R., M. B. PODLISNY, D. S. WITKER, T. OLTERSDORF, L. H. YOUNKIN, D. J. SELKOE & S. G. YOUNKIN. 1989. The beta-amyloid protein precursor of Alzheimer's disease has soluble derivatives found in human brain and cerebrospinal fluid. Proc. Natl. Acad. Sci. USA **86:**6338–6342.

13. ESCH, F. S., P. S. KEIM, E. C. BEATTIE, R. W. BLACHER, A. R. CULWELL, T. OLTERSDORF, D. MCCLURE & P. J. WARD. 1990. Cleavage of amyloid beta peptide during constitutive processing of its precursor. Science **248:**1122–1124.

14. SMALL, D. H., R. D. MOIR, S. J. FULLER, S. MICHAELSON, A. I. BUSH, Q. X. LI, E. A. MILWARD, C. HILBICH, A. WEIDEMANN, K. BEYREUTHER & C. L.

MASTERS. 1991. A protease activity associated with acetylcholinesterase releases the membrane-bound form of the amyloid protein precursor of Alzheimer's disease. Biochemistry **30:**10795–10799.

15. SISODIA, S. S. 1992. Beta-amyloid precursor protein cleavage by a membrane-bound protease. Proc. Natl. Acad. Sci. USA **89:**6075–6079.

16. SMALL, D. H., V. NURCOMBE, R. MOIR, S. MICHAELSON, D. MONARD, K. BEYREUTHER & C. L. MASTERS. 1992. Association and release of the amyloid protein precursor of Alzheimer's disease from chick brain extracellular matrix. J. Neurosci. **12:**4143–4150.

17. NARINDRASORASAK, S., D. LOWERY, P. GONZALEZ-DEWHITT, R. A. POORMAN, B. GREENBERG & R. KISILEVSKY. 1991. High affinity interactions between the Alzheimer's beta-amyloid precursor protein and the basement membrane form of heparan sulfate proteoglycan. J. Biol. Chem. **266:**12878–12883.

18. CARDIN, A. D. & H. J. WEINTRAUB. 1989. Molecular modeling of protein-glycosaminoglycan interactions. Arteriosclerosis **9:**21–32.

The βA4 Amyloid Protein Precursor in Human Circulation[a]

ASHLEY I. BUSH,[b,d] KONRAD BEYREUTHER,[c]
AND COLIN L. MASTERS[b]

[b] Department of Pathology, The University of Melbourne and Mental Health
Research Institute of Victoria, Victoria Australia
[c] Center for Molecular Biology, University of Heidelberg, Heidelberg, Germany

ABSTRACT: βA4, the principal constituent of the brain amyloid collections in Alzheimer's disease, is derived from a much larger precursor, the amyloid protein precursor (APP). APP exists in the blood as full-length, potentially amyloidogenic forms in platelets, and as an attenuated species in plasma and T-lymphocytes. Studies of circulating APP facilitate the elaboration of the function of this protein, as well as the elucidation of its processing in health and disease.

Our understanding of the molecular basis for the pathophysiology of Alzheimer's disease (AD) has advanced rapidly over the last decade. Much of that understanding has come from elaborating the role played by βA4, the 4.2 kD peptide found to be the principal constituent of the cerebral amyloid deposits which are the pathological hallmark of the disease. βA4 is derived from a much larger precursor protein, whose function is still uncertain. The amyloid protein precursors, constitute a complex family of membrane-bound and soluble glycoproteins that are derived by alternate splicing of a gene on chromosome 21 yielding more than ten isoforms, some of which contain a Kunitz-type protease inhibitory (KPI) insert. Considerable controversy exists as to whether βA4 accumulation is itself neurotoxic, or whether βA4 amyloidogenesis is merely an epiphenomenon of an alternative neuronal lesion. However, the discoveries of mutations of APP linked to the autosomal dominant conditions of familial Alzheimer's disease (FAD) and hereditary cerebral hemorrhage with amyloidosis-Dutch (HCHWA-D), have established the

[a] Professor Masters is supported by funds from the Victorian Health Promotion Foundation and the Aluminium Development Council. Professor Beyreuther is supported by the Deutsche Forschungsgemeinschaft and the Bundesministerium für Forschung und Technologie. Dr. Bush is the recipient of the National Health and Medical Research Council Post-graduate Medical Scholarship and the Harkness Fellowship of the Commonwealth Fund of New York.

[d] *Send correspondence to:* Dr. Ashley I. Bush, Laboratory for Genetics and Aging, Massachusetts General Hospital East, 6th floor, Building 149, 13th Street, Charlestown, MA 02129 USA; TEL: 617-726-5746; FAX: 617-726-5736.

centrality of the biochemistry of βA4 and APP in the pathogenesis of AD. These clinically linked mutations occur related to the βA4 domain of APP but represent <3% of all FAD cases.[1] Linkage of early- and late-onset FAD pedigrees to loci on chromosomes 14 and 19, respectively, may lead to the identification of novel elements in the APP/βA4 processing pathway whose disruption leads to amyloid formation.

Most cases of AD are sporadic, with the proportion of FAD cases being ≈5%. AD also invariably occurs in Down's syndrome (DS) where pathological changes, accelerated by some thirty years, are associated with increased APP mRNA and protein levels.[2] Hence, βA4 amyloid formation in AD is a common feature of a group of clinically associated dementing diseases. The elaboration of the processing pathways for APP will be necessary to help delineate the neurotoxic mechanisms involved in this pathogenetically heterogeneous disorder.

PROCESSING OF APP

APP undergoes considerable post-translational modification and once produced, the intact holoprotein is believed to be handled by more than one cellular processing pathway. In the neuron, the APP is anterogradely transported to synaptic endings where it colocalizes with synaptophysin in vesicles.[3] APP may be stored in a soluble pool in these vesicles, as is the case with platelet α-granules,[4] or it may be released from the plasma membrane. An unidentified APP "secretase" has been described which cleaves APP at residue 16 of the βA4 domain rendering the products incapable of forming βA4 amyloid. Although several candidate proteases for the processing of APP have been proposed, an association between an APP-cleaving protease activity and clinical AD has yet to be shown.

The translation frame is such that βA4 could not be the product of an aberrant alternative splicing event. Hence, at least four mechanisms could lead to the generation of βA4. Each of these mechanisms could yield an abnormal soluble product which may be manifested in biological fluids such as the media of cultured cell lines, cerebrospinal fluid (CSF) and plasma.

Aberrant cleavage of APP may be caused by a defect in the constitutive proteolysis that renders amyloid formation impossible by cleaving APP within the βA4 domain.[5] Failure of the proteolytic mechanism which cleaves APP within the βA4 domain may permit APP to become a substrate for an alternative, βA4-generating, pathway. Just how the integral transmembrane forms of APP could be cleaved within the transmembrane domain to yield the carboxyl terminus of the βA4 monomer is difficult to imagine.

Conversely, there may be a modification to the APP molecule itself which then results in an alteration of the constitutive proteolysis. This mechanism is possible in the FAD syndromes associated with a mutation within the βA4 domain of APP. The processing of APP into various potentially amyloidogenic fragments is also influenced by phosphorylation.

A third mechanism could involve an increase in APP substrate overwhelming the constitutive pathway and providing APP for an amyloidogenic pathway. This mechanism is likely in Down's syndrome (DS) where an extra copy of chromosome 21 is associated with an increased expression of APP and the premature deposition of βA4.[2] No such duplication of chromosome 21 has been observed in sporadic AD cases.

A fourth possible mechanism is that constitutive processing of APP could yield soluble βA4 fragments[6,7] and that post-processing, a pathogenic event occurs which impels the soluble βA4 towards polymerization and aggregation. Soluble βA4 may precipitate into insoluble complexes as a product of elevated concentration,[8] or they may become more self-aggregating and polymerize as a consequence of oxidative stress.[9]

The biochemical status of the blood is of great interest in the study of Alzheimer's disease for several reasons. Clinical medicine is greatly aided by peripheral markers of pathological conditions. A biochemical marker ideally serves to facilitate diagnosis of a disorder and also serves to monitor the progress of the disorder or its response to therapeutic intervention. Alzheimer's disease lacks such a clinical biochemical marker, which leaves clinicians to rely upon clinical diagnosis by exclusion, a process that causes a false positive rate of approximately 15%. Also, the effect of any therapeutic intervention can be monitored only by observation of the clinical response of the patient, with no assay of objective antemortem biochemical phenomena that relates to the pathophysiology. Blood sampling is a safe and convenient way of probing for a peripheral biochemical manifestation of disease.

Another reason for studying the blood in AD is the possibility that the substrate for βA4 amyloidogenesis has a hematogenous origin. APP, with βA4 intact, exists in the circulation where it is found in platelets.[4] The localization of βA4 deposits within the media of meningeal blood vessels outside of brain tissue in sporadic AD and in HCHWA-D is similar to that of some systemic amyloid deposits which arise from circulating proteins (for example, serum AA protein in secondary and amyloidosis; cystatin C in hereditary cerebral hemorrhage with amyloidosis-Icelandic type; and transthyretin in familial amyloidotic polyneuropathy). The association of vascular malformations with βA4 congophilic angiopathy, and the observation of βA4 deposition in skin, also indicate that a circulating form of APP is a likely substrate source for these collections.

A further reason for studying APP metabolism in blood is to gain insight into central (brain) processing events that may be represented in the periphery. If the same lesion of brain APP metabolism in AD is present in the metabolism of the peripheral protein, this would provide a conveniently accessible means of studying the lesion. Even information concerning the constitutive metabolism of peripheral APP would enrich our understanding of the nature of the abnormal central processing in AD.

Our laboratories have studied the metabolism of APP in the human circulation. Such studies have aimed to 1) determine the location and function of APP in the blood, 2) elucidate environmental or nutritional factors which may alter the levels of APP production, and 3) determine whether the abnormalities of APP metabolism evident in the brain in AD are reflected in the blood. We have described APP in lymphocytes, platelets and plasma.

APP IN LYMPHOCYTES

The finding of low levels of APP were initially described in a proportion of lymphocytes.[4] A very large increase in soluble APP secretion was observed in T-lymphocytes upon activation,[10] but only low levels in the resting state. L-APP, which lacks the 18 residues encoded by exon 15, has increased expression in non-adherent T-lymphocytes and lowered expression in adherent T-lymphocytes.[11] This indicates that the function of exon 15 concerns cell contact or adhesiveness. These findings also indicate that APP plays a role in the immune response.

APP IN PLATELETS

The human platelet, which carries out a number of biochemical processes that also occur in the brain, has been proposed as a peripheral model for neurons. The demonstration of abnormalities of function, morphology and metabolism of platelets in Parkinson's disease, Huntington's disease and depression suggests that disease-specific abnormalities in the brain could be reflected in the platelet. There are associations between abnormal platelet membrane proliferation and fluidity and AD, and between megakaryocytic leukemia and Down's syndrome. Also, the deficiency of oxidative phosphorylation in the brain in AD, is manifested in the platelet.[12]

We found carboxyl-terminal attenuated APP as the predominant form of platelet APP and released during platelet activation and degranulation.[4] This soluble species has been identified as protease nexin-II[13] and as the coagulation factor XIa inhibitor,[14] hence the APP species must contain the protease inhibitor domain. Messenger RNAs for APP_{695}, APP_{751} and APP_{770} have been isolated from platelets. Importantly, full-length APP is found in platelets as a minor species associated with platelet membranes, but which might be shed during platelet activation.[4] So far, there has been no report identifying a detectable quantitative or qualitative abnormality in platelet APP in AD. Technique refinements may allow detection of differences between isoforms which correlate to the development or progression of AD.

The concentration of APP in the platelet indicates that it may have an important physiological role in events associated with coagulation. A breach of the vascular endothelial wall sets off a cascade of events which include the activation and aggregation of circulating platelets and the degranulation of the glycoprotein contents of their α-granules—substrates for the coagulation cascade (such as vWF, fibrinogen, fibronectin, thrombospondin, factor V, high molecular weight kininogen, β-thromboglobulin, prothrombin, platelet factor 4), protease inhibitors (α-2-macroglobulin, α-1-antitrypsin, C1 − inhibitor and α-2-antiplasmin), as well as numerous growth factors (such as PDGF, FGF, EGF and TGF-β), the dual roles for which are the local repair of the defect and the promotion of reparative tissue proliferation. It is possible that forms of APP released by the platelet may have a growth factor-related function. APP has been shown to promote the growth of cultured fibroblasts and neurons. It is more likely, however, that the serine protease inhibitor-containing forms of APP may be released by the platelet to participate in the coagulation cascade by inhibiting activated coagulation pathway enzymes. The protease inhibitor region of APP has been shown to inhibit coagulation factor Xa. The 120 kDa form of APP released by platelets has been found to inhibit coagulation factor XIa.[14] A third possible role for APP in the platelet is to modulate cell-cell contact. The breach in a disrupted endothelial surface is first remedied by the aggregation of platelets into the haemostatic plug. APP has been proposed to modulate cell adhesiveness and participate in the extracellular matrix. Hence, a physiological role for secreted APP in clot formation is likely.

APP IN PLASMA AND SERUM

Our laboratory has reported a relative increase in the 130 kDa form and decrease in the 65 and 42 kDa forms of APP in the plasma of moderately to severely demented AD patients.[15] Plasma APP was assayed by western blot following enrichment by heparin-Sepharose chromatography. These observations may form the basis for a peripheral biochemical marker for AD. Prospective studies are required to determine the predictive value of the plasma APP profile for clinical or pathological outcome but these may take many years to complete. It is anticipated that the proportion of 130 kDa or 42 kDa APP in plasma may predict individuals who are likely to develop βA4 amyloid deposition although it is not expected that the test could accurately predict which individual will dement or predict when dementia will occur because the quantity of βA4 deposition does not always correlate with neuropsychological deficit. It is certainly possible to have abundant βA4 deposition in the brain without evidence of cognitive decline.

Our observations are consistent with an increased production of fully-processed 130 kDa KPI-containing APP in AD plasma. Human plasma contains forms of APP of similar size to those released by the platelet. These data together with the observation of APP in megakaryocytes,[4] indicate that the platelet may be the major source of circulating APP. Our estimate of the concentration of 130 and 110 kDa plasma APP agrees with other estimates of plasma KPI-containing APP of similar molecular weight[16] suggesting, like others,[17] that KPI-containing APP may be the predominant form in plasma. Several lines of evidence support the possibility that an overproduction of Kunitz protease inhibitor (KPI)-containing APP or an increase in the ratio of KPI-containing APP to APP_{695} is associated with βA4 amyloidogenesis. A recent study has described a 2- to 3-fold increase in the levels of 133 kDa APP holoprotein in AD and aged brain,[18] are consistent with an increased production of fully processed KPI-containing 130 kDa. KPI-containing forms of APP are present in the dystrophic neurites of amyloid plaques. Although there is not yet a clear consensus, reports are accumulating that the proportion of KPI-containing APP mRNA relative to non-KPI-containing APP mRNA is increased in sporadic AD. A strong linear relation between increased APP_{751}/APP_{695} mRNA ratio and increased plaque density in hippocampus and entorhinal cortex has been reported.[19] Increased mRNA and expression of KPI-containing APP released by lymphoblastoid cells from familial Alzheimer's disease cases has also been shown to be accompanied by aberrant intra-βA4 proteolysis. Finally, it has been reported that transgenic mice over-expressing KPI-containing APP_{751} in the brain rapidly develop βA4 immunoreactive deposits.

There is substantially more APP in serum than in plasma (A. I. Bush, K. Beyreuther, and C. L. Masters, unpublished observations), presumably released by platelet degranulation during clotting. Rumble *et al.*[2] employed a radioimmunoassay for the carboxyl terminus of APP to find a 50% in APP levels in the sera of Down's syndrome subjects, but found no such elevation in AD.

APP co-purified upon heparin-Sepharose chromatography of plasma with a Zn^{2+}-stimulated serine protease. Its identity may yield clues to the role of APP in blood and the nature of APP processing in general. This finding raises a possible role for zinc in the physiology of APP. Zinc is important in the regulation of platelet aggregation where it acts through the fibrinogen receptors, platelet membrane glycoproteins IIb and IIIa. Furthermore, high molecular weight kininogen, an essential cofactor in the initiation of the intrinsic coagulation pathway, has an obligate requirement of zinc (50 mM) for binding to platelets, as do other plasma proteins.[20] Coagulation factor XIIa cleaves the zymogen prekallikrein into kallikrein, which, in turn, cleaves the factor XII into its active form, factor XIIa. This positive feedback loop is dependent upon the presence of zinc (50–100 mM).[20] APP in its association with coagulation enzymes and platelet activity, may also require Zn^{2+} as a functional cofactor.

REFERENCES

1. TANZI, R. E., G. VAULA, D. M. ROMANO, M. MORTILLA, T. L. HUANG, R. G. TUPLER, W. WASCO, B. T. HYMAN, J. L. HAINES, B. J. JENKINS, M. KALAITSIDAKI, A. C. WARREN, M. C. MCINNIS, S. E. ANTONARAKIS, H. KARLINSKY, M. E. PERCY, L. CONNOR, J. GROWDON, D. R. CRAPPER-MCLACHLAN, J. F. GUSELLA & P. H. ST GEORGE-HYSLOP. 1992. Assessment of amyloid β-protein precursor gene mutations in a large set of familial and sporadic Alzheimer disease cases. Am. J. Hum. Genet. **51**:273–282.

2. RUMBLE, B., R. RETALLACK, C. HILBICH, G. SIMMS, G. MULTHAUP, R. MARTINS, A. HOCKEY, P. MONTGOMERY, K. BEYREUTHER & C. L. MASTERS. 1989. Amyloid A4 protein and its precursor in Down's syndrome and Alzheimer's disease. N. Engl. J. Med. **320**:1446–1452.

3. SCHUBERT, W., R. PRIOR, A. WEIDEMANN, H. DIRCKSEN, G. MULTHAUP, C. L. MASTERS & K. BEYREUTHER. 1991. Localization of βA4 precursor protein at central and peripheral synaptic sites. Brain Res. **563**:184–194.

4. BUSH, A. I., R. N. MARTINS, B. RUMBLE, R. MOIR, S. FULLER, E. MILWARD, J. CURRIE, D. AMES, A. WEIDEMANN, P. FISCHER, G. MULTHAUP, K. BEYREUTHER & C. L. MASTERS. 1990. The amyloid precursor protein of Alzheimer's disease is released by human platelets. J. Biol. Chem. **265**:15977–15983.

5. SISODIA, S. S. 1992. Beta-amyloid precursor protein cleavage by a membrane-bound protease. Proc. Natl. Acad. Sci. USA **89**:6075–6079.

6. HAASS, C., M. G. SCHLOSSMACHER, A. Y. HUNG, C. VIGO-PELFREY, A. MELLON, B. L. OSTASZEWSKI, I. LIEBERBURG, E. H. KOO, D. SCHENK, D. B. TEPLOW & D. S. SELKOE. 1992. Amyloid β-peptide is produced by cultured cells during normal metabolism. Nature **359**:322–325.

7. SHOJI, M., T. E. GOLDE, J. GHISO, T. T. CHEUNG, S. ESTUS, L. M. SHAFFER, X-D. CAI, D. M. MCKAY, R. TINTNER, B. FRANGIONE & S. G. YOUNKIN. 1992. Production of the Alzheimer amyloid β protein by normal proteolytic processing. Science **258**:126–129.

8. BURDICK, D., B. SOREGHAN, M. KWON, J. KOSMOSKI, M. KNAUER, A. HENSCHEN, J. YATES, C. COTMAN & C. GLABE. 1992. Assembly and aggregation properties of synthetic Alzheimer's A4/β amyloid peptide analogs. J. Biol. Chem. **267**:546–554.

9. DYRKS, T., E. DYRKS, T. HARTMANN, C. MASTERS & K. BEYREUTHER. 1992. Amyloidogenicity of βA4 and βA4-containing amyloid protein precursor fragments by metal-catalyzed oxidation. J. Biol. Chem. **267**:18210–18217.

10. MÖNNING, U., G. KÖNIG, R. PRIOR, H. MECHLER, U. SCHREITER-GASSER, C. L. MASTERS & K. BEYREUTHER. 1990. Synthesis and secretion of Alzheimer

amyloid βA4 precursor protein by stimulated human peripheral blood leucocytes. FEBS Lett. **277**:261–266.

11. KÖNIG, G., U. MÖNNING, C. CZECK, R. PRIOR, R. BANITI, U. SCHREITER-GASSER, J. BAUER, C. L. MASTERS & K. BEYREUTHER. 1992. Identification and expression of a novel alternative splice form of the βA4 amyloid precursor protein (APP) mRNA in leucocytes and brain microglial cells. J. Biol. Chem. **267**:10804–10809.

12. PARKER, W. D., JR., C. M. FILLEY & J. K. PARKS. 1990. Cytochrome oxidase deficiency in Alzheimer's disease. Neurology **40**:1302–1303.

13. VAN NOSTRAND, W. E., A. H. SCHMAIER, J. S. FARROW & D. D. CUNNINGHAM. 1990. Protease nexin-II (amyloid β-protein precursor): A platelet α-granule protein. Science **248**:745–748.

14. SMITH, R. P., D. A. HIGUCHI & G. J. BROZE, JR. 1990. Platelet coagulation factor XI_a-inhibitor, a form of Alzheimer amyloid precursor protein. Science **248**:1126–1128.

15. BUSH, A. I., S. WHYTE, L. D. THOMAS, T. G. WILLIAMSON, C. J. VAN TIGGELEN, J. CURRIE, D. H. SMALL, R. D. MOIR, Q-X. LI, B. RUMBLE, U. MÖNNING, K. BEYREUTHER & C. L. MASTERS. 1992. An abnormality of plasma amyloid protein precursor in Alzheimer's disease. Ann. Neurol. **32**:57–65.

16. VAN NOSTRAND, W. E., A. H. SCHMAIER, J. S. FARROW, D. B. CINES & D. D. CUNNINGHAM. 1991. Protease nexin-2/amyloid β-protein precursor in blood is a platelet-specific protein. Biochem. Biophys. Res. Commun. **175**:15–21.

17. PODLISNY, M. B., A. L. MAMMEN, M. G. SCHLOSSMACHER, M. R. PALMERT, S. G. YOUNKIN & D. J. SELKOE. 1990. Detection of soluble forms of the β-amyloid precursor protein in human plasma. Biochem. Biophys. Res. Commun. **167**:1094–1101.

18. NORDSTEDT, C., S. E. GANDY, J. ALAFUZOFF, G. L. CAPORASO, K. IVERFELDT, J. A. GREBB, B. WINBLAD & P. GREENGARD. 1991. Alzheimer β/A4 amyloid precursor protein in human brain: Aging-associated increases in holoprotein and in a proteolytic fragment. Proc. Natl. Acad. Sci. USA **88**:8910–8914.

19. JOHNSON, S. A., T. MCNEILL, B. CORDELL & C. E. FINCH. 1990. Relation of neuronal APP-751/APP-695 mRNA ratio and neuritic plaque density in Alzheimer's disease. Science **248**:854–857.

20. GUSTAFSON, E. J., D. SCHUTSKY, L. C. KNIGHT & A. H. SCHMAIER. 1986. High molecular weight kininogen binds to unstimulated platelets. J. Clin. Invest. **78**:310–318.

Expression of L-APP mRNA in Brain Cells[a]

RUPERT SANDBRINK[b,f], RICHARD BANATI[c],
COLIN L. MASTERS[d], KONRAD BEYREUTHER[b], AND
GERHARD KÖNIG[e]

[b] *Zentrum für Molekulare Biologie Heidelberg, Universtität Heidelberg,*
   D-69120 Heidelberg Germany
[c] *Max-Planck-Institute für Psychiatrie, Abteilung Neuromorphologie,*
   Am Klopferspitz 18a, D-82452 Planegg-Martinsried, Germany
[d] *Department of Pathology, University of Melbourne, Parkville, Victoria 3052*
   Australia
[e] *Miles Inc., Institute of Dementia Research, West Haven, Connecticut 06516 USA*

ABSTRACT: Several reports addressed the issue of how the alternative splicing of exon 7 and 8 in the APP pre-mRNA is regulated in different tissues. Of special interest here was the potential involvement of exon 7 containing APP splice isoforms, since this exon codes for a serine protease inhibitor and is therefore of putative relevance for amyloidogenic catabolism of the precursor protein. The recent identification of a third alternative splice site in close proximity to the βA4-amyloid portion in the APP gene which may also increase APP amyloidogenicity, allowed us to investigate its regulation in cells of the central nervous system. With our assay, we were able to resolve six different APP isoforms of the eight potential isoforms which can be generated from the three alternatively spliced exons 7, 8, and 15. We demonstrate here that, in addition to rat brain microglia cells, astrocyte-enriched cultures also skip the novel alternative 3′-splice site in front of exon 15, generating L-APP mRNA. Neurons are the only cells in the central nervous system which seem to use the 3′-splice site of intron 14 nearly 100%. Interestingly, this very 3′-splice site is the only one present in the APP gene that completely matches the consensus sequence for the branchpoint sequence proposed for introns. We would therefore suggest that neurons lack a specific splicing factor which inhibits the use of the rather strong 3′-splice site in front of exon 15. It remains to be shown whether this is also the case for neurons in Alzheimer's disease.

[a] Supported through the Metropolitan Life Foundation, the SFB's 317 and 258, the BMFT and the Fonds der Chemischen Industrie. C. L. Masters is supported by a grant from the National Health and Medical Research Council of Australia.

[f] *Send correspondence to:* Rupert Sandbrink, Zentrum für Molekulare Biologie Heidelberg, Im Neuenheimer Feld 282, D-69120 Heidelberg, Germany; TEL: 49-6221-566848; FAX: 49-6221-565891.

INTRODUCTION

The gene for the βA4-amyloid protein precursor (APP) contains 19 exons out of which 16 are constitutively and 3 are alternatively spliced to give rise to transmembrane β/A4-amyloid protein precursors.[1–3] Exon 7, coding for a domain with considerable homology to a serine protease inhibitor of the Kunitz-type (KPI), is contained in nearly all APP splice forms found in peripheral organs.[4,5] Exon 8 codes for a domain which shows some homology to an antigen found on rat thymocytes, which raised speculations that it could play a role in neuro-immune interaction.[6] This exon was shown to be present in APP transcripts less often than exon 7 and is used mostly together in combination with exon 7.[2,7] Although it has been established that both exons are differentially spliced in neurons and peripheral organs, it should be mentioned that neurons as well as non-neuronal cells do have the capacity to use all three alternative 3'-splice sites in front of exon 7, 8, and 9.

We recently identified a third alternatively used splice site in the APP gene, involving the 54 bp large exon 15.[3] This exon codes for 18 amino acids which precede the βA4 region of APP by 16 amino acids. We therefore suggested that alternative splicing of exon 15 may influence the pathway leading to the liberation to the βA4 subunit.[3] The APP transcripts excluding exon 15 were discovered in peripheral leukocytes, and therefore denoted leukocyte-derived APP (L-APP) mRNA. In peripheral leukocytes, L-APP transcripts coding for the KPI-domain (exon 7) were shown to be the predominant L-APP transcripts (APP733 mRNA).[8] Splicing of exon 15 therefore appears to be independent by the control of the splice site decision made at exons 7 and 8.

The finding of detectable L-APP m-RNA expression in biopsy rat brain allowed us to address the open question of L-APP expression in cells of the central nervous-system in more detail. For this we used perfused brain material as well as primary cell cultures from rat brain. Under conditions where either neuronal cells survive and non-neuronal cells do not proliferate, or conditions where astroglial and microglial cells proliferated and neurons died, we assayed for L-APP mRNA expression. A quantitative polymerase chain reaction from reverse transcribed RNA (RT-PCR) was designed with primer pairs allowing to analyze the region between exon 6 and 16 of the APP gene (FIG. 1).[7,9] This strategy enabled us to distinguish between most of the APP splice isoforms generated by alternative splicing of exons 7, 8, and 15.

RESULTS AND DISCUSSION

In our initial experiments we tested the PCR amplification rate of the different products for different cycling times within a cDNA pool from perfused rat hippocampus (FIG. 1). As shown in FIGURE 2, the amplification

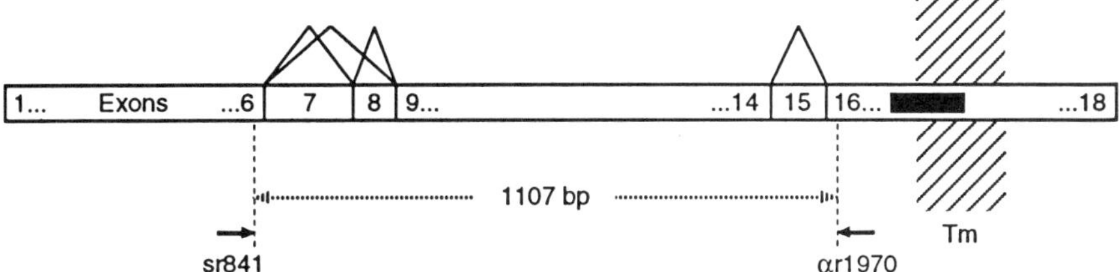

FIGURE 1. RT-PCR assay to detect APP mRNA isoforms. The primer pair ar1970(24b)/sr841(22b) was designed to encompass exon 7/8 and exon 15 alternative splice sites. The sizes of the corresponding RT-PCR products are: 1153bp for APP770, 1099bp for APP752, 1096bp for APP751, 1042bp for APP733, 985bp for APP714, 928bp for APP695, and 874bp for APP677. The antisense primer αr1970 was radioactively labeled on its 5′-end with polynucleotide kinase and [γ-^{33}P]ATP to a specific activity of 0.2μCi/pmol primer. 2μg of total RNA were reverse transcribed with oligo-dT (17mer) and SuperScript reverse transcriptase (BRL) according to the manufacturers protocol. For the PCR 1/100 of this "cDNA pool" was used. Reaction conditions were as following: 200 nM of sense primer, 160 nM of antisense primer and 40 nM of labeled antisense primer, 0.2 mM dNTP, 2.5U Taq polymerase (Boehringer Mannheim) with buffer conditions from the Taq polymerase supplier. The PCR was performed with a "Hot-start"; cycle conditions were 94°C for 1 min, 55°C for 1 min, 72°C for 2.5 min (2 sec extension per cycle). The RT-PCR products were resolved on denaturing polyacrylamide gel electrophoresis and subsequent autoradiography. For quantitation of individual bands, gels were analyzed on a phosphor-imager (Molecular Dynamics). Tm denotes the transmembrane region, the black bar the βA4-sequence in APP.

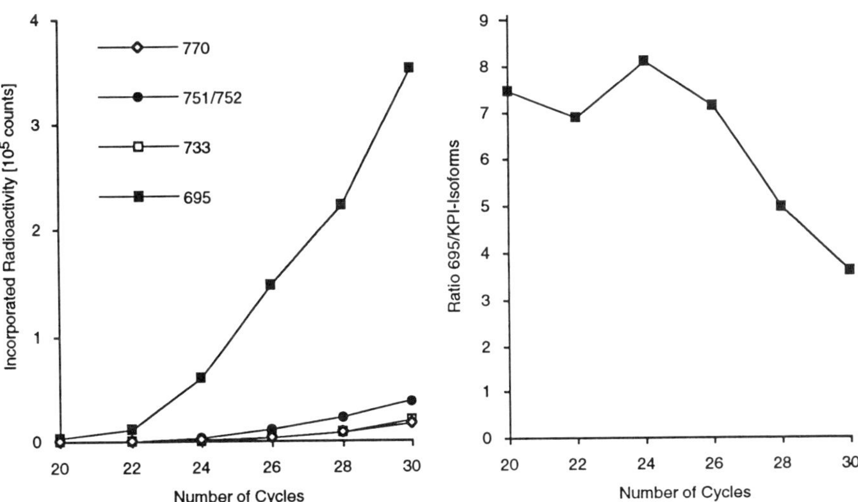

FIGURE 2. Incorporation of radioactivity as a function of the number of PCR cycles on hippocampal cDNA pool. (*Left*) Amount of incorporated radioactivity depending on cycle number. (*Right*) Ratio of APP695 mRNA to KPI encoding APP mRNA-isoforms as a function of PCR cycle number. Up to a total number of 26 PCR cycles the 695/KPI ratio remained constant, indicating a similar amplification rate for all APP isoforms.

efficiency remained constant through 26 cycles which is in good accordance with the results obtained by Golde *et al.* (1990). From this, we concluded that we can indeed use our RT-PCR protocol with the chosen primer pair for a quantitative RNA analysis to compare the relative amounts of APP transcripts within different tissue samples. Furthermore, hippocampus of rat brain (Sprague Dawley, 1 year of age) showed the typical neuronal APP splicing pattern with a predominant amount of APP695 mRNA of more than 90%, and a relative amount of exon 7 containing splice isoforms (APP751/752 mRNA) of about 6.7% (FIG. 2). Regarding the exon 15 missing L-APP mRNA isoforms, we can clearly detect the L-ARP733 mRNA to about 2%.

To compare neuronal with non-neuronal cells of the central nervous system primary cultures of rat septal cells were prepared. More than 95% pure neuronal cultures were obtained when the septal cells were plated on poly-DL-ornithine coated dishes and kept in serum-free medium with cytosine-arabinoside for 8 days (Spd8 −, + araC).[10] A rather mixed culture of neurons, astrocytes and some microglial cells could be obtained by plating the cells on poly-ornithine coated dishes and cultivating them in serum containing medium (5% FCS) without cytosine arabinoside (Spd8 +, − araC). Highly purified microglial cells were obtained from newborn rat brain as described previously and cultured for 3 weeks without further stimulation.[11] A more than 95% pure astrocytic culture (GFAP +) was obtained by culturing rat postnatal (P6) cerebellar cells onto uncoated dishes, shaking them after a period of 2 weeks for several hours and subsequently cultivating them in serum containing medium without cytosine arabinoside for more than 6 weeks.

The results obtained for the primary septal neurons are consistent with the known splice pattern for primary neuronal cultures which predominantly expressed APP695 mRNA (89.9%) (TABLE 1).[12] The KPI-domain encoding

TABLE 1. Relative Distribution of APP mRNA-Isoforms in Different Primary Cell Cultures of Rat Brain Cells

APP mRNA	Spd8-, + araC	Spd8 +,-araC	Astrocytes[a]	Microglia[b]
770	2.4	33.7	40.6	21.2
751/752	3.8	21.4	41.5	33.5
733	n.d.	5.0	11.4	20.1
714	3.8	2.8	2.8	5.0
695	89.9	34.4	2.5	13.7
677	n.d.	2.8	1.4	6.5

Abbreviations: Spd8-, + araC: septal cells, 8 days *in vitro* in serum-free medium, 2·M cytosine-arabinoside; Spd8-, + araC: septal cells, 8 days *in vitro* in medium plus 5% fetal calf serum, no cytosine-arabinoside.
[a] Astrocyte-enriched cultures (≥95% pure).
[b] More than 99% pure microglial cells.

isoforms APP751 together with L-APP752, the only transmembrane APP isoforms which cannot be resolved separately in our assay, made up approximately 3.8% of total APP transcripts. APP770 mRNA represented 2.4% of total APP, whereas the APP714 mRNA made up 3.8% of total APP transcripts. APP splice isoforms missing exon 15, such as L-APP677 or APP733 mRNA were not detectable in neuronal cultures (TABLE 1). Thus, under our experimental conditions, neurons appear to be unable to skip the 3′-splice site in front of exon 15.

A completely different picture is seen in more than 99% pure rat microglial cells. Here the KPI-domain encoding L-APP733 transcript made up 20.1% of total APP transcripts (TABLE 1). The shortest transmembrane encoding transcript L-APP677 mRNA was present with 6.5%, compared to 13.7% of APP695 mRNA. The dominant splice isoforms were the KPI-domain encoding APP751/L-APP752 mRNA's with together 33.5% of total APP mRNA (TABLE 1). It can therefore be suggested that exon 15 skipping occurs with a frequency of roughly 40 to 50% in these cells, irrespective of the splice site selection that occurred further upstream on the APP hnRNA.

Cultures highly enriched for astrocytes showed amounts of 40.6% APP770 and 41.5% APP751/L-APP752 mRNA, whereas the APP695 mRNA accounted for 2.5% of total APP transcripts (TABLE 1). Interestingly, we were able to observe considerable amounts of L-APP733 mRNA (11.4%) and very weak, but detectable L-APP677 mRNA (1.4%). We can hereby confirm our previous observation of L-APP733 protein expression in these rat astrocyte-enriched cultures.[8] Together with our finding of L-APP mRNA expression in a rat astroglioblastoma cell line (F98; data not shown), we can conclude that exclusion of exon 15 seems to occur to a considerable extent in proliferating astrocytes. L-APP expression may be used to distinguish neuronal and astrocytic/microglial APP mRNA in brain.

The mixed neuronal cultures, finally, show a more complicated APP splice pattern. As expected already from the RNA yield, which was increased by a factor of 4, we did observe a strong proliferation of non-neuronal premitotic cells, mainly of astrocytes as judged by morphology. Indeed, APP695 mRNA content was reduced to 34.4%, whereas the KPI-encoding APP751/L-APP752 mRNA's and APP770 mRNA were increased to 21.4% and 33.7%, respectively (TABLE 1). In these cultures L-APP733 as well as L-APP677 mRNA were detected in significant amounts, indicating the non-neuronal proliferation.

Taken together, neurons (as shown for septum derived neurons) seem to be the only cells of the central nervous system which use exon 15 constitutively in their APP mRNA isoforms. Together with our previous observations of only very weak L-APP expression in perfused rat brain, it can be inferred that the 3′-splice site of intron 14 is not used alternatively in neurons. Interestingly, this is the only 3′-splice site in the APP gene that has a 100% homology to the consensus sequence proposed for branchpoint sequences in introns.[13] Thus, the "cis-requirements" for constitutive usage of exon 15 are optimal. One explanation to resolve the superficial contradiction of the observed alternative splicing of exactly this exon in leukocytes, microglia, and also astrocytes could be the presence of a specific splicing factor which inhibits accessibility or the strength of this 3′-splice site in front of exon 15, thereby leading to the exclusion of exon 15 in the APP mRNA. According to this model, neurons and other peripheral cells which do not show L-APP expression would lack such a factor; exon 15 would therefore always be included. In AD, where gliosis compensates in late stages for neuronal loss, we would expect detectable levels of L-APP expression in brain, as remains to be shown.

REFERENCES

1. Kang, J., H. G. Lemaire, A. Unterbeck, J. M. Salbaum, C. L. Masters, K. H. Grzeschik, G. Multhaup, K. Beyreuther, B. Müller-Hill. 1987. The precursor of Alzheimer's disease amyloid A4 protein resembles a cell-surface receptor. Nature **325:**733–736.

2. Weidemann, A., G. König, D. Bunke, P. Fischer, J. M. Salbaum, C. L. Masters & K. Beyreuther. 1989. Identification, biogenesis, and localization of precursors of Alzheimer's disease A4 amyloid protein. Cell **57:**115–126.

3. König, G., U. Mönning, C. Czech, R. Prior, R. B. Banati, U. Schreiter-Gasser, J. Bauer, C. L. Masters & K. Beyreuther. 1992. Identification and differential expression of a novel alternative splice isoform of the βA4 amyloid precursor protein (APP) mRNA in leukocytes and brain microglial cells. J. Biol. Chem. **267:**10804–10809.

4. Tanzi, R. E., A. I. McClatchey, E. D. Lamperti, L. Villa-Komaroff, J. F. Gusella & R. L. Neve. 1988. Protease inhibitor domain encoded by an amyloid protein precursor mRNA associated with Alzheimer's disease. Nature **331:**528–530.

5. Neve, R. L., E. A. Finch & L. R. Dawes. 1988. Expression of the Alzheimer amyloid precursor gene transcripts in the human brain. Neuron **1:**669–677.

6. Müller-Hill, B. & K. Beyreuther. 1989. Molecular biology of Alzheimer's disease. Ann. Rev. Biochem. **58:**287–307.

7. Golde, T. E., S. Estus, M. Usiak, L. H. Younkin & S. G. Younkin. 1990. Expression of β amyloid protein precursor mRNAs: Recognition of a novel alternative spliced form and quantitation in Alzheimer's disease using PCR. Neuron **4:**253–267.

8. Mönning, U., G. König, R. B. Banati, H. Mechler, C. Czech, J. Gehrmann, U. Schreiter-Gasser, C. L. Masters & K. Beyreuther. 1992. Alzheimer βA4-amyloid protein precursor in immunocompetent cells. J. Biol. Chem. **267:**23950–23956.

9. Lemaire, G., J. M. Salbaum, G. Multhaup, J. Kang, R. M. Bayney, A.

UNTERBECK, K. BEYREUTHER & B. MÜLLER-HILL. 1989. The PreA4695 precursor protein of Alzheimer's disease A4 amyloid is encoded by 16 exons. Nucl. Acids Res. **17**:517–522.

10. BREWER, G. J. & C. W. COTMAN. 1989. Survival and growth of hippocampal neurons in defined medium at low density: Advantages of a sandwich culture technique or low oxygen. Brain Res. **494**:65–74.

11. BANATI, R. B., D. HOPPE, K. GOTTMANN, G. W. KREUTZBERG & H. A. KETTENMANN. 1991. Subpopulation of bone marrow-derived macrophage-like cells shares an unique ion channel pattern with microglia. J. Neurosci. Res. **30:** 593–600.

12. LEBLANC, A. C., H. Y. CHEN, L. AUTILIO-GAMBETTI & P. GAMBETTI. 1991. Differential APP gene expression in rat cerebral cortex, meninges, and primary astroglial, microglial and neuronal cultures. FEBS Lett. **292**:171–178.

13. KRAINER, A. R. & T. MANIATIS. 1988. RNA splicing. *In* Transcription and Splicing. B. D. Hames & D. M. Glover, Eds. 131–143. IRL Press. Oxford.

The Amyloid Precursor Protein in Ischemic Brain Injury and Chronic Hypoperfusion[a]

R. N. KALARIA[b], S. U. BHATTI, W. D. LUST, AND G. PERRY

Departments of Neurology, Neurosciences, Neurological Surgery, and Pathology, Case Western Reserve University, Cleveland, Ohio 44106 USA

ABSTRACT: We studied changes in the spatial and temporal distribution of the β amyloid precursor protein (APP) of Alzheimer's disease (AD) in experimental ischemic brain injury. Rats with repeated reversible occlusions of one middle cerebral artery showed striking APP reactivity in astrocytic processes in perifocal regions and adjacent white matter. APP reactive dystrophic axons and neurons were also evident in the cortex and hippocampus ipsilateral to the MCA occlusion. Such changes were similarly apparent in animals subjected to partial forebrain ischemia induced by bilateral occlusion of the carotid arteries. Our studies suggest that focal ischemic insults or chronic hypoperfusion leads to increased accumulation or induction of APP in surviving cellular elements that may relate to the processes involved in β amyloid deposition in AD.

INTRODUCTION

Extracellular β amyloid deposition in the brain is a common feature of the pathological lesions in AD.[1] The β protein portion can be released as a soluble fragment from the precursor, which upon fibrillar formation and subsequent accumulation may be directly toxic to neurons and possibly other brain cells including endothelial cells.[2] However, the mechanism(s) or sequelae of events by which this occurs is not established.

Recent reports suggest changes in expression or induction of APP in brain cells after intrathecal or intraparenchymal injections of excitotoxins.[3–6] These studies indicate the rapid induction of APP particularly in reactive astrocytes[3] and hippocampal neurons[4] subsequent to neuronal damage. More recent studies demonstrate the rapid appearance of diffuse APP immunoreactivity in damaged axons and reactive glial cells following needle stab injury.[7] It is

[a] This work was supported by the University Hospitals Alzheimer Center and the USPHS grants AG08012 and AG10030 (RNK), and AG07552 and AG09287 (GP).
[b] *Send correspondence to:* Dr. R. N. Kalaria, Department of Neurology, University Hospitals of Cleveland, 2074 Abington Road, Cleveland, Ohio 44106 USA; TEL: (216) 844-4846; FAX: (216) 844-3160.

possible that ischemic brain injury or chronic hypoperfusion (oligemia) also induces changes in APP reactivity. The cellular distribution of APP in such injury or states has not been fully evaluated. We studied changes in the immunocytochemical distribution of APP in brains of rats subjected to focal cerebral ischemia by unilateral reversible middle cerebral artery (MCA) occlusion and to partial forebrain ischemia by bilateral carotid (2-V) occlusion.[8] We used well-characterized antibodies to different peptide amino- and carboxyl-terminal fragments of APP to demonstrate accumulation of the protein in cells following ischemia or oligemia.

RESULTS AND DISCUSSION

Rats subjected to MCA occlusion showed marked reduction in cerebral blood flow demarcating the infarcted cortex which exhibited pallor upon H and E staining indicating neuronal necrosis in the ischemic area. We noted altered patterns of APP-immunoreactivity in both focal and partial forebrain ischemia as observed in the reversible MCA and the 2-V occlusion models.[8] The changes in cellular reactivity were most strikingly evident in astroglial processes but also apparent in neurons as early as 3 days in the MCA and 3 weeks in the 2-V occlusion rats. We frequently observed staining in fibrillary structures resembling dystrophic neurities and hypertrophic neurons in the ipsilateral cortex. In the rats subjected to chronic hypoperfusion APP-reactivity was observed in perivascular glial processes and in white matter, and superficial layers of the cortical ribbon below the glial limitans. The observed changes presumably reflect increased localization of APP in reactive glia in the perifocal regions of ischemic damage and in other regions such as the white matter. These observations suggest that localized ischemic insults or chronic hypoperfusion can lead to increased expression of APP in surviving brain cells that may relate to APP mobilization in AD.

Our findings are relevant to the recent studies of Kogure and colleagues[9] who demonstrated the induction of the mRNA for the Kunitz inhibitor domain-containing APP in rats subjected to persistent focal ischemia. While the total amounts of APP mRNA did not change, the peak effect was observed 4 days after the ischemic insult.[9] They are also relevant to recent observations[10] on the accumulation of APP along with ubiquitin (a heat shock protein) in dystrophic axons in infarcted brain tissue from humans. The neuronal accumulation of APP also parallels that in AD in which neurons and their processes are predominantly the only structures noted to accumulate APP although astrocytes exhibited APP-immunoreactivity.[11] While there are limitations, these cellular aspects suggest ischemia or oligomeia can be useful to study APP mobilization. These observations in APP mobilization may be responsible for the rapid induction of multiple diffuse plaques, stained by β/A4 protein antibodies in brains of human subjects following head trauma.[12] Although the early events leading to APP mobilization after any injury are unknown, it is probable that the expression of APP during ischemic injury is regulated by released cytokines such as interleukin or activated heat shock proteins (HSP70), which appear to act as promoters of the APP gene.[13,14]

Several mechanisms may be responsible for the increased cellular localization and origin of APP in neurons and astrocytes in ischemic injury. First, APP production is increased or turnover decreased in vulnerable neurons and astrocytes within or adjacent to infarcted regions. Second, APP may be released by neurons upon degeneration and subsequently taken up by astrocytes surrounding the infarcted region. Third, APP derived from blood cells such as platelets[15] or the circulation through damaged vasculature may be taken up by perivascular astrocytes. In summary, it remains to be determined which of these mechanisms is operative and whether the observed changes represent alterations in APP mRNA within the cells involved. Nevertheless, these observations emphasize that cerebral hypoperfusion, commonly manifest in aging and pronounced in AD, may affect APP accumulation and metabolism in vivo that may be germane to β amyloid deposition.

ACKNOWLEDGMENTS

We thank Drs. I. Lieberburg (Athena Neurosciences) and E. Shelton (Syntex Research) for providing some of the antibodies to APP.

REFERENCES

1. SELKOE, D. 1991. The molecular pathology of Alzheimer's disease. Neuron **6:** 1–8.
2. KALARIA, R. N. 1992. The blood-brain barrier and microcirculation in Alzheimer's disease. Cerebrovasc. Brain Metab. Rev. **4:**226–260.
3. SIMAN, R., J. P. CARD, R. B. NELSON & L. G. DAVIS. 1989. Expression of β-amyloid precursor protein in reactive astrocytes following neuronal damage. Neuron **3:**275–285.
4. KAWARABAYASHI, T., M. SHOJI, Y. HARIGAYA, H. YAMAGUCHI & S. HIRAI. 1991. Expression of APP in the early stage of brain damage. Brain Res. **563:** 334–338.
5. SHIGEMATSU, K., P. L. McGEER, D. G. WALKER, T. ISHII & E. G. McGEER. 1992. Reactive microglial/macrophages phagocytose amyloid precursor protein produced by neurons following neural damage. J. Neurosci. Res. **31:**443–453.
6. NAKAMURA, Y., M. TAKEDA, H. NIIGAWA, S. HARIGUCHI & T. NISHIMURA. 1992. Amyloid β-protein precursor deposition in rat hippocampus lesioned by ibotenic acid injection. Neurosci. Lett. **136:**95–98.

7. OTSUKA, N., M. TOMONAGA & K. IKEDA. 1991. Rapid appearance of β-amyloid precursor protein immunoreactivity in damaged axons and reactive glial cells in rat brain following needle stab injury. Brain Res. **568:**335–338.

8. SETA, K., C. R. CRUMRINE, T. S. WHITTINGHAM, W. D. LUST & D. W. MCCANDLESS. 1992. Experimental models of human stroke. *In* Neuromethods, Vol. 22. Animal models of neurological disease II. A. Boulton, G. Baker and R. Butterworth, Eds. 1–50. The Humana Press. New York.

9. ABE, K., R. E. TANZI & K. KOGURE. 1991. Selective induction of Kunitz-type protease inhibitor domain-containing amyloid precursor protein mRNA after persistent focal ischemia in rat cerebral cortex. Neurosci. Lett. **125:**172–174.

10. COCHRAN, E., B. BACCI, Y. CHEN, A. PATTON, P. GAMBETTI & L. AUTILIO-GAMBETTI. 1991. Amyloid precursor protein and ubiquitin immunoreactivity in dystrophic axons is not unique to Alzheimer's disease. Am. J. Pathol. **139:** 485–489.

11. CRAS, P., M. KAWAI, S. SIEDLAK, P. MULVIHILL, P. GAMBETTI, D. LOWERY, P. GONZALEZ-DEWHITT, B. GREENBERG & G. PERRY. 1990. Neuronal and microglial involvement in β-amyloid protein deposition in Alzheimer's disease. Am. J. Pathol. **137:**241–246.

12. ROBERTS, G. W., S. M. GENTLEMAN, A. LYNCH & D. I. GRAHAM. 1991. βA4 amyloid protein deposition in brain after head trauma. Lancet **338:**1422–1423.

13. GRIFFIN, W. S. T., L. C. STANLEY, C. L. LING, L. WHITE, V. MACLEOD, L. J. PERROT, C. L. WHITE III & C. ARAOZ. 1989. Brain interleukin 1 and S-100 immunoreactivity are elevated in Down syndrome and Alzheimer disease. Proc. Natl. Acad. Sci. USA **86:**7611–7615.

14. GOLDGABER, D., H. W. HARRIS, T. HLA, T. MACIAG, R. J. DONNELLY, J. S. JACOBSEN, M. P. VITEK & D. C. GAJDUSEK. 1989. Interleukin 1 regulates synthesis of amyloid β-protein precursor mRNAs: Recognition of a novel alternatively spliced form and quantitation in Alzheimer's disease using PCR. Proc. Natl. Acad. Sci. USA **86:**7606–7610.

15. GARDELLA, J. E., G. A. GORGONE, P. C. MUNOZ, J. GHISO, B. FRANGIONE & P. D. GOREVIC. 1992. β-Protein precursor expression in human platelets and a megakaryocyte cell line: Possible implications for the origin of cerebral amyloidosis in Alzheimer's disease. Lab. Invest. **67:**303–313.

Heat-shocked Neuronal PC12 Cells Reveal Alzheimer's Disease–associated Alterations in Amyloid Precursor Protein and Tau

G. JOHNSON, L. M. REFOLO, AND W. WALLACE[a]

Molecular Geriatrics, Inc., Lake Bluff, Illinois 60044 USA and
Laboratory of Biochemical Genetics, National Institute of Mental Health,
Washington, D.C. 20032 USA

ABSTRACT: The Alzheimer's disease (AD) brain contains many abnormal protein modifications. These include the abnormal processing of amyloid precursor protein (APP) to form the amyloidogenic β/A4 peptide and the abnormal phosphorylation of tau to form A68, the major constituent of the neurofibrillary tangle. In addition, many of the biochemical alterations found in the AD brain are also found in heat-shocked or stressed cells. We used heat-shocked neuronal PC12 cells to investigate the effects of stress on APP and tau. We found that by simply exposing neuronal PC12 cells to an elevated temperature (45°C) for 30 minutes, they exhibited several features characteristic of the heat shock response. These included a 45% reduction in total protein synthesis, the induction of heat shock protein (hsp) 72, and increased phosphorylation of the protein synthesis initiation factor eIF-2 α. The heat-shocked cells also exhibited alterations in the metabolism and phosphorylation of APP. Under heat shock conditions, we found two additional APP-like polypeptides not present in controls and a significant decrease in the phosphorylation state of APP. We also found that an A68-like protein is formed in neuronal PC12 cells when subjected to elevated temperature. This A68-like protein was formed with heat shock even in the absence of protein synthesis, suggesting that its production occurred post-translationally. The tau/A68 polypeptides were identified as phosphoproteins, and the phosphorylation of tau to form A68 was reversed with recovery of the cells from heat shock. Immunoprecipitation of lysates from heat shocked cells with antibodies to hsp72/73 resulted in co-precipitation of tau, but not A68 with hsp72 indicating a stable complex formation between these two proteins. These results suggest that heat shock proteins may play either a protective or promoting role in the formation of A68 and/or the amyloidogenic C-terminal fragment of APP.

BACKGROUND

Biochemical characterization of postmortem AD tissue has shown a number of protein alterations associated with the disease. In order to investigate

[a] *Send correspondence to:* W. Wallace, Laboratory of Biochemical Genetics, NIMH Neuroscience Center, St. Elizabeth's Hospital, 2700 Martin Luther King Jr. Avenue, Washington, D.C. 20032 USA; TEL: (202) 373-6076; FAX: (202) 373-6087.

altered gene expression in AD, we previously isolated and assayed proteins synthesized by polysomes from postmortem tissues to determine whether these changes occur pre- or post-translationally. We noted two prominent differences in AD polysome function: AD polysomes translated less efficiently, synthesizing lower amounts of total protein, even though the levels of mRNA showed no reduction;[1] and several proteins synthesized by AD polysomes were not among the proteins synthesized by polysomes from age-matched control tissues.[2] Subsequently, we identified some of these AD-associated proteins using two-dimensional (2D) electrophoresis and immuno-detection as heat shock proteins of 72kD and 73kD (hsp72 and hsp73). These results indicated that AD tissues actively synthesized elevated levels of various heat shock proteins. We showed that hsp accumulated in the brains of AD patients.[2] Hamos *et al.* further showed that hsps accumulate in senile plaques and neurofibrillary tangles.[3]

The increased presence of hsp in postmortem tissues is not the only evidence that AD brain undergoes a heat shock–like response. Reduced protein synthesis, increased ubiquitination of protein, breakdown of neuronal cytoskeleton, and altered phosphorylation of certain proteins are all common to both AD brain and heat shocked cells. The heat shock response is actually a cellular response to a wide variety of stresses. The similarities in the biochemistry of the AD brain and heat-shocked cells lead us to propose that degenerating neurons in AD are undergoing an "AD-stress" response.

One function of many heat shock proteins including hsp72, is that of a molecular chaperone which co-translationally mediates the processing of nascent polypeptides.[4] Heat shock proteins facilitate appropriate polypeptide folding, subunit assembly, and translocation across organelle membranes. The AD brain is characterized by a number of apparently abnormally processed proteins such as the β/A4 peptide (derived from amyloid precursor protein, APP)⋅ and A68 (an abnormally phosphorylated form of the microtubule-associated protein, tau). Because hsp functions in the early events of protein processing, we wanted to determine the cause and effect relationship between the induction of hsp and the disrupted processing of APP and tau.

RESULTS

We used neuronal (nerve growth factor-treated) PC12 cells as a model system to investigate the response of neurons to stress and to compare this response to the biochemistry of the AD brain.[6,7] Neuronal PC12 cells were radiolabeled, incubated at either 37°C (control cells) or 45°C (heat-shocked cells) for 30 minutes, lysed, and proteins were analyzed. We found that after a 30-minute exposure to elevated temperature, total protein synthesis was reduced by 45% as determined by incorporation of [^{35}S] methionine into trichloroacetic acid-precipitable material. Two-dimensional analysis of the [35S]-labeled proteins showed that, despite an overall reduction in protein synthesis, the level of hsp72 was significantly increased. Heat-shocked and control PC12 cells were labeled with [32P] orthophosphate to examine the effects of heat shock on protein phosphorylation. Although there was a slight (20%) decrease in total protein phosphorylation, the protein synthesis initiation factor eIF-2a showed a significant increase in phosphorylation state.

We then investigated stress-related alterations in the synthesis and phosphorylation of APP.[6] Immunoprecipitates of [35S]-labeled cell lysates using antibody to the C-terminal portion of APP revealed an increased overall synthesis of APP and the appearance of two additional polypeptides at approximately 95kD and 120kD in the heat shocked cells. Analysis of [32P]-labeled immunoprecipitates of APP revealed a 70% reduction in the phosphorylation state of APP in the heat-shocked cells.

We also examined the content of tau and A68 in heat shocked neuronal PC12 cells.[7] Immunoprecipitates of [35S]-labeled cell lysates using two different antibodies to tau (ALZ50 or tau-2) revealed a single polypeptide (62kD) in control cells while a second polypeptide (68kD) was present under condition of heat shock. Based on electrophoretic mobility, we identified the 62kD protein as the normal form of tau and the 68kD protein as the abnormally phosphorylated A68. Cells treated with cycloheximide during heat shock resulted in a 50% inhibition of protein synthesis; however, A68 was still formed. Both tau and A68 were identified as phosphoproteins by immunoprecipitation of [32P]-labeled lysates with ALZ50 and tau-2. Using a modified procedure which did not disrupt co-translational complexes, control and heat shocked lysates were immunoprecipitated with antibody to either tau or hsp72/73. Two-dimensional analysis of [35S]-labeled immunoprecipitates from control cells revealed a single polypeptide of approximately 70kD with antibody to hsp72/73. A doublet of approximately 62kD was immunoprecipitated with antibody to tau. In heat-shocked cells, immunoprecipitation with hsp72/73 antibody resulted in the presence of both the hsp polypeptide (70kD) and the tau doublet (62kD). However, no polypeptide at 68kD, representing the abnormally phosphorylated form of tau, co-precipitated with antibody to hsp72/73.

DISCUSSION

These results showed that with heat shock of neuronal cells, tau undergoes an abnormal phosphorylation thus transforming it to an A68-like protein. Under these conditions, normal tau complexes with hsp72, while the A68 form of tau does not. We propose that heat shock-induced hsp72 protects tau from abnormal phosphorylation and transformation to A68. We suggest that hsp72 associates with tau co-translationally and remains associated for the duration of heat shock, thereby protecting newly synthesized tau from abnormal phosphorylation. On the other hand, mature tau, which is synthesized prior to heat shock, does not associate with hsp72 and is therefore vulnerable to a heat shock-induced alteration which may permit abnormal phosphorylation and the production of A68. Similarly, induction of hsp72 may play a protective role in the AD brain. However, abnormal protein modifications still occur in AD. These AD modifications may be the result of: 1) overwhelmed hsp due to the chronic nature of neurodegeneration, 2) abnormal modification of only mature proteins that do not associate with hsp and are therefore not protected, or 3) a faulty hsp function in AD. It is of interest to note that the region of chromosome 14 that has been recently linked to FAD includes a gene for a 70kD heat shock protein.[5] We are currently investigating the association of hsp with APP to determine if it has a similar protective role.

We speculate that heat shock proteins may act as endogenous agents preventing the abnormal protein modifications that characterize AD. Induction of heat shock proteins either prior to the "AD-stress" or at increased levels may reduce the formation of senile plaques and neurofibrillary tangles.

REFERENCES

1. LANGSTROM, N. S., J. P. ANDERSON, H. G. LINDROOS, B. WINBLAD & W. C. WALLACE. 1989. Alzheimer's disease-associated reduction of polysomal mRNA translation. Mol. Brain Res. **5:**259–269.

2. PEREZ, N., J. SUGAR, S. CHARYA, G. JOHNSON, C. MERRIL, L. BIERER, D. PERL, V. HAROUTUNIAN & W. WALLACE. 1991. Increased synthesis and accumulation of heat shock 70 protein in Alzheimer's disease. Mol. Brain Res. **11:** 249–254.

3. HAMOS, J. E., B. OBLAS, D. PULASKI-SALO, W. J. WELCH, D. G. BOLE & D. A. DRACHMAN. 1991. Expression of heat shock protein in Alzheimer's disease. Neurology **41:**354–359.

4. WELCH, W. J., L. A. MIZZEN & A. P. ARRIGO. 1989. Structure and function of mammalian stress proteins. *In* Stress-Induced Proteins. M. L. Pardue, J. R. Feramisco & S. Lindquist, Eds. Liss. New York.

5. SCHELLENBERG, G. D., T. D. BIRD, E. M. WIJSMAN, H. T. ORR, L. ANDERSON, E. NEMENS, J. A. WHITE, L. BONNYCASTLE, J. L. WEBER, M. E. ALONSO, H. POTTER, L. L. HESTON & G. M. MARTIN. 1992. Genetic linkage evidence for a familial Alzheimer's disease locus on chromosome 14. Science **258:**668–671.

6. JOHNSON, G., L. M. REFOLO, C. R. MERRIL & W. WALLACE. 1993. Altered expression and phosphorylation of amyloid precursor protein in heat-shocked neuronal PC12 cells. Mol. Brain Res. **19:**140–148.

7. WALLACE, W., G. JOHNSON, J. SUGAR, C. R. MERRIL & L. M. REFOLO. 1993. Reversible phosphorylation of tau to form A68 in heat-shocked neuronal PC12 cells. Mol. Brain Res. **19:**149–155.

Alzheimer's Disease Families with Amyloid Precursor Protein Mutations[a]

M. N. ROSSOR,[b,c,f] S. NEWMAN,[b,c] R. S. J. FRACKOWIAK,[c,d]
P. LANTOS,[e] AND A. M. KENNEDY[b]

[b] Dementia Research Group, St. Mary's Hospital, London, United Kingdom
[c] The National Hospital for Neurology and Neurosurgery, London,
United Kingdom;
[d] MRC Cyclotron Unit, London, United Kingdom
[e] The Department of Neuropathology, Institute of Psychiatry,
London, United Kingdom

ABSTRACT: Early onset Familial Alzheimer's Disease (FAD) is an autosomal dominant disease with apparent complete penetrance. It is genetically heterogeneous with some families carrying mutations in the amyloid precursor protein (APP) gene which segregate with the disease. In addition, there is allelic heterogeneity with four mutations associated with FAD. Three mutations have been reported at APP 717, just distal to the C-terminus of the β-amyloid domain, APP 717 val-ile, APP 717 val-phe, and APP 717 val-gly, which are associated with autopsy-proven Alzheimer's disease (AD). APP 670/671 lies at the N terminus of the β-amyloid domain and is associated with clinically diagnosed FAD in two Swedish families. FAD tends to have prominent myoclonus and this is shared by the cases with APP mutations. In two unrelated UK families with APP 717 val-ile mutations there was early prominent memory impairment with dyscalculia proceeding to generalized cognitive impairment with a lack of insight. There was a late development of a gait disturbance with extrapyramidal features in some members. Positron emission tomography (PET) with fluorodeoxyglucose demonstrated posterior bitemporal biparietal hypometabolism in one case. Magnetic resonance imaging (MRI) showed generalized cerebral atrophy particularly affecting the temporal lobes and hippocampus. At autopsy, a single case showed extensive β-amyloid deposition with congophilic angiopathy and widespread senile plaques and neurofibrillary tangles. The cytoskeletal pathology associated with abnormally phosphorylated tau was similar to cases of sporadic AD. In addition, there were widespread cortical and subcortical Lewy bodies. A single family with the APP 717 val-gly mutation also showed prominent myoclonus, lack of insight, and seizures, PET, in a single case, showed classical biparietal bitemporal hypometabolism. Autopsy, in a single case, showed diffuse deposits of β-amyloid throughout the cortex with frequent neuritic plaques and neurofibrillary tangles. No other inclusion bodies were seen. There was severe congophilic angiopathy. The age at onset of APP mutations is around 50 years of age by contrast to other early onset FAD pedigrees.

[a] Support for this work was received from the Medical Research Council, Research Into Aging, and the Kirkwood Memorial Trust.
[f] Send correspondence to: M. N. Rossor, Department of Neurology, St. Mary's Hospital, Praed Street, London W2 1NY United Kingdom; TEL: 44-071-725-1264; FAX: 44-071-725-1422.

INTRODUCTION

Familial clustering of Alzheimer's disease (AD) has been observed for over 50 years and more recently large pedigrees with hereditary Alzheimer's disease have been identified.[1] In each instance the disease behaves as an autosomal dominant with apparent full penetrance and equal male and female transmission. However, the question of incomplete penetrance is difficult to assess since there is a selection bias in studies towards families with full penetrance. Late onset cases of Familial Alzheimer's Disease (FAD) are difficult to assess since coincidental disease and early death censors such pedigrees. Differences have been sought both clinically and neuropathologically between FAD and sporadic AD but no consistent differences have been found. Within the FAD group variable clinical patterns have been observed which include additional pyramidal, cerebellar and extrapyramidal features, early or late onset, associated white matter changes, anterior horn cell disease and neuropathological differences such as those with tangles and no plaques.[2,3] The phenotypic heterogeneity in FAD is believed to reflect the underlying genetic heterogeneity and such studies have been advanced considerably by the demonstrations of mutations in the APP gene. The first mutation to be described in one UK and one US family was a valine to isoleucine substitution at position 717 of the APP transcript.[4] Subsequently, two other mutations at the same site were reported APP 717 val-phe[5] and APP 717 val-gly.[6] These APP 717 mutations lie just outside the C-terminus of the β/A4 amyloid domain. Recently, a double mutation at APP 670/671 resulting in a lysine methionine to asparagine leucine double substitution has been described in two, probably related, Swedish families with NINCDS clinically diagnosed Alzheimer's disease.[7] This mutation at APP 607/671 lies at the N terminus of the β/A4 amyloid domain. Further evidence of allelic heterogeneity at the APP locus is provided by mutations at APP 692 and 693 which are associated with a different clinical phenotype. APP 693 glu-gln is associated with hereditary cerebral hemorrhage with amyloidosis of Dutch type.[8] These patients present with recurrent cortical hemorrhage due to a severe congophilic angiopathy. There is some cognitive impairment with diffuse parenchymal amyloid deposition but no neuritic plaques or neurofibrillary tangles. Recently, APP 692 ala-gly has been described in one family with a variable phenotype; members present with either presenile progressive dementia or with recurrent cerebral hemorrhage.[9]

APP mutations appear to be a very rare cause of FAD. Screening of the Dementia Research Group Family Resource uncovered only one other family with APP 717 val-ile of early onset cases screened.[10]

APP 717 VALINE-ISOLEUCINE

There are now 7 pedigrees reported in the literature; the original UK and US families,[4] 3 Japanese families,[11,12] and a further UK family;[10] additionally, a Canadian family of Irish ancestry, originally reported as Toronto 3,[13] has now been demonstrated to have the APP 717 val-ile mutation.[14] The clinical features in the two UK families are those of an early memory impairment and dyscalculia with a variable decline in other cognitive function leading to a severe dementia. Insight is strikingly absent. Dyscalculia is also an early feature noted in the Canadian family.[13] Of interest is the early appearance of a number of non-cognitive symptoms, such as vertigo, fatigue, and change in personality. Myoclonus is present and late features include a gait disturbance with rigidity and occasional seizures. Positron emission tomography in one case showed posterior biparietal bitemporal hypometabolism and an MRI scan showed cerebral cortical atrophy with prominent changes in the temporal lobe. Modest white matter changes consistent with age were noted.

Neuropathology in the original index case of the UK family revealed extensive β–amyloid protein deposition both in brain parenchyma and as vascular deposits leading to a congophilic angiopathy. Neurofibrillary tangles, neuritic senile plaques and neuropil threads were widespread. Immunostaining with antibodies to β-amyloid, tau, phosphorylated neurofilament epitopes and ubiquitin together with fractionation and western blot analysis confirm the abnormally phosphorylated form of tau seen in sporadic Alzheimer's disease.[15] In addition, cortical and subcortical Lewy bodies were seen and associated clinical features. In this particular case gait disturbance and prominent extra pyramidal features were seen. However, this has not been a consistent feature with this mutation and other reported cases have not shown Lewy bodies. The mean ages at onset in the two UK families are 49.4 years and 50.5 years.

APP 717 VALINE-GLYCINE

A single UK family has been reported with this mutation.[6] Early memory impairment and visuospatial dysfunction and lack of insight accompanied the progression to a generalized dementia. Myoclonus was particularly prominent and there was an early appearance of seizures.[16] PET scanning in a single individual showed biparietal bitemporal hypometabolism and MRI scanning cortical atrophy without white matter changes. A single member has come to autopsy who was shown to have diffuse deposits of β-amyloid throughout the cortex with neuritic senile plaques and neurofibrillary tangles in all cortical regions and hippocampus and amygdala. There was a severe congophilic angiopathy but no Lewy bodies were seen. The median age at onset was 52 years for this pedigree.

DISCUSSION

APP 717 val-ile and APP 717 val-gly share common features of early myoclonus, seizures and lack of insight with a similar age at onset in the early 50s. The single reported pedigree with the APP 717 valine-phenylalanine mutation had an earlier age at onset of 43 years and a mean death at 50 years. The common mode of presentation is reported to be with memory disturbance and the available neuropathology is of widespread senile plaques and neurofibrillary tangles but a mild angiopathy. Plaques with large amyloid cores were prominent in the hippocampus.[17,18] The available clinical details on the APP 670/671 pedigrees indicate a mean age at onset of 55 years with memory impairment.[7] There is no neuropathology available.

It is too early to state whether individual APP 717 mutations have a characteristic phenotype. In general the APP mutations have an age at onset of around 50 years although this is reported to be slightly earlier in the APP 717 val-phe pedigree.[17] This is in contrast to the earlier age at onset to the other non-APP linked early onset FAD cases.[19] The neuropathology shows no striking differences from other cases of Alzheimer's disease with the exception of a single index case of APP 717 val-ile case with widespread Lewy bodies. Imaging shows the characteristic features both on PET and MRI imaging. In both affected and at-risk individuals with APP mutations we have not demonstrated white matter changes which might relate to the congophilic angiopathy and we have not been able to confirm the claim that white matter changes may be an early feature on MRI.[20]

REFERENCES

1. ROSSOR, M. N. 1992. Familial Alzheimer's Disease. *In* Unusual Dementias. M. N. Rossor, Ed. Balliere Tindall **1:3**, pp. 517–534.
2. VAN BOGAERT, M. & E. SMELDT. Sur les formes familiales précoces de la malady Alzheimer. 1940. Monatssch. Psychiatr. Neurol. **102:**249–301.
3. BIRD, T. D., D. SUMI & E. J. NEMENS. 1989. Phenotypic heterogeneity in Familial Alzheimer's Disease: A study of 24 kindreds. Ann. Neurol. **25:**2–21.
4. GOATE, A., M. C. CHARTIER-HARLIN, M. MULLAN, *et al.* 1991. Segregation of a missense mutation in the amyloid precursor protein gene with Familial Alzheimer's Disease. Nature **349:**704–706.
5. MURRELL, J., M. FARLOW, B. GHETTI, *et al.* 1991. A mutation in the amyloid precursor protein associated with hereditary Alzheimer's Disease. Science **254:** 97–98.
6. CHARTIER-HARLIN, M. C., F. CRAWFORD, H. HOULDEN, *et al.* 1991. Early-onset Alzheimer's Disease caused by mutations at codon 717 of the beta-amyloid precursor protein gene. Nature **353:**844–846.
7. MULLAN, M., F. CRAWFORD, K. AXELMAN, H. HOULDEN, L. LILIUS, B. WIN-BLAD & L. LANNFELT. 1992. A pathogenic mutation for probable Alzheimer's

Disease in the APP Gene at the N-Terminus of β-amyloid. Nature Genet. **1:** 345–347.

8. LEVY, E., M. D. CARMEN, I. J. FERNANDEZ-MADRID, *et al.* 1990. Mutation of the Alzheimer Disease amyloid gene in hereditary cerebral haemorrhage, Dutch-type. Science **248:**1124–1126.

9. HENDRIKS, L., C. M. VAN DUIJN, P. CRAS, *et al.* 1992. Presenile dementia and cerebral haemorrhage linked to a mutation at codon 692 of the β-amyloid precursor protein gene. Nature Genet. **337:**218–221.

10. FIDANI, L., K. ROOKE, M. C. CHARTIER-HARLIN, D. HUGHES, R. TANZI, M. MULLAN, P. ROQUES, M. ROSSOR & J. HARDY. 1992. Screening for mutations in the open reading frame and promotor of the β-amyloid precursor protein gene in Familial Alzheimer's Disease: Identification of a further family with APP 717 VAL-ILE. Human Mol. Genet. **1:**165–168.

11. HARDY, J., M. MULLAN, M. C. CHARTIER-HARLIN, *et al.* 1991. Alzheimer's Disease; A new nosology. Lancet **327:**1342–1343.

12. NARUSE, S., S. IGARASHI, KOBAYASHI *et al.* 1991. Missense mutation of Valine to isoleucine in exon 17 of amyloid precursor protein gene in Japanese Familial Alzheimer's Disease. Lancet **337:**978–979.

13. KARLINSKY, H., E. MADRICK, J. RIDGELEY, *et al.* 1991. A Family with multiple instances of definite, probable and possible early-onset Alzheimer's Disease. Br. J. Psychiatr. **159:**1524–1530.

14. KARLINSKY, H., G. VALUA, J. L. HAINES, *et al.* 1992. Molecular and prospective phenotypic characterization of a pedigree with Familial Alzheimer's Disease and a missense mutation in codon 717 of the β-amyloid precursor protein gene. Neurology **42:**1445–1453.

15. LANTOS, P. L., P. J. LUTHERT, D. HANGER, B. H. ANDERTON, M. MULLAN & M. ROSSOR. 1992. Familial Alzheimer's Disease with the amyloid precursor protein position 717 mutation and sporadic Alzheimer's Disease have the same cytoskeletal pathology. Neurosci. Lett. **137:**221–224.

16. KENNEDY, A. M., S. NEWMAN, A. McCADDON, J. BALL, P. ROQUES, M. MULLAN, J. HARDY, M. C. CHARTIER-HARLIN, R. S. J. FRACKOWIAK, E. K. WARRINGTON & M. W. ROSSOR. 1993. Familial Alzheimer's Disease: A pedigree with a missense mutation in the amyloid precursor protein gene (APP 717 Valine-Glycine). Brain **116:**309–324.

17. FARLOW, M. R., J. MULL, S. ZELDENRUST, B. GHETTI & M. BENSON. 1992. Clinical, neuropathological and molecular genetic characteristics of a family with early-onset Alzheimer's Disease. Neurology **42**(Suppl. 3):720.

18. GHETTI, B., J. MURRELL, M. D. BENSON & M. R. FARLOW. 1992. Spectrum of amyloid beta-protein immunoreactivity in hereditary Alzheimer's Disease with a guanine to thymine missense change of position 1924 of the APP Gene. Brain Res. **571:**133–139.

19. MULLAN, M., A. M. KENNEDY & M. N. ROSSOR. The age at onset in familial early onset Alzheimer's disease correlates with genetic aetiology. In submission.

20. SAGAWA, K., S. KAWAKATSU & S. TOTSUKA. 1992. MRI finding in an offspring of an individual with Familial Alzheimer's Disease. Dementia **3:**186–188.

Search for the Genes Responsible for Familial Alzheimer's Disease

WILMA WASCO, JEFFREY PEPPERCORN, AND
RUDOLPH E. TANZI[a]

*The Laboratory of Genetics and Aging, Department of Neurology, Massachusetts
General Hospital, Harvard Medical School, Charlestown,
Massachusetts 02129 USA*

ABSTRACT: Inherited or Familial Alzheimer's Disease (FAD) has clearly been
shown to be a genetically heterogeneous disorder. Mutations in the gene on
chromosome 21 encoding the β–amyloid protein precursor (APP) have been
shown to be linked to 2–3% of FAD kindreds examined around the world. A
late onset FAD locus has been mapped to a region of chromosome 19 in which
a recently isolated APP-like gene, APLP1 has also been localized, making this
gene a strong candidate to harbor a late-onset FAD defect. More recently, a
major FAD locus has been mapped to the long arm of chromosome 14. The
chromosome 14 locus appears to be mainly linked to the gene defect in early
onset FAD pedigrees. Besides the FAD loci on chromosome 21, 19, and 14, at
least two other loci must exist since the gene defect in some early- and late-
onset FAD pedigrees do not appear to segregate with markers from any of these
autosomes. As different gene defects responsible for various forms of FAD are
discovered, perhaps, a common basis for the etiology of this devastating disorder
can be discerned.

INTRODUCTION

Alzheimer's disease (AD) is clearly one of the prevailing health problems
in the USA and will have an even greater impact as the proportion of elderly
in the population increases. There is currently no effective treatment for preventing or delaying the progression of AD. A major difficulty in developing
rational therapies for the disorder is the lack of knowledge of its primary
cause(s). While the identification of specific environmental agents causing
human neurodegenerative diseases can be a daunting task, in at least some
cases of AD the primary cause lies not in the environment but in the genome
of the affected individual. In a small proportion of families, FAD results from
an inherited defect in the chromosome 21 gene, APP, encoding the precursor
of the β/A4 peptide that deposits in AD senile plaques.[1–4] However, the

[a] *Send correspondence to:* Dr. Rudolph E. Tanzi, The Laboratory of Genetics and Aging, Department of Neurology, Massachusetts General Hospital, Harvard Medical School, Charlestown,
MA 02129 USA.

absence of any amino acid alteration in APP in most (>97%) FAD kindreds and the absence of genetic linkage to chromosome 21 in most of these kindreds suggested that one or more loci located elsewhere in the genome can cause or predispose to FAD.[5,6]

Genetic linkage analysis has proved to be a powerful technique for identifying the chromosomal locations of genes causing human disease, but the ease with which it can be applied varies greatly, depending on the nature of the disorder. When we first attempted genetic linkage analysis in FAD, it was with the anticipation that it would be quite difficult, given the late onset of the disorder and consequent limited informativeness of most pedigrees and, an even greater hindrance, the limited informativeness of most restriction fragment length polymorphism (RFLP) markers. Consequently, we concentrated on the chromosome 21 because it was a strong candidate, given the similar neuropathology of Down's syndrome.

Fortunately, the outlook for scanning the remainder of the genome has changed dramatically in the past few years for two major reasons. First, the FAD pedigrees which we, and others, have been banking since 1982 have increased in number, and with age, they have increased in genetic informativeness as additional family members have aged and become affected. We have now identified several pedigrees capable of individually yielding significant positive lod scores for linkage. Second, and of even greater import, is the development and validation of an easy-to-use, abundant, and highly informative new class of genetic markers. The recognition that simple sequence repeats (SSR), such as (dGdT)n, frequently vary in length and are present at least every 100,000 bp throughout the genome has led to the rapid elaboration of these new marker systems.[7] They are typed by polymerase chain reaction amplification of the simple sequence repeat using flanking unique primers and the resulting allelic products are viewed directly on polyacrylamide gels. The markers frequently display heterozygosity greater than 0.8 with as many as 15 alleles and more. Within the past year, they have largely replaced the much more cumbersome, expensive, and less informative RFLP markers. In fact, individual laboratories designated for each chromosome are currently generating simple sequence repeat markers of greater than 80% heterozygosity and 5−10 cm spacing across the whole genome. It is anticipated that these "index" markers, most of which will be available within the next two years, will form a standard battery, accessible to all via their primer sequences, for detecting linkage of disease genes in any region of the genome.

APP AND THE APP-LIKE GENE FAMILY IN FAMILIAL ALZHEIMER DISEASE

In 1987, genetic linkage analysis implicated chromosome 21 as the location of a putative defective gene for FAD.[8] Subsequently, a comprehensive collaborative study in 1990[9] showed that the chromosome 21 linkage was applicable to only a small subset of FAD kindreds. Meanwhile, the remaining pedigrees appeared to involve genetic defects on other chromosomes. Over the last two years, a portion of the chromosome 21-linked families have been found to possess missense mutations in APP, the gene encoding the precursor of the β/A4 peptide.[1-4] In a recently published study, we have determined that mutations in APP are involved in less than 3% of FAD kindreds.[6] Therefore, the genetic defect in approximately 97% of FAD pedigrees has remained unlinked and involve a defect(s) on an autosome(s) other than chromosome 21. In agreement with this assessment, a set of late-onset FAD families has been linked to chromosome 19.[10]

The identity of the putative chromosome 19 FAD gene defect remains unknown; however, we recently identified an APP-like protein, APLP1 that maps to chromosome 19q and represents a candidate gene for this locus.[11] Recent evidence indicates that APP is a member of a highly conserved family of proteins. An APP-like protein, APPL, was isolated from Drosophila.[12] Recently, Luo *et al.*[13] demonstrated a functional homology between APPL and human APP. Transgenes expressing human APP695 or Drosophila APPL were equally capable of rescuing a fast phototaxis defect in mutant Drosophila lacking the APP1 gene. We have isolated mouse and human cDNAs encoding a novel member of the APP-like gene family, APLP.

APLP1 resembles a membrane-associated glycoprotein with a predicted structure that is highly similar to that of APP. APLP1 is 43% identical and 66% similar to APP, and virtually all of the identified domains and motifs that characterize APP are present in APLP1. Specifically, an N-terminal cysteine-rich region consisting of 12 cysteines, a zinc-binding motif, and acidic-rich domain, an alternatively-transcribed Kunitz protease inhibitor domain, potential N-glycosylation sites, a cytoplasmic clathrin-binding domain, and several phosphorylation sites are significantly conserved. Interestingly, although APP and APLP1 have very similar hydrophilicity profiles throughout, APLP1 does not contain a β/A4 domain.

The lack of β/A4 in APLP1 indicates that APLP1 would not serve as substrate for β-amyloid formation. However, the overall conservation of amino acid sequence and domain structure within APP, APPL, and APLP implies that they may share common functions and be processed similarly. It is also conceivable that APP and APLP1 interact with the same sets of enzymes, and that an alteration in, or the overproduction of APLP could affect the overall maturation and metabolism of APP. In fact, changes in the level of processing of APLP1 could have profound effects on APP and, ultimately, the generation of β/A4 and amyloid. It is also possible that factors or events leading to the up-regulation of APLP1 might also result in increased expression of APP shuttling more APP into the amyloidogenic pathway.

The notion of APLP1 interfering with APP metabolism or expression would require that they are produced in the same sets of cells. We have performed *in situ* hybridization studies that demonstrate virtually identical regional distribution and cellular specificity for APP and APLP1 in rat brain and human hippocampal formation. In addition, both APP and APLP1 mRNAs are localized to the neuronal cell soma and apical and basal dendrites, indicating that both of these genes may produce messages that are directly translated at nerve terminals where these proteins may both play a role in synapse formation. At the immunohistochemical levels, both APP and APLP1 are visualized in association with intracellular organelles including the Golgi apparatus[11] where they are most likely undergoing maturation.

We have mapped APLP1 to the long arm of chromosome 19 in the same general vicinity that has been postulated to contain the late-onset FAD gene defect.[10,14] We are currently screening the APLP1 gene for the presence of mutations in late onset FAD patients and attempting to isolate other APP-related genes. Along these lines, we have recently isolated a second APP-like gene, APLP2 which is presently being characterized.

A NOVEL FAD LOCUS ON CHROMOSOME 14

The recent explosion of the number of FAD pedigrees available for analysis combined with the development of the easily typed, highly informative simple sequence repeat (SSR) markers, has made it feasible to begin a total genome search for other loci causing FAD. Using SSR technology, we and others have recently discovered genetic linkage to a major FAD gene defect on chromosome 14 in the vicinity of the markers D14S43 and D14S53 in the region 14q24.[5,15] The peak multipoint lod-score obtained with these markers in our pedigree set is $z = 23.4$. This clearly indicates the existence of a major FAD locus on chromosome 14 and the linkage appears to be strongest in the early-onset pedigrees. Of the pedigrees we have tested for linkage to both chromosome 14, six have individually provided significant lod-scores ($> +3.0$) on their own.

Previous analysis of the chromosome 14-linked pedigrees for chromosome 19 and 21 markers has given a strong positive lod score in only one pedigree, FAD4. This pedigree of Italian origin yields a highly significant lod score of 2.9 to chromosome 21 markers, but shows a clear crossover with, and contains no mutations in the APP gene.[6] Although the possibility that two gene defects (on chromosomes 14 and 21) cause FAD in this pedigree, it is more likely that the linkage to chromosome 21 in FAD4 is either spurious or due to non-random sorting of a particular chromosome 21 with the chromosome 14 harboring the gene defect in this pedigree. In support of the later possibility, in Robertsonian translocations involving chromosomes 21, chromosome 14 is associated 95% of the time.

A number of candidate genes have been mapped to the implicated region of chromosome 14 (14q24) including an HSP70 gene family member and the oncogene cFOS. With respect to the amyloid hypothesis of FAD, both of these loci represent strong candidate genes. The APP promoter contains an AP-1 transcriptional element which would confer transcriptional regulation via cFOS and cJUN. Overexpression of APP as a result of abnormal cFOS could result in a situation similar to that in Down's syndrome where overproduction of APP (due to trisomy 21) presumably results in accelerated formation of amyloid. Members of the HSP70 family act as molecular chaperonins, which by binding to APP or the β/A4 peptide may serve to prevent amyloid formation. It is, of course, possible that the chromosome 14 locus is a gene which has nothing to do with amyloid formation. We are currently attempting to define flanking markers for the chromosome 14 locus by recombination analysis. In addition, the DNA comprising the linked region is being isolated in Yeast Artificial Clones (YACs) with which cDNAs and expressed sequences will be obtained, characterized, sequenced, and analyzed for potential mutations associated with FAD.

REFERENCES

1. CHARITER-HARLIN, M.-C., F. CRAWFORD, H. HOULDEN, A. WARREN, D. HUGHES, L. FIDANI, A. GOATE, et al. 1991. Early-onset Alzheimer's disease caused by mutations at codon 717 of the β-amyloid precursor protein gene. Nature **353**:884–886.
2. GOATE, A. M., M. C. CHARTIER-HARLIN, M. C. MULLAN, J. BROWN, F. CRAWFORD, L. FIDANI, A. GUIFFRA, A. HAYNES, et al. 1991. Segregation of a missense mutation in the amyloid precursor protein gene with familial Alzheimer's disease. Nature **349**:704–706.
3. HENDRIKS, L., C. M. VANDUIJN, P. CRAS, M. CRUTS, W. VAN HUL, F. VAN HARKSKAMP, A. WARREN, M. G. McINNIS, S. E. ANTONARAKIS, J. J. MARTIN, A. HOFMAN & C. VAN BROECKHOVEN. 1992. Presenile dementia and cerebral haemorrhage linked to a mutation at codon 692 of the β-amyloid precursor protein gene. Nature Genet. **1**:218–221.
4. MURRELL, O., M. FARLOW, B. GHETTI & M. BENSON. 1991. A mutation in the amyloid precursor protein associated with hereditary Alzheimer's disease. Science **254**:97–99.
5. SCHELLENBERG, G. D., T. D. BIRD, E. M. WIJSMAN, H. T. ORR, L. ANDERSON, E. NEMENS, J. A. WHITE, L. BONNYCASTLE, J. L. WEBER, M. E. ALONSO, H. POTTER, L. L. HESTON & J. MARTIN. 1992 Genetic linkage evidence for a familial Alzheimer's disease locus on chromosome 14. Science **258**:668–671.
6. TANZI, R. E., G. VAULA, D. M. ROMANO, M. MORTILLA, T. L. HYANG, R. G. TUPLER, W. WASCO, B. T. HYMAN, J. L. HAINES, B. J. JENKINS, M. KALAITSIDAKI, A. C. WARREN, M. G. McINNIS, S. E. ANTONARAKIS, H. KARLINSKY, M. E. PERCY, L. CONNOR, J. GROWDON, D. R. CRAPPER-McLACHLAN, J. F. GUSELLA & P. H. ST. GEORGE-HYSLOP. 1992. Assessment of amyloid β protein

precursor gene mutations in a large set of familial and sporadic Alzheimer disease cases. Am. J. Hum. Genet. **51:**273–282.

7. WEBER, J. L. & P. E. MAY. 1989. Abundant class of human DNA polymorphisms which can be typed by the polymerase chain reaction. Am. J. Hum. Genet. **44:**388–396.

8. ST. GEORGE-HYSLOP, P. H., R. E. TANZI, R. J. POLINSKY, J. L. HAINES, L. NEE, P. C. WATKINS, R. H. MYERS, *et al.* 1987. The genetic defect causing familial Alzheimer's disease maps on chromosome 21. Science **235:**885–889.

9. ST. GEORGE-HYSLOP, P. H., J. L. HAINES, L. A. FARRER, R. POLINSKY, C. VAN BROECKHOVEN, A. GOATE, D. R CRAPPER-MCLACHLAN, H. ORR, A. C. BRUNI, S. SORBI, I. RAINERO, J. F. FONCIN, D. POLLEN, J. M. CANTU, R. TUPLER, N. VOSKRESENSKAYA, R. MAYEUX, J. GROWDON, L. NEE, H. BACKHOVENS, J. J. MARTIN, M. ROSSOR, M. J. OWEN, M. MULLAN, M. E. PERCY, H. KARLINSKY, S. RICH, L. HESTON, M. MONTESI, M. MORTILLA, N. NACMIAS, G. VAULA, J. F. GUSELLA, J. A. HARDY & the FAD COLLABORATIVE GROUP. 1990. Genetic linkage studies suggest that Alzheimer's disease is not a single homogeneous entity. Nature **347:**194–197.

10. PERICAK-VANCE, M. A., J. L. BEBOUT, P. C. GASKELL, L. H. YAMAOKA, W-Y. HUNG, M. J. ALBERTS, A. P. WALKER, *et al.* 1991. Linkage studies in familial Alzheimer's disease; Evidence for chromosome 19 linkage. Am. J. Hum. Genet. **48:**1034–1050.

11. WASCO, W., K. BUPP, M. MAGENDANTZ, J. GUSELLA, R. E. TANZI & F. SOLOMON. 1990. Identification of a mouse brain cDNA that encodes a protein related to the Alzheimer-associated amyloid β precursor protein. Proc. Natl. Acad. Sci. USA **87:**2405–2408.

12. ROSEN, D. R., L. MARTIN-MORRIS, L. LUO & K. WHITE. 1989. A Drosophila gene encoding a protein resembling the human β-amyloid protein precursor. Proc. Natl. Acad. Sci. USA **86:**2478–2482.

13. LUO, L., T. TULLY & K. WHITE. 1992. Human amyloid precursor protein ameliorates behavioral deficit of flies deleted for APP1 gene. Neuron **4:** 595–605.

14. WASCO, W., J. D. BROOK, J. F. GUSELLA, D. E. HOUSMAN & R. E. TANZI. 1993. The amyloid precursor-like gene maps to the long arm of chromosome 19. Genomics **15:**237–239.

15. ST. GEORGE-HYSLOP, P. H., J. HAINES, E. ROGAEV, M. MORTILLA, G. VAULA, M. PERICAK-VANCE, J.-F. FONCIN, M. MONTESI, A. BRUNI, S. SORBI, I. RAINERO, L. PINESSI, D. POLLEN, R. POLINSKY, L. NEE, J. KENNEDY, F. MACCIARDI, E. ROGAEVA, Y. LIANG, N. ALEXANDEROVA, W. LUKIW, K. SCHLUMPF, R. TANZI, T. TSUDA, L. FARRER, J.-M. CANTU, R. DUARA, L. AMADUCCI, L. BERGAMINI, J. GUSELLA, A. ROSES & D. CRAPPER-MCLACHLAN. 1992. Genetic evidence for a novel familial Alzheimer's disease locus on chromosome 14. Nature Genet. **2:**330–334.

Microtubule-associated Protein Tau, Paired Helical Filaments, and Phosphorylation[a]

E.-M. MANDELKOW,[b] J. BIERNAT, G. DREWES, B. STEINER,
B. LICHTENBERG-KRAAG, H. WILLE, N. GUSTKE,
AND E. MANDELKOW

Max-Planck-Unit for Structural Molecular Biology, D-22603 Hamburg, Germany

ABSTRACT: This paper summarizes our recent studies on microtubule-associated protein tau and its pathological state resembling that of the paired helical filaments of Alzheimer's disease. The Alzheimer-like state of tau protein can be identified and analyzed in terms of certain phosphorylation sites and phosphorylation-dependent antibody epitopes. It can be induced by protein kinases which tend to phosphorylate serine or threonine residues followed by a proline; this includes mitogen-activated protein kinase (MAPK) and glycogen-synthase kinase 3 (GSK-3). Both of these are tightly associated with microtubules as well as with paired helical filaments. Structurally, tau appears as a rod-like molecule; it tends to self-associate into dimers whose monomers are antiparallel. Constructs of truncated tau made up of antiparallel dimers of the microtubule binding domain can be assembled into paired helical filaments *in vitro*.

INTRODUCTION

The neurofibrillary tangles (NFTs) found in brain tissue of Alzheimer patients are composed largely of paired helical filaments (PHFs), which are in turn made up mainly of an insoluble form of the microtubule-associated protein tau. This protein normally stabilizes microtubules in axons and thus helps to maintain axonal transport, but in PHFs it is abnormally phosphorylated, aggregated, and perhaps modified in other yet unknown ways.[1,2] In this paper, we review recent experiments in which we have addressed the following questions: Can we identify the differences between normal and pathological tau? Can we induce them *in vitro* and thereby study the causes

[a] This work was supported by Bundesministerium für Forschung und Technologie (BMFT) and the Deutsche Forschungsgemeinschaft (DFG).
[b] *Send correspondence to:* E.-M. Mandelkow, Max-Planck-Unit for Structural Molecular Biology, c/o DESY, Notkestrasse 85, D-22603 Hamburg, Germany; TEL: 49-40-89982810; FAX: 49-40-891314.

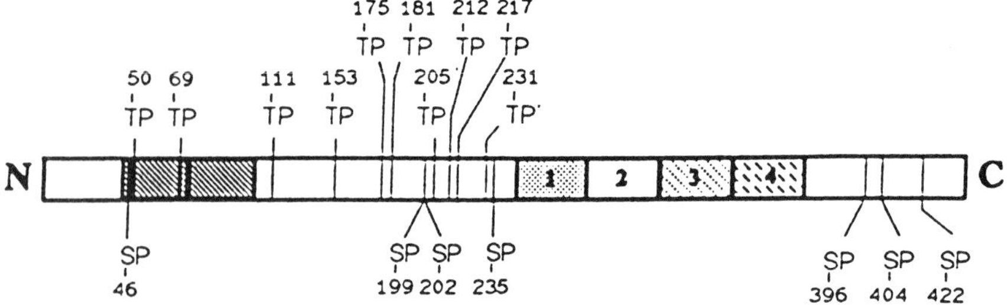

FIGURE 1. Location of the phosphorylatable Ser-Pro and Thr-Pro motifs in tau protein. The diagram shows the isoform htau40 (441 residues), the largest of the six human tau isoforms described in ref. 7. It contains two 29-mer inserts near the N-terminus *(shaded)* and four 31-residue repeats in the microtubule-binding region (labeled 1–4).

of the pathological transformation? What are the structural and biochemical consequences of the transformation?

METHODS

Methods have been described previously. Briefly, PHFs were prepared following Greenberg and Davies.[3] For construction of recombinant tau proteins by PCR and expression in *E. coli,* see Steiner *et al.*[4] and Biernat *et al.,*[5] using derivatives of the pET-3 vector[6]; the constructs were derived from the six human tau isoforms,[7] and the numbering of residues follows that of htau40 (441 residues, FIG. 1). For radioactive labeling, separation of labeled tryptic peptides, and phosphopeptide sequencing, see Steiner *et al.,*[4] using the sequencing procedures of Meyer *et al.*[8] For binding studies of tau to taxol-stabilized microtubules, see Gustke *et al.*[9] For preparation of kinase activity from brain and its use in tau phosphorylation, see Biernat *et al.*[5] and Lichtenberg-Kraag *et al.*[10] MAP kinase and GSK-3 from brain were prepared following Drewes *et al.*[11] and Mandelkow *et al.*[12] For determination of phosphorylation sensitive antibody epitopes see Biernat *et al.*[5] and Lichtenberg-Kraag *et al.*[10] For electron microscopy of tau, chemical crosslinking, and assembly of synthetic paired helical filaments see Wille *et al.*[13]

RESULTS AND DISCUSSION

Phosphorylation Sites and Antibody Epitopes of Tau Protein

Since tau protein from PHF's is abnormally phosphorylated and has a reduced electrophoretic mobility,[14] we searched for a protein kinase that would affect these parameters. Several widely used kinases were tested; CaM kinase induced a clear shift by phosphorylating a single site (Ser 416 in the htau40 numbering[4]). However, the phosphorylated protein did not react with PHF-specific antibodies. Other kinases such as PKC or cdc2 were even less effective with regard to electrophoretic mobility or PHF-antibodies.[4,11] However, a kinase activity prepared from brain extract conferred Alzheimer-like characteristics to tau protein in the presence of the phosphatase inhibitor, okadaic acid. The kinase activity incorporated up to 6 Pi into tau, caused a mobility shift in brain tau as well as all recombinant tau isoforms, and induced an Alzheimer-like immunoreactivity with several antibodies.[5,10] All antibodies that distinguished between PHF tau and normal tau were phosphorylation sensitive, either in a positive sense (*i.e.*, reacting with phosphorylated epitopes of PHFs and of recombinant tau, for example AT8 and SMI31), or in a negative sense (*i.e.*, reacting only with normal and unphosphorylated tau, for example TAU1 and SMI33; FIGS. 2 and 3). These results also showed that the Alzheimer-like kinase activity was already present in normal brain and not generated by a pathological condition.

The epitopes of the antibodies and the phosphorylation sites which controlled their reactivities were determined by a combination of phosphopeptide sequencing and site directed mutagenesis (FIG. 2). Most epitopes involved phosphorylatable serines followed by prolines. An example is the epitope of the PHF-specific antibody AT8 which includes phosphorylated Ser 199 and Ser 202, and TAU1 whose epitope is complementary in that it requires these two serines in an unphosphorylated form (and therefore reacts with normal tau but not with PHF-tau). In addition to antibody epitopes, all Ser-Pro

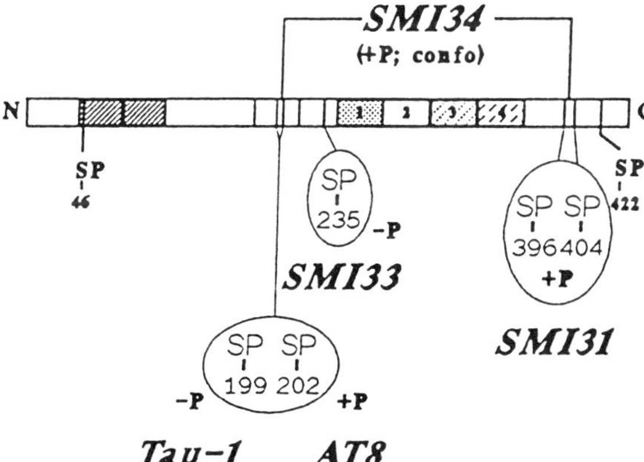

FIGURE 2. Location of epitopes of some antibodies that distinguish between normal and pathological tau. Antibodies AT8, SMI31, SMI34, SMI35, SMI310 require phosphorylation of their epitopes. Antibodies TAU1 and SMI33 require unphosphorylated epitopes.

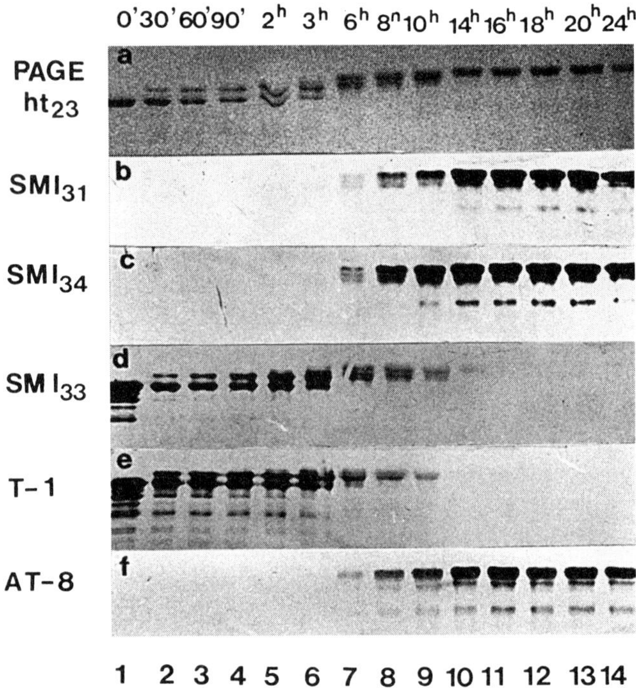

FIGURE 3. Time course of phosphorylation of htau23 (a, SDS-PAGE), and immunoblots with several antibodies (b–e). Note that the Alzheimer-like immunoreactivity appears around 6 hours (stage 2 phosphorylation).

motifs in recombinant tau have now been found to be phosphorylatable by the kinase activity from brain, as well as several other residues.[9] Most sites are clustered in the vicinity of residue 200 or 400 (*i.e.,* flanking the region of internal repeats which bind to microtubules).

The phosphorylation causes a gel shift in several characteristic stages (FIG. 3). Starting from the original unphosphorylated state we distinguish three main stages with several substages. The PHF-life immunoreactivity is detectable from stage 2 onwards. Conversely, other antibodies reacting with normal tau lose their reactivity during stage 2. By these criteria, tau acquires its Alzheimer-like state during stage 2 of the phosphorylation.[10]

The Structure and Interactions of Tau

The interaction between tau and microtubules can be assayed by measuring how much of tau can be co-sedimented with taxol-stabilized microtubules.

The most conspicuous effect of the phosphorylation of tau by the kinase activity from brain is the decrease in binding capacity from about 1 tau per 2 tubulin dimers to 1 tau per 6 tubulin dimer (*i.e.,* by a factor of about three[9]). This confirms that phosphorylation can reduce the interaction between microtubules and tau, and could therefore be responsible for a destabilization of microtubules. In the cell this would cause a loss in axonal transport, since microtubules provide the tracks for vesicle traffic driven by motor proteins.

A prominent aspect of abnormal tau is its assembly into the PHFs in Alzheimer brains. Because of their poor solubility, it has been difficult to analyse their assembly properties. We therefore investigated the structure of recombinant tau and its assembly properties by electron microscopy. The protein is usually difficult to visualize because of its low contrast; the method we found most useful was glycerol spraying combined with rotary shadowing at very shallow angles. All tau isoforms are thin and rod-like; the isoform htau23 has an average length of 35 nm,[13] whereas the microtubule-binding domain of internal repeats (constructs K11 or K12) are only about 25 nm long. In addition, tau has the ability to form antiparallel dimers. This can be visualized structurally by labeling the protein with an antibody that binds near one end. Tau dimers show up as rods with two labels at both ends.

The capacity to form antiparallel dimers is preserved even in the recombinant microtubule-binding domain. The dimers can be crosslinked covalently by chemical modification. This is particularly clear in the case of constructs containing only repeats 1, 3 and 4 (*i.e.,* the three repeats present in htau23; see FIG. 1). In this case there is only one cysteine (Cys 322) which can be crosslinked to the same Cys of a second molecule by PDM. This covalent dimer can be isolated cromatographically and imaged by electron microscopy. It also forms antiparallel dimers whose length is similar to that of the monomer, indicating that the crosslinked cysteines of repeat 3 must be roughly at the center of the microtubule-binding domain.[13] These results imply that tau molecules could interact with one another on the surface of a microtubule and, since the microtubule-binding region of tau is flanked by clusters of phosphorylatable serines, one could imagine that the interaction is regulated by phosphorylation. This would explain why phosphorylation affects the stoichiometry of binding.

Another significant consequence is that dimers of the repeat domain are capable of further assembly into the filaments shown in FIGURE 4. They share certain key features of the paired helical filaments isolated from Alzheimer tissue. They can be either of uniform diameter, *ca.* 20 nm, or the diameter can vary between 8 and 15 nm, with an axial periodicity of *ca.* 75–80 nm;[13] compare these with the twisted and straight PHFs of Crowther.[15]

Our working hypothesis is therefore the antiparallel dimers of the repeat region of tau are crosslinked by the cysteines in repeat 3 and thus form the core of the PHF's. It is not clear at present how this might be regulated by

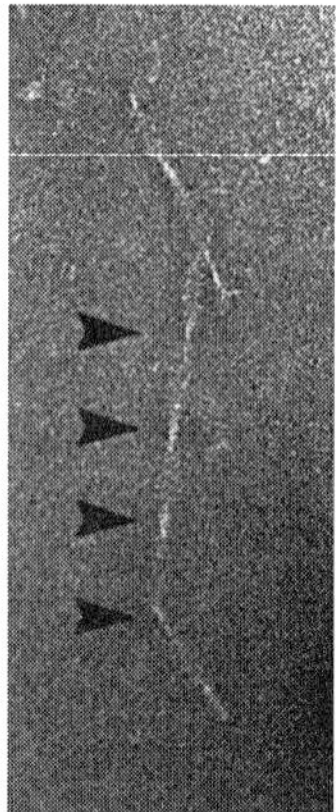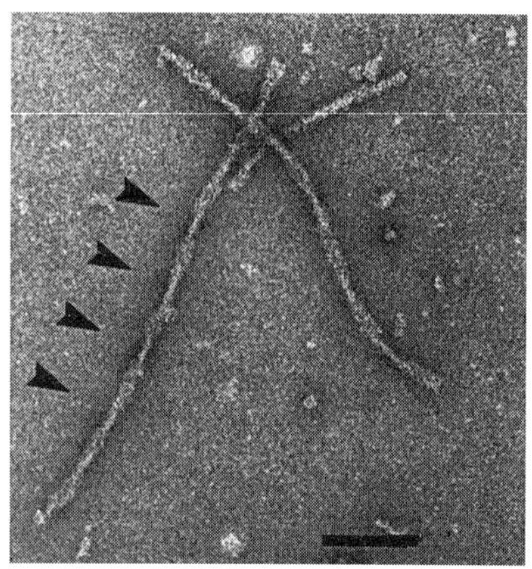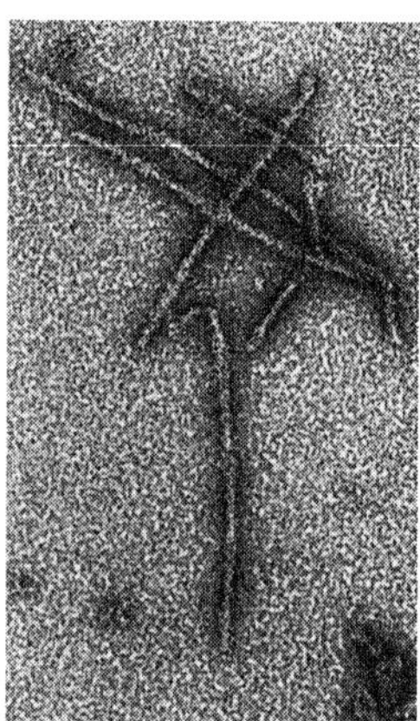

FIGURE 4. Synthetic paired helical filaments assembled from tau construct K12. Note the crossover periodicity of about 75–80 nm, and the tendency to aggregate into bundles; Bar = 100 nm.

phosphorylation. So far, we have not been able to assemble bona fide PHFs from complete tau variants (such as htau23). It is possible that these molecules do not have the proper conformation for polymerization, and that this conformation can only be brought about by abnormal phosphorylation. This hypothesis remains to be tested.

Kinases Inducing the Alzheimer-like Immunoreactivity

We mentioned above that abnormal phosphorylation of tau occurs predominantly at Ser-Pro motifs (judging by PHF-specific antibodies) and that the corresponding kinase(s) are present in normal brain tissue. This meant that we had to search for a proline-directed kinase in brain tissue; it also explained why our earlier searches had failed[4]: PKA, PKC, casein kinase, and CaM kinase are not proline-directed kinases.

A number of Pro-directed kinases are known.[16] We initially tested the cell cycle kinase p34(cdc2) which can be complexed with different regulatory subunits (cyclins), but this did not cause appreciable phosphorylation, nor the reactivity with PHF-specific antibodies.[11] The next attempt was MAP kinase.[17] The enzyme (Mr = 42 kDal) was prepared from porcine brain and met the criteria required for abnormal phosphorylation[11]: it induced the immunoreactivity with PHF-specific antibodies; it incorporated between 12–15 Pi into the tau molecule; and it phosphorylated Ser-Pro as well as Thr-Pro motifs in all recombinant isoforms tested (FIG. 1). Moreover, when PHFs from Alzheimer brains were dephosphorylated with alkaline phosphatase they lost their immune reactivity, but regained it when re-phosphorylated with MAP kinase. Another Pro-directed kinase in brain is GSK-3 (α and β isoforms, 51 and 45 kDal[18]). When this was tested on tau protein, both isoforms yielded qualitatively similar results as MAP kinase. The degree of phosphorylation was considerably lower, but the Ser-Pro motifs that affect the reactivity of PHF-specific antibodies (FIG. 2) were phosphorylated with similar kinetics and efficiency.[12]

It may be significant that both MAP kinase and GSK-3 are involved in cellular signal transduction pathways. This suggests that an abnormal regulation of signal transduction may be important in the generation of the disease. Moreover, MAP kinase and GSK-3 not only transformed tau into the Alzheimer-like state in solution, they also appeared to be physically associated with microtubules, as well as with PHFs from Alzheimer brain tissue.[12] Thus, any dysregulation of these kinases or their corresponding phosphatases could affect tau protein directly. The nature of these interactions are at present unknown, but they will have to be explored in order to unravel the cascade of events that leads to the deposition of PHFs during Alzheimer's disease.

ACKNOWLEDGMENTS

We would like to thank Dr. M. Goedert for clones of human tau; Dr. W. Studier for the pET expression vector; and Drs. J. Dingus, R. Vallee, L. Binder, and M. Mercken for antibodies. Phosphopeptide sequencing was done in collaboration with Dr. H. E. Meyer (Universiteit Bochum). Brain tissue was a gift of Dr. B. Crain and K. Dole (K. Bryan Alzheimer Disease Research Center, Duke University).

REFERENCES

1. KOSIK, K. S. 1992. Science **256:**780–783.
2. LEE, V. & J. TROJANOWSKI. 1992. Curr. Opin. Neurobiol. **2:**653–656.
3. GREENBERG, S. & P. DAVIES. 1990. Proc. Natl. Acad. Sci. USA **87:**5827–5831.
4. STEINER, B., E.-M. MANDELKOW, J. BIERNAT, N. GUSTKE, H. E. MEYER, B. SCHMIDT, G. MIESKES, H. D. SÖLING, D. DRECHSEL, M. W. KIRSCHNER, M. GOEDERT & E. MANDELKOW. 1990. EMBO J. **9:**3539–3544.
5. BIERNAT, J., E.-M. MANDELKOW, C. SCHRÖTER, B. LICHTENBERG-KRAAG, B. STEINER, B. BERLING, H. E. MEYER, M. MERCKEN, A. VANDERMEEREN, M. GOEDERT & E. MANDELKOW. 1992. EMBO J. **11:**1593–1597.
6. STUDIER, W. F., A. H. ROSENBERG, J. J. DUNN & J. W. DUBENDORFF. 1990. Meth. Enzymol. **185:**60–89.
7. GOEDERT, M., M. SPILLANTINI, R. JAKES, D. RUTHERFORD & R. A. CROWTHER. 1989. Neuron **3:**519–526.

8. MEYER, H. E., E. HOFFMANN-POSORSKE & L. M. G. HEILMEYER. 1991. Meth. Enzymol. **201:**169–185.
9. GUSTKE, N., B. STEINER, E.-M. MANDELKOW, J. BIERNAT, H. E. MEYER, M. GOEDERT & E. MANDELKOW. 1992. FEBS Letters **307:**199–205.
10. LICHTENBERG-KRAAG, B., E.-M. MANDELKOW, J. BIERNAT, B. STEINER, C. SCHRÖTER, N. GUSTKE, H. E. MEYER & E. MANDELKOW. 1992. Proc. Natl. Acad. Sci. USA **89:**5384–5388.
11. DREWES, G., B. LICHTENBERG-KRAAG, F. DÖRING, E.-M. MANDELKOW, J. BIERNAT, J. GORIS, M. DORÉE & E. MANDELKOW. 1992. EMBO J. **11:** 2131–2138.
12. MANDELKOW, E.-M., G. DREWES, J. BIERNAT, N. GUSTKE, J. VAN LINT, J. R. VANDENHEEDE & E. MANDELKOW. 1992. FEBS Lett. **314:**315–321.
13. WILLE, H., G. DREWES, J. BIERNAT, E.-M. MANDELKOW & E. MANDELKOW. 1992. J. Cell Biol. **118:**573–584.
14. GRUNDKE-IQBAL, I., K. IQBAL, Y. TUNG, M. QUINLAN, H. WISNIEWSKI & L. BINDER. 1986. Proc. Natl. Acad. Sci. USA **83:**4913–4917.
15. CROWTHER, R. A. 1991. Biochim. Biophys. Acta **1096:**1–9.
16. HUNTER, T. 1991. Meth. Enzym. **200:**3–37.
17. STURGILL, T. & J. WU. 1991. Biochim. Biophys. Acta **1092:**350–357.
18. WOODGETT, J. R. 1991. TIBS **16:**177–181.

Transgenic Animal Models for Alzheimer's Disease[a]

KEN-ICHIRO FUKUCHI[b], CHARLES E. OGBURN,
ANNETTE C. SMITH, DENNIS D. KUNKEL,
CLEMENT E. FURLONG, SAMIR S. DEEB, DAVID NOCHLIN,
S. MARK SUMI, AND GEORGE M. MARTIN[b]

*Departments of Pathology, Neurosurgery, and Medicine, University of Washington,
Seattle, Washington 98195 USA*

ABSTRACT: The neuropathology of Alzheimer's disease is characterized by the deposition of abnormal protein aggregates. The main constituent of the deposition is β-amyloid protein. A seminal role of this protein is supported by the discovery of point mutations in the gene of its precursor protein in certain forms of familial Alzheimer's disease. *In vitro* (cultured neuronal cells), overexpression of the precursor protein or a part of the precursor leads to degeneration of neurons, suggesting neurotoxicity of its derivatives. At this time, all of the reported transgenic mice bearing DNA construct for the precursor or a part of the precursor, however, have not developed convincing pathological changes similar to what is observed in patients with Alzheimer's disease. This interesting discrepancy between *in vitro* and *in vivo* suggests suppressors *in vivo* which ameliorate β-amyloid precursor protein derivative-mediated neurotoxicity.

ALZHEIMER'S DISEASE (AD) AND β/A4 AMYLOID PROTEIN (Aβ)

AD is a neurodegenerative disorder characterized by progressive loss of memory and cognitive functions and is the most common cause of dementia over age 60. The characteristic pathological changes include neurofibrillary tangles and the deposition of abnormal protein aggregates termed amyloid in the form of neuritic plaques (NP) and cerebrovascular amyloidosis (CVA). Losses of synapses and of neurons are also observed. The precise roles and origins of such pathological markers in the etiology of the disease is unknown. Correlations between these pathological markers and cognitive impairment in AD is controversial. Compelling evidence that Aβ and its precursor protein

[a] This work was supported by grant AG10917 from the National Institutes of Health (GMM) and by grant II RG-90-098 from the Alzheimer's Associations, Inc. (KF).

[b] *Send correspondence to:* Drs. G. M. Martin and K. Fukuchi, Department of Pathology SM-30, University of Washington, Seattle, WA 98195 USA; TEL: (206) 543-5088 (GMM) or (206) 543-9362 (KF); FAX: (206) 685-8356.

(βPP) play a seminal role in the pathogenesis of AD comes from the discovery of constitutional mutations in the βPP gene in some families with AD of early onset type.[1]

β/A4 AMYLOID PRECURSOR PROTEIN

The Aβ is derived from a larger precursor protein (βPP), which is a tyrosine-sulfated O- and N-glycosylated integral membrane protein, and consists of 39–42 amino acids extending from the extracytoplasmic to the transmembrane domains of βPP. Seven alternatively spliced βPP mRNA transcripts encoding for 365, 543, 695, 714, 751, 752 or 770 amino acids (AA) have been identified. Except for βPP-365 and βPP-543 mRNA, these transcripts contain the Aβ sequence. Five transcripts (βPP-365, -543, -751, -752, and -770) contain a 56-AA domain homologous to the Kunitz family of serine protease inhibitors. Among them, mRNA coding for 695 AA is a major form in brain. To assess levels of expression of these mRNA species for βPP in the AD brain, *in situ* hybridization, Northern blot, dot blot and polymerase chain reaction (PCR) analyses have been performed. Although this information is very important for determination of a DNA construct to study amyloidogenicity and neurotoxicity of βPP by its overexpression in transgenic mice, the results of the experiments, however, are inconsistent and no consensus has been reached regarding the correlation between the disease status and the levels of specific mRNAs for βPP.

Aβ is a main component of β-amyloid. βPP is transported to a cytoplasmic membrane and then relatively rapidly cleaved to yield a secreted extracellular domain and a relatively long-lived, approximately 11-kDa membrane-bound COOH-terminal fragment. Since this cleavage by "βPP secretase" takes place near the middle of Aβ (at residues between 15–17 AA of Aβ), this secretory pathway cannot produce amyloidogenic fragments.[2,3] Recently Younkin's group found an alternative endosomal/lysosomal pathway.[4,5] In the latter pathway, multiple COOH-terminal fragments of βPP are produced by lysosomal proteases and some of the fragments contain intact Aβ. Therefore, these COOH-terminal fragments are potentially amyloidogenic. Although several candidate proteases have been claimed as a βPP secretase, proteases involved in these proteolytic pathways of βPP are yet to be defined. We also found that overproduction of COOH-terminal fragments of βPP in COS cells (an African green monkey kidney cell line), P19 cells (a mouse embryonic carcinoma cell line), and SK-N-SH cells (a human neuroblastoma cell line), results in multiple COOH-terminal fragments of βPP and that some of the fragments (16 and 14 kDa) are neurotoxic and contain intact Aβ.[6,7]

AMYLOIDOGENICITY AND NEUROTOXICITY OF Aβ AND COOH-TERMINAL FRAGMENTS OF βPP

Synthetic peptides homologous to Aβ (Aβ AA 1-28, 12-28, 1-42) form amyloid-like fibrils comparable to those isolated from amyloid plaque cores from AD brain. Amyloidogenicity (aggregate or fibril formation) of Aβ is thus well-documented. Toxicity of the peptide is, however, controversial. Yankner *et al.*[8] reported that β/A4 was neurotrophic to undifferentiated hippocampal neurons at low concentrations (0.1–10 nM) and neurotoxic to mature neurons at higher concentrations (1 mM). Other investigators could not reproduce the experiments. Neurotoxicity and amyloidogenicity of Aβ *in vivo* need further evaluation. Our experiments address these questions by neurotransplantation of P19 cells overproducing βAP.

A COOH-terminal fragment of βPP (an approximately 100 AA COOH-terminal residue) self-aggregates to form high molecular mass in an in vitro translation system. The overproduction of the fragment in cultured cells leads to fibril formation and to deposition of the aggregates and the aggregates can be detected by immunoblot analysis.[6] Yankner *et al.*[9] reported neurotoxicity of a COOH-terminal fragment of βPP by overexpression of the DNA construct in PC12 cells which produce a high molecular aggregated mass (>110 kDa) of the fragment detectable on immunoblot analysis of the conditioned medium. Although we observed neurotoxicity of COOH fragments of βPP in neuronally differentiating P19 cells in which the fragments were overexpressed, toxicity was related to the 15- and 14-kDa COOH-terminal fragments.[6] The difference could be explainable by the differences of the cell lines and of the DNA constructs. Using the identical cell culture system (neuronally differentiating P19 cells), Yoshikawa *et al.*[10] also demonstrated that overexpression of full-length cDNA constructs for βPP-695, -751 and -770 led to degeneration of P19-derived neurons. These transformed P19 cells were treated with dimethyl sulfoxide to induce differentiation of the cells into muscle cells. The proteolysis of βPP in the muscle cells is similar to that observed in neuronal P19 cells but the 15- and 14-kDa fragments did not affect the survival of muscle cells. Furthermore, when a DNA construct for the COOH-terminal fragment was introduced into a morphologically heterogeneous neuroblastoma cell line (SK-N-SH, consisting of neuronal and non-neuronal cells), selective neurotoxicity of the fragments was observed.[7] The neurotoxicity of βPP derivatives using cultured neurons and their DNA constructs, therefore, seems to be well-established.

TRANSGENIC MICE BEARING DNA CONSTRUCTS FOR βPP OR A PART OF βPP

Five papers have been published on transgenics overproducing βPP or a part of βPP. Wirak *et al.*[11] produced transgenic mice bearing a DNA construct that encodes the 42-AA β-amyloid protein, regulated by the human βPP gene promoter. Levels of mRNA from the transgene were lower than those of the endogenous mouse βPP mRNA, determined by S1 nuclease protection analysis. In 1-year-old transgenic mice, accumulation of Aβ in the dendrites of some hippocampal neurons was observed. Jucker *et al.*,[12] however, found that laminin-binding protein-like immunoreactive granules increased with age in the brains of C57BL/6 mice and to a lesser extent in C3H mice and that these granules were stained with polyclonal antisera directed against Aβ, somatostatin, and neurotensin. Because of the report of "pseudoamyloid" age-associated inclusions in mice by Jucker *et al.*,[12] the work of Wirak *et al.*[11] was retracted.

Quon *et al.*[13] established transgenic mice overproducing βPP-751 under the control of the rat neural-specific enolase (NSE) promoter. Expression of mRNA from the transgenes were detected by PCR. Increased βPP-751 was also demonstrated by Western blot analysis compared to nontransgenic littermates. The cortical and hippocampal brain regions of the transgenic mice (3- to 15-month-old) displayed extracellular β-amyloid immunoreactive deposits varying in size (<5 to 50 μm) and abundance. These deposits were also occasionally found in the thalamus and striatum. The deposits were stained by silver salts, infrequently by thioflavin S, but not by Congo red. These authors also reported that transgenics overproduce βPP-695 under the control of NSE promoter did not develop the β-amyloid deposits. These results suggest that changes in ratios of neuronal βPP isoforms (especially increase of βPP-751) may lead to amyloidogenesis. Much more complete analysis of these transgenic mice, however, is necessary for acceptance as models for AD.

Overexpression of a COOH-terminal region of the βPP in transgenic mice was first reported by Sandhu *et al.*[14] They used the JC viral early region promoter to direct the expression of 100-AA COOH-terminal residues in transgenic mice. JC virus is a human papovavirus with brain-specific tissue tropism. Brain-specific expression of mRNA from the transgene was detected by PCR. Although increased immunoreactivity for Aβ was reported in the cerebral cortex and hindbrain of transgenic mice, absolute levels of identifiable transgene products and detailed histochemical studies of the transgenic mice have not been demonstrated.

Kawabata *et al.*[15] also overexpressed 100-AA COOH-terminal residues of βPP under the control of the human Thy-1 gene promoter. Brain-specific expression of mRNA from the transgene was demonstrated by Northern blotting and in situ hybridization. Extracellular diffuse amyloid deposits were found in the hippocampus of 4- and 8-month-old transgenic mice. At 8 months of age, dense-core plaques, NT, and neuritic dystrophy in the hippocampal formation, amyglaloid complex, and neocortex were visualized by silver staining. Dystrophic neurities were also visualized with Alz-50 antibody. Subsequent studies of the additional transgenic mice did not replicate the initial observations. Biochemical studies of the animals showed no evidence of the transgene products.[16] The other paper has been retracted.

Other lines of transgenic mice overproducing COOH-terminal 104-AA of βPP were reported by Kammesheidt *et al.*[17] The cDNA was placed under the control of the brain dystrophin promoter and mRNA from the transgene was detected by PCR. The 4- and 6-month-old transgenic mice showed accumulation of Aβ immunoreactive material in the neuronal cell body and neuropil in the hippocampus. Positive staining of thioflavin S was also found in the cerebrovasculature in the animals. These thioflavin X positive materials were not stained by antibodies against Aβ. Obvious protein products from the transgene have, however, not been demonstrated.

We have established four lines of transgenic mice overproducing a COOH-terminal fragment of βPP. In our transgenic animals, the cDNA for the signal sequence (17 AA) of βPP + the COOH-terminal 99 AA of βPP was placed under the control of a cytomegalovirus enhancer and a chick β-actin promoter. The levels of expression of the transgene were determined by Northern blot and Western blot analysis of the tissues from a 3-month-old transgenic mouse. High levels of expression of mRNA from the transgene were observed in virtually all tissues examined, including brain. On the Western blot, high levels of expression of approximately 14-kDa protein products from the transgene were observed only in lung, muscle, intestine, liver, and kidney of a transgenic mouse, but no corresponding fragments were found in a control mouse. A 2- to 3-fold increase of the COOH-terminal fragments were found in the brain of the transgenic mouse as compared to the control. Immunohistochemical and histopathological studies revealed no significant differences between transgenic mice (6-, 12- and 13-months old) and C57BL6/J age-matched control mice. Deposit-like immunostaining for Aβ was occasionally observed in cortex, hippocampus, and brain vessels of both transgenic mice and control mice. Therefore, we could not conclude that these positive immunoreactivities for Aβ were due to transgene expression. Although the transgenic mice produced substantial protein products from the transgene, no neuronal degeneration was found in the 13-month-old transgenic animal. This interesting discrepancy between our results *in vivo* (transgenic animals) and *in vitro* (P19 cultured cells), in which substantial neurotoxicity was observed, suggests that the COOH-terminal fragment-mediated neurotoxicity can be suppressed in the transgenic mice. As discussed above, there are as yet no transgenic models showing pathological changes comparable to what is observed in AD. It may, however, be too early to conclude that these transgenic mice do not develop such pathological lesions, since animal models for familial amyloidotic polyneuropathy type I, transgenic mice carrying a mutant human transthyretin gene, consistently develop amyloid deposition after one year of age in the alimentary tract and other tissues but, curiously, not in the peripheral nerve of transgenic mice; also, in humans, the disease takes between 20 to 45 years of age to develop the first symptoms of amyloid deposition. These results suggest that the accumulations of amyloid may be related to intrinsic biological aging rather than chronological time, and thus provides encouragement that, despite the short life spans of rodent species and the limited careers of human investigators, important aspects of the pathogenesis of a number of late-onset human genetic disorders of relevance to the pathobiology of aging (including AD) might be modeled in mice.

ACKNOWLEDGMENT

We thank J. Garr for preparing the manuscript.

REFERENCES

1. HARDY, J. 1992. Framing β-amyloid. Nature Genet 1:233–234.
2. ESCH, F. S., P. S. KEIM, E. C. BEATTIE, R. W. BLACHER, A. R. CULWELL, T. OLTERSDORF, D. MCCLURE & P. J. WARD. 1991. Cleavage of amyloid β peptide during constitutive processing of its precursor. Science 248:1122–1124.
3. SISODIA, S. S., E. H. KOO, K. BEYREUTHER, A. UNTERBECK & D. L. PRICE. 1991. Evidence that β-amyloid protein in Alzheimer's disease is not derived by normal processing. Science 248:492–495.
4. ESTUS, S., T. E. GOLDE, T. KUNISHITA, D. BLADES, D. LOWERY, M. EISEN, M. USIAK, X. QU, T. TABIRA, B. D. GREENBERG & S. G. YOUNKIN. 1992. Potentially amyloidogenic, carboxyl-terminal derivatives of the amyloid protein precursor. Science 255:726–728.
5. GOLDE, T. E., S. ESTUS, L. H. YOUNKIN, D. J. SELKOE & S. G. YOUNKIN. 1992. Processing of the amyloid protein precursor to potentially amyloidogenic derivatives. Science 255:728–730.
6. FUKUCHI, K., K. KAMINO, S. S. DEEB, A. C. SMITH, T. DANG & G. M. MARTIN. 1992. Overexpression of amyloid precursor protein alters its normal processing and is associated with neurotoxicity. Biochem. Biophys. Res. Commun. 182:165–173.
7. FUKUCHI, K., K. KAMINO, S. S. DEEB, C. E. FURLONG, J. A. SUNDSTROM, A. C. SMITH & G. M. MARTIN. 1992. Expression of a carboxy-terminal region of the β-amyloid precursor protein in a heterogeneous culture of neuroblastoma cells: evidence for altered processing and selective neurotoxicity. Mol. Brain Res. 16:37–46.
8. YANKNER, B. A., L. K. DUFFY & D. A. KIRSCHNER. 1990. Neurotrophic and neurotoxic effects of amyloid β protein: reversal by tachykinin neuropeptides. Science 250:279–280.
9. YANKNER, B. A., L. R. DAWES, S. FISHER, L. VILLA-KOMAROFF, M. L. OSTER-GRANITE & R. L. NEVE. 1989. Neurotoxicity of a fragment of the amyloid precursor associated with Alzheimer's disease. Science 245:417–420.

10. YOSHIKAWA, K., T. AIZAWA & Y. HAYASHI. 1992. Degeneration in vitro of post-mitotic neurons overexpressing the Alzheimer's amyloid protein precursor. Nature **359:**264–67.

11. WIRAK, D. O., R. BAYNEY, T. V. RAMABHADRAN, R. P. FRACASSO, J. T. HART, P. E. HAUER, P. HSIAU, S. K. PEKAR, G. A. SCANGOS, B. D. TRAPP & A. J. UNTERBECK. 1991. Deposits of amyloid β protein in the central nervous system of transgenic mice. Science **253:**323–325.

12. JUCKER, M., L. C. WALKER, L. J. MARTIN, C. A. KITT, H. K. KLEINMAN, D. K. INGRAM & D. L. PRICE. 1992. Age-associated inclusions in normal and transgenic mouse brain. Science **255:**1443–1445.

13. QUON, D., Y. WANG, R. CATALANO, J. M. SCARDINA, K. MURAKAMI & B. CORDELL. 1991. Formation of β-amyloid protein deposits in brains of transgenic mice. Nature **352:**239–241.

14. SANDHU, F. A., M. SALIM & S. B. ZAIN. 1991. Expression of the human β-amyloid protein of Alzheimer's disease specifically in the brains of transgenic mice. J. Biol. Chem. **266:**21331–21334.

15. KAWABATA, S., G. A. HIGGINS & J. W. GORDON. 1991. Amyloid plaques neuro-fibrillary tangles and neuronal loss in brains of transgenic mice overexpressing a C-terminal fragment of human amyloid precursor protein. Nature **354:**476–478.

16. PRICE, D. L., L. C. WALKER, L. J. MARTIN & S. S. SISODIA. 1992. Amyloidosis in aging and Alzheimer's disease. Am. J. Pathol. **141:**767–772.

17. KAMMESHEIDT, A., F. M. BOYCE, A. F. SPANYOANNIS, B. J. CUMMINGS, M. ORTEGON, C. COTMAN, J. L. VAUGHT & R. L. NEVE. 1992. Deposition of β/A4 immunoreactivity and neuronal pathology in transgenic mice expressing the carboxyl-terminal fragment of the Alzheimer amyloid precursor in the brain. Proc. Natl. Acad. Sci. USA **89:**10857–10861.

Transgenic Mice Expressing Human β-APP751, But Not Mice Expressing β-APP695, Display Early Alzheimer's Disease-like Histopathology[a]

L. S. HIGGINS[b], R. CATALANO, D. QUON, AND B. CORDELL

Scios Nova Inc., Mountain View, California 94043 USA

ABSTRACT: Mice transgenic for the 751 amino acid isoform of the human β-amyloid precursor protein (β-APP) driven by the rat neuron specific enolase (NSE) promoter (NSE:β-APP751) show features of early Alzheimer's disease (AD) pathology. These features, which were evident in multiple pedigrees, include: 1) preamyloid deposits which stain with antibodies that are specific for the β-amyloid peptide and stain AD amyloid deposits and plaques, and 2) neuronal soma and processes which stain with an antibody (Alz50) that detects abnormal isoforms of tau which are characteristic of AD. The quality and distribution of both types of immunoreactivity revealed in the NSE:β-APP751 mouse brains most closely resemble those seen in brains of young adults with Down's syndrome. Both structures are rarely, if ever, observed in brains from mice transgenic for the 695 amino acid isoform of β-APP (NSE:β-APP695) or in wild type mice.

INTRODUCTION

Two major histological characteristics of AD are amyloid plaques and neurofibrillary tangles (NFT). AD plaques contain β-amyloid (β/A4), a ~4kD protein derived from a precursor protein, β-APP.[1] Identical structures are observed in brain tissues of individuals with trisomy 21, or Down's syndrome (DS), all of whom invariably develop AD.[2,3] Therefore, DS brain tissue is extremely useful in elucidating the possible temporal progression of amyloid plaque and NFT formation in AD. However, an understanding of AD has been hampered by the lack of a small animal model, which would allow for experimental manipulation. In an effort to develop a workable model, we have

[a] This research is supported by grant RO1 AG10655-01 to B. C. and by Marion Merrell Dow, Inc.
[b] *Send correspondence to:* Dr. L. S. Higgins, Scios Nova Inc., 2450 Bayshore Parkway, Mountain View, CA 94043 USA; TEL: (415) 966-1550; FAX: (415) 968-2438.

generated transgenic mice which are programmed for neuronal expression of human β-APP751 or β-APP695.

RESULTS AND DISCUSSION

β-Amyloid Immunoreactive Deposits

β/A4 immunohistochemistry was performed using monoclonal antibody mAb 4.1 on midline coronal brain sections of NSE:β-APP751, NSE:β-APP695, and wild type (WT) mice as well as on AD and DS brain sections. The epitope this antibody recognizes resides in the first seventeen amino acids of the β/A4 peptide and has been used for specific, competable staining of extracellular classic plaques as well as smaller deposits and diffuse preamyloid in AD brain.[4] In contrast, brain sections from a 16-year-old DS individual display only diffuse preamyloid β/A4 immunoreactive deposits. Diffuse β/A4 immunoreactive deposits are detected in NSE:β-APP751 mouse brains when stained with mAb 4.1, and are rarely seen in NSE:β-APP695 or WT brains (TABLE 1). The deposits are about 5–30 μm in diameter and have a cotton-like appearance or occasionally a more dense morphology; neither is punctuated by neuritic structures evident in mature plaques. Some are in proximity to neuronal soma, while others appear isolated in the neuropil. The deposits appear extracellular and are structurally similar to those observed in the brains of young adult DS individuals, as well as to the immature preamyloid and small deposits in AD brain. Similar results are obtained when mouse brains are immunostained with anti-β/A4 rabbit sera 2332 and 2333. Consistent with the preamyloid nature of the NSE:β-APP751 deposits, they are also detected by methenamine silver. It is interesting that sections from

TABLE 1. Frequency of β/A4 Immunoreactive Deposits in Brains from Transgenic and Wild Type Mice

% Sections Positive for β/A4 Immunoreactive Deposits (n)		
NSE:β-APP751	NSE:β-APP695	Wild Type
27%[a] (122)	1% (68)	5% (107)

NSE:β-APP751 set included 33 animals from six independent pedigrees; NSE:β-APP695 set included 20 animals from four pedigrees; 18 wild type mice were included from the strain used to create the transgenic pedigrees. Three or more midline coronal sections were stained from each animal. Three investigators independently scored the sections with close agreement. Sections with at least one deposit were scored positive. Most, but not all, deposits were observed in the hippocampus and cortex.
[a] Significantly different from values for NSE:β-APP695 and WT, $p <$ 0.01 (two tailed).

animals homozygous for the transgene were positive for β/A4 immunoreactive deposits at twice the rate of sections from hemizygous mice.

Increase in Deposits with Age

The relationship of β/A4 deposit frequency to age was determined for mice within a single NSE:β-APP751 pedigree (F10) that expresses the transgene at a relatively high level. The old animals, which were at the end of the natural life span of this strain, had twice the frequency of positive sections as young animals (TABLE 2). In general, the quality of the deposits was similar between the groups, but a single old animal had multiple large immunoreactive structures with a dense, mature appearance.

TABLE 2. βA4 Immunoreactive Deposits Are More Frequent In Old NSE:β-APP751 Mice

Age (months)	% Sections Positive (n)
2–3	29% (35)
22	49% (35)

Three midline coronal sections were stained for each of 12 old and 12 young animals of the F10 pedigree and scored blind by two investigators. Sections with at least one β/A4 immunoreactive deposit were scored positive. The values are statistically different, $p > 0.01$ (one tailed).

Alz50 Immunoreactivity

Numerous neuropil threads and neurofibrillary tangles are revealed in AD brain tissue by immunoreactivity to the monoclonal antibody Alz50, which detects aberrant isoforms of tau. Alz50 stained brain sections from a young DS adult show sparsely distributed immunoreactive neurons and processes with a punctate appearance rather than the dense fibrillar nature of mature NFT.

In a survey of mouse brain tissue, abnormal Alz50 reactivity was defined in the study as the presence of stained neurons. NSE:β-APP751 brain sections stained with Alz50 often revealed stained neurons and processes, as well as fields of punctate staining of the neuropil. These structures were rarely or

TABLE 3. Frequency of Alz50 Immunoreactivity in Mouse Brains

% Sections with Abnormal Alz50 Staining (n)		
NSE:β-APP751	NSE:β-APP695	Wild Type
42%[a] (52)	0% (30)	6% (53)

NSE:β-APP751 set included 15 animals representing three independent pedigrees; NSE:β-APP695 set included 10 animals from three independent pedigrees; wild type included 12 animals. Three or more midline coronal sections were immunostained from each animal. All stained soma and most processes were observed in the cerebral cortex and in the amygdala. Occasional processes were also seen in the hippocampus. A concordance of 79% was obtained for animals positive for Alz50 and β/A4 immunoreactivity.

[a] Significantly different from values for NSE:β-APP695 and WT, $p < 0.01$ (two tailed).

never seen in NSE:β-APP695 or WT animals (TABLE 3). As in the case of β/A4 immunoreactivity, Alz50 staining of NSE:β-APP751 mouse brains most closely resembles staining in the young adult DS brain and not the late-stage AD brain.

ACKNOWLEDGMENTS

We thank P. Davies and V. Lee for generously providing antibodies, and are grateful to G. Murphy and W. G. Ellis for tissue samples.

REFERENCES

1. KANG, J., H.-G. LEMAIRE, A. UNTERBECK, J. M. SALBAUM, C. L. MASTERS, K.-H. GRESHIK, G. MULTHAUP, K. BEYREUTHER & B. MULLER-HILL. 1987. The precursor protein of Alzheimer's disease amyloid A4 protein resembles a cell-surface receptor. Nature **325:**733–736.
2. BURGER, P. C. & F. C. VOGEL. 1973. The development of the pathological changes of Alzheimer's disease and senile dementia in patients with Down's syndrome. Am. J. Pathol. **73:**457–476.
3. MANN, D. M. A. 1988. The pathological association between Down syndrome and Alzheimer disease. Mech. of Ageing Dev. **43:**99–136.
4. QUON, D., Y. WANG, R. CATALANO, J. M. SCARDINA, K. MURAKAMI & B. CORDELL. 1991. Formation of β-amyloid protein deposits in brains of transgenic mice. Nature **352:**239–241.

Experimental Induction of β-Amyloid Plaques and Cerebral Angiopathy in Primates[a]

H. F. BAKER[b], R. M. RIDLEY[b,e], L. W. DUCHEN[c], T. J. CROW[b], AND C. J. BRUTON[b,d]

[b] Division of Psychiatry, Clinical Research Centre, Harrow HA1 3UJ
United Kingdom
[c] Department of Neuropathology, Institute of Neurology, National Hospital,
Queen Square, London WC1N 3BG United Kingdom
[d] MRC Department of Neuropathology, Runwell Hospital, Wickford,
Essex SS1 17QE United Kingdom

ABSTRACT: Moderate numbers of amyloid plaques with associated argyrophilic dystrophic neurites and cerebral amyloid angiopathy (CAA) but no neurofibrillary tangles (NFTs) were found in the brains of 3 middle-aged common marmosets *(Callithrix jacchus)* inoculated intracerebrally (i.c.) 6–7 years earlier with brain tissue from a patient with early onset Alzheimer's disease. The plaques and vascular amyloid stained positively with antibodies to β(A4)-protein. The brains of 3 age-matched control marmosets from the same colony did not show these neuropathological features. β-amyloid plaques and CAA (but no spongiform encephalopathy) were also found in the brain of a marmoset inoculated with brain tissue from a patient with prion disease with concomitant β-amyloid plaques and CAA. An occasional β-amyloid plaque was found in the brains of two marmosets inoculated with brain tissue from elderly patients. No β-amyloid plaques nor CAA were found in 6 other marmosets who were older than the inoculated marmosets, 10 further marmosets who were slightly younger but who had been inoculated several years previously with brain tissue which did not contain β-amyloid, and 10 younger marmosets who had been subjected to various neurosurgical procedures. These results suggest that β-amyloidosis is a transmissible process.

INTRODUCTION

Cerebral amyloidosis is characterized by the deposition of fibrillar protein of varying composition. In Alzheimer's disease (AD), the characteristic amyloid plaques and vascular amyloid deposits immunostain with antibodies to

[a] This work was supported by the Medical Research Council, U.K.
[e] *Send correspondence to:* Dr. R. M. Ridley, Division of Psychiatry, MRC Clinical Research Centre, Watford Road, Harrow, Middlesex HA1 3UJ U.K.; TEL: 44-081-869-3518; FAX: 44-081-869-3511.

β-amyloid (β/A4), a 4 kD protein subfragment of amyloid precursor protein (APP). The amyloid deposits sometimes seen in human and animal prion diseases immunostain with antibodies to prion protein (PrP) which derives from an abnormal isoform of normal host-coded prion protein. Experimental transmission of prion diseases results in the conversion of the new host's prion protein to the abnormal form by what is thought to be an autocatalytic process. In the context of our transmission studies with prion diseases, we also inoculated marmosets i.c. with brain tissue from several patients with β-amyloid plaques and angiopathy, one of whom had early onset AD.

MATERIALS AND METHODS

Laboratory-bred common marmosets were used. Their natural lifespan in captivity is in excess of 12 years and maximum longevity is more than 16 years. Thus, the experimental animals reported here (aged 6–9 years) cannot be regarded as elderly.

Animals were inoculated i.c. under general anaesthesia using stereotaxic placements according to our standard procedures.[1] The inocula consisted of 10% weight/volume homogenates of fresh cerebral tissue in 0.85% sterile saline taken from cases described below. With the exception of some animals in the supplementary experiment (see below), all the animals were behaviorally normal when killed for histology. Formalin-fixed sections were stained with hematoxylin-eosin, hematoxylin-van Gieson, luxol fast blue-cresyl violet, Congo red, and modified Glees' silver impregnation for axons. Sections were also stained by the immunoperoxidase method using antibodies to β-protein, tau protein and PrP, after pretreatment with formic acid. Positive and negative controls were included for each immunostain.

In experiment 1, three marmosets, inoculated i.c. 6–7 years earlier with brain tissue from a patient (case 1) with early onset, neuropathologically verified AD (*i.e.*, β-amyloid plaques, CAA, and neurofibrillary tangles) were healthy when killed for histology aged 8–9 years. Their brains were compared with those of three healthy age-matched control monkeys with no previous surgery.

In experiment 2, 8 marmosets inoculated i.c. about 5 years previously with brain tissue from four suspected cases of prion disease (cases 2–5) or from 1 elderly control (case 6) were healthy when killed for histology aged 6–7 years. Case 2 (aged 62 years) had a diagnosis of Gerstmann-Sträussler-Scheinker disease (GSS) with concomitant β-amyloidosis. The brain showed spongiform encephalopathy (SE), PrP plaques, and β-amyloid plaques and CAA. There were some neurofibrillary tangles (NFTs). Case 3 (a cousin of case 2) had a diagnosis of atypical prion dementia based on a codon 102 mutation in the prion gene, and minimal neuropathological change. Case 4 (aged 79 years) and case 5 (aged 81 years) were diagnosed as Creutzfeldt-Jakob disease (CJD). Both brains showed mild SE, some PrP-plaques and a few β-amyloid plaques but no NFTs.

The brains of a further 26 marmosets used in other experiments were available for supplementary neuropathological examination. Of these, 6 were older than the animals in experiments 1 and 2, 10 were slightly younger but had been inoculated some years previously with brain tissue from cases of GSS, BSE, scrapie and suspected CJD. None of the donor brains contained β-amyloid deposits. All except two of these animals inoculated with suspected CJD material developed neurological signs and SE. The remaining 10 animals were young (2–3 years); 8 had received neurotoxic lesions of cholinergic nuclei.

RESULTS

All three animals inoculated with tissue from case 1 and one of two animals inoculated with tissue from case 2 showed moderate numbers of neuritic plaques using silver stains. There were also vascular amyloid deposits in all these animals. There were no NFTs. The amyloid plaques and the vascular amyloid immunostained with antibodies to β-protein. Cases 1 and 2 had both had substantial numbers of β-amyloid plaques and marked β-amyloid angiopathy. An occasional plaque was seen in one animal inoculated with tissue from case 4 and in one of two animals with tissue from the elderly control (case 6). No β-amyloid plaques or angiopathy were found in 6 animals which were older than those in experiments 1 and 2, nor in 10 marmosets which were slightly younger but which had received inoculations of brain tissue several years previously, nor in 10 younger animals subjected to various neurological procedures.

In the four animals which developed moderate β-amyloidosis, lesions were found only in grey matter including all regions of cerebral cortex and amygdala. They were not found in deep grey nuclei, brainstem or cerebellum. With β-protein antibody immunostaining, a dense, solidly stained area was present at the centre of those plaques with fibrillar processes radiating out from it; the plaque periphery was composed of a delicate network of lightly stained threads. The distribution of these plaques was not related to the inoculation sites; they were found scattered throughout cortex in all the sections examined. Vascular β-amyloid was found in meningeal vessels over the entire cerebral hemispheres and within intracortical vessels. Arterioles as well as capillaries were involved. No immunostained vessels were present in white matter.

DISCUSSION

These results suggest that the β-amyloidosis found in four marmosets was not age-related, was not caused by non-specific aspects of neurosurgery, and was not the consequence of other neurodegeneration (SE); rather, they suggest that the formation of β-amyloid plaques and CAA is a process that can be transmitted by i.c. inoculation. It should be stressed that it is the process of β-amyloidosis not Alzheimer's disease which has been transmitted in this experiment. The animals were not debilitated and their brains did not show NFTs.

In some respects, the transmissibility of the β-amyloidosis process resembles the phenomenon of transmission seen in prion diseases. In experimental transmission of prion diseases, it is argued that when the abnormal isoform of prion protein is introduced into the recipient animal it induces the new host's normal protein to convert to the abnormal form. Amyloid fibrils (SAFS) composed of the abnormal form of prion protein can be prepared from affected brains in both naturally occurring cases of prion disease and in animals after experimental transmission. In sporadic cases of prion disease, it seems likely that the conversion of normal prion protein to the abnormal form is a probabilistic or stochastic event which occurs at a low level but that the presence of the abnormal form then acts as a catalyst for conversion of more normal protein. In the inherited forms of prion disease, where a mutation in the PrP gene has been identified, this probability may be increased because of differences in the amino acid sequence of the normal protein. Similarly, it may be postulated that the conversion of soluble β-protein into an insoluble amyloidogenic β-pleated sheet conformation may be a stochastic event occurring at a low level in normal aged brains. The probability of this happening may be enhanced by mutations in the APP gene on chromosome 21 which alter the primary sequence of the protein, or by an over-production of the precursor protein as in trisomy-21 Down's cases, or as a result of head trauma as seen in brain-damaged boxers. The presence of some of the insoluble forms of β-protein may act as a catalyst or seed for the conversion of more protein to the insoluble form and lead to the initially slow but accelerating amyloid plaque formation. The demonstration that the brains of monkeys contained amyloid plaques and CAA some years after inoculation with brain tissue containing β-amyloid provides evidence to support this model of amyloidosis.

REFERENCE

1. BAKER, H. F., L. W. DUCHEN, J. M. JACOBS & R. M. RIDLEY. 1990. Spongiform encephalopathy transmitted experimentally from Creutzfeldt-Jakob and familial Gerstmann-Sträussler-Scheinker diseases. Brain **113:**1891–1909.

The Age of Biosenescence and the Incidence of Cerebral β-Amyloidosis in Aged Captive Rhesus Monkeys[a]

H. UNO[b,d] AND L. C. WALKER[c]

[b] *Regional Primate Research Center and Department of Pathology and Laboratory Medicine, School of Medicine, University of Wisconsin, Madison, 53706 USA*
[c] *Department of Pathology, Neuropathology Laboratory, The Johns Hopkins University School of Medicine, Baltimore, Maryland 21205 USA*

ABSTRACT: Autopsy surveillance of 186 rhesus monkeys aged 20 to 36 years revealed that development of major geriatric diseases such as emphysema, coronary sclerosis, and cancer increased rapidly after the age of 25 years, and nearly 70% of the monkeys in each cohort group died by 30 years. According to our 12-year longitudinal survey, the age of biosenescence in captive rhesus monkeys begins around 25 years and the maximum longevity is 36 years. The incidence of cerebral β-amyloidosis associated with plaque formation and cerebral angiopathy was observed in 51 brains of rhesus monkeys aged 25 to 36 years. Lesions were found in 31 of 51 aged brains (60%) and 6 monkeys over 34 years of age were all severely affected. Despite the size of the plaque, nearly all of them showed immunopositive β-amyloid. Cerebral angiopathy coexisted in 10 of 31 plaque-positive brains. The basal prefrontal gyrus was the most common site and contained the highest density of plaques, followed by the amygdala region. The amyloid in the liver, spleen, adrenal and pancreatic islets in visceral amyloidosis showed no positivity to the β-amyloid demonstrated in the brain. As in aged human brains, the incidence of age-dependent cerebral β-amyloidosis in captive rhesus monkeys showed great individual variation.

The occurrence of cerebral β-amyloidosis, the deposition of amyloid-β protein (ABP) in senile plaques and meningeal and cerebral vessel walls of nonhuman primates, has been widely reported.[1–7] Although the neurofibrillar tangles are generally absent in the aged monkey brain, a complete homology of amyloid precursor protein (APP) and essential similarities of the plaques and angiography in monkey and human brains suggests that the

[a] This research and maintenance of the aging rhesus monkey colony were supported by NIH Grant RR00167 and the National Institute of Aging.
[d] *Send correspondence to:* H. Uno, M.D., Ph.D., Wisconsin Regional Primate Research Center, 1223 Capitol Court, Madison, WI 53715-1299 USA; TEL: (608) 263-3529; FAX: (608) 263-4031.

aging process in the monkey brain would be a good model of human Alzheimer's disease and other cerebral amyloidosis.[8]

During the past 10 years, the population in our aging colony of rhesus monkeys (aged over 20 years) had an annual average of 93 live animals and 15 deaths. Among this population a complete cessation of menses and ovarian folliculogenesis occurred around 26 years of age. By 30 years of age 50 to 70% of each cohort group had died, and maximum longevity was 36 years.

Autopsy surveillance of 186 cases of monkeys aged 20 to 36 years revealed that major geriatric pathology of organs increased rapidly after 26 years (postmenopausal age); over 50% of animals manifested emphysema and coronary sclerosis and 30% developed cancers of the colon and other organs. Cerebral disorders with paralysis and MRI-detectable multiple infarctions were found in only four cases. Together with other geriatric symptoms such as loss of motility, cataracta, tooth decay, arthritic disorders, and dried teleangiectatic skin, we defined the age of biosenescence in captive rhesus monkeys as that period beginning around 25 years of age.

Although spontaneously developed systemic amyloidosis in rhesus monkeys occurred in various age groups, 5 of 11 cases were encountered in animals aged 25 to 28 years. Amyloid deposition in the pancreatic islets in 6 aged monkeys was usually found in postmortem study, but a few cases were known to have hyperglycemia associated with low insulin levels. The islets showing a varying rate of endocrine cell depletion contained diffuse or focal deposition of amyloid. Ultrastructurally, the amyloid in both systemic and islet amyloidosis contained bundles of filaments and was largely found in the perisinusoidal or pericapillary space.

In the present study, we examined the presence of senile plaques and cerebral angiopathy in 51 brains of rhesus monkeys aged 25 to 36 years. The sections of the basal prefrontal, hippocampal with entorhinal, front-parietal gyri, and the amygdala were examined by both the silver-impregnation method and immunocytochemistry with amyloid-β protein antibody (10D5). Using the same antibody, the liver, spleen, and adrenal gland with systemic amyloidosis in 5 cases and the pancreas with amyloid deposits in the islets in 6 cases of aged monkeys were examined in the presence of ABP for such visceral amyloid. Immuno-staining of amyloid precursor protein was performed in the brain section containing large numbers of plaques and amyloid angiopathy. Ultrastructural observations were also aimed at the plaques and cerebral vessels.

There was a substantial rate of individual variation in the incidence and regional density of the plaques with or without cerebral angiopathy. Surprisingly, 20 of 51 aged brains had no detectable plaque formations and angiopathy in examined brain regions. Among 31 plaque-positive cases, 21 were found in brains aged 25 to 30 years (56% positive) and 10 in ages over 31 years (71% positive). Overall sexual differences were 7 positive cases in 10 male (70%) and 22 positive cases in 41 female brains (53%). The density of plaques per 1 mm^2 area of section varied greatly in each region and individual. However, the basal prefrontal gyri (area 10, 11, 25) generally contained the highest incidence and density of plaques; approximately 30% of brains showed an average of 12 plaques per 1 mm^2. The amygdala was the next highest region and the hippocampal and pre- and post-central (area 4.3-1.) gyri contained sporadic plaques.

Most plaques consisted of swollen neurites associated with diffuse or nodular amorphous mass demonstrated by immunopositive ABP and ultrastructural amyloid filaments. Some of the plaques were closely associated with dilated vessels surrounded by an amyloid cuff. Cerebral or meningeal amyloid angiopathy coexisted in 10 out of 31 plaque-positive brains. Immunopositive ABP densely surrounded by perivascular walls and ultrastructural amyloid mass occupied the intercellular space of vascular smooth muscles.

Although APP could not be detected in the plaques or cerebral vessels of these brain sections, this negative finding was considered to be largely due to the tissues being kept in formalin solution for a long period of time.

Four out of five cases of systemic amyloidosis had senile plaques in the brain. The amyloid masses in the liver, spleen, and adrenal glands of these five cases showed no immunopositive ABP. Three out of six cases of pancreatic islet amyloidosis had plaques. ABP was demonstrated in the capillary endothelial cells of the islet which contained the amyloid deposit, but not in the capillaries of normal islets and interlobular tissues.

In conclusion, as in the human senescent brain, cerebral β-amyloidosis was not the ubiquitous outcome in rhesus monkeys of the senescent age group. However, of six monkeys reaching the age of maximum longevity, 34 to 36 years, all had a rather high density of plaque formation, although none displayed amyloid angiopathy. This may suggest that ABP in the plaques was derived directly from APP in degenerated neurites, but not entirely from the vascular source.

It is generally accepted that the amyloid protein in systemic amyloidosis has different components than ABP. Indeed, the present study showed no presence of ABP in visceral amyloidosis. Although specificity and cross-reactivity with other peptides in the islet cells have not been confirmed, the capillary endothelial cells in the amyloid-laden islet of the pancreas showed positive immuno-reactivity to ABP.

The cerebral β-amyloidosis of aged monkeys appears to be a useful model for histogenesis of the senile plaques and amyloidogenesis in the plaques or in the perivascular space of the cerebral vessels.

REFERENCES

1. WISNIEWSKI, H.M., B. GHETTI & R. D. TERRY. 1973. Neuritic (senile) plaques and filamentous changes in aged rhesus monkeys. JNEN **32:**566–584.

2. STRUBLE, R. G., D. L. PRICE JR., L. C. CORK & D. L. PRICE. 1985. Senile plaques in cortex of aged normal monkeys. Brain Res. **361:**267–275.

3. PRICE, D. L., L. C. CORK, R. G. STRUBLE, C. A. KITT, D. L. PRICE, JR., J. LEHMANN & J. C. HEDREEN. 1985. Neuropathological, neurochemical and behavioral studies of the aging nonhuman primate. *In* Behavior and Pathology of Aging in Rhesus monkeys. 113–135. Alan R. Liss, Inc. New York.

4. IWATA, T. 1986. Studies on senile changes in the brains in monkeys (Macaca fuscata). I. On Senile Plaque. Acta Sch. Med. Univ. Gifu **34:**540–550.

5. WALKER, L. C. & C. A. KITT. 1987. Senile plaques in aged squirrel monkeys. Neurobiol. Aging **8:**291–296.

6. CORK, L. C., C. MASTERS, K. BEYREUTHER & D. L. PRICE. 1990. Development of senile plaques. Relationships of neuronal abnormalities and amyloid deposits. Am. J. Pathol. **137:**1383–1392.

7. UNO, H., C. THIEME, P. ALSUM, R. RICHARDSON & W. D. HOUSER. 1991. Incidence of senile plaque in brains of aged rhesus monkeys. Lab. Investigation **64:**103A.

8. HEDREEN, J. C., L. S. RASKIN, M. D. APPLEGATE, D. L. PRICE & J. C. TRON-COSO. 1990. A quick silver method for senile plaques and a comparison of eight methods for the demonstration of senile plaques. Neuropathol. Exp. Neurol. **49:**308.

9. TOMLINSON, B. E., G. BLESSED & M. ROTH. 1968. Observations on the brains of non-demented old people. J. Neurol. Sci. **7:**331–356.

10. DAYAN, A. D. 1970. Quantitative histological studies on the aged human brain. Acta. Neuropathol. **16:**85–102.

Cholinergic and Non-cholinergic Synaptic Mechanisms in the Aged Rat Hippocampus[a]

B. POTIER, Y. LAMOUR, AND P. DUTAR[b]

*Laboratoire de Physiopharmacologie du Système Nerveux INSERM U 161,
75014 Paris, France*

ABSTRACT: We compared age-related alterations in the electrophysiological and pharmacological properties of CA1 hippocampal pyramidal neurons in three strains of rats (Sprague-Dawley, Fisher 344 and Wistar) at 3–4 and 25–32 months of age, using the *in vitro* slice preparation. The most consistent age-related alterations were: a decrease in membrane excitability, a decrease in the amplitude and duration of inhibitory postsynaptic potentials and a decreased sensitivity to the effect of the cholinergic agonist carbachol. In contrast, no consistent alterations in calcium-dependent events were observed in these strains of rats. The age-related changes in the duration of the after-hyperpolarization (AHP) were different (and even opposite) depending on the strain studied. Our results show that age-related changes observed in a given strain are not necessarily present in all strains of the same species.

INTRODUCTION

One of the main questions in studies of age-related alterations in laboratory animals is: how general can our conclusions be? In other words, to what extent observations made in a given species can be generalized to other species and specially to man? One way to answer this difficult question is to compare age-related alterations in different species or at least in different strains within the same species. Unfortunately, cross-species comparisons or even comparison between strains are rare in the literature. No studies comparing the electrophysiological properties of central neurons in different strains of aged rats are currently available. The present experiment was designed to compare the age-related changes in electrophysiological and pharmacological properties of CA1 pyramidal hippocampal neurons in three different strains of rats: Sprague-Dawley, Wistar, and Fisher 344.

[a] This work was supported by grants from Bayer Pharma France and MGEN.
[b] *Send correspondence to:* Dr. P. Dutar, Laboratoire de Physiopharmacologie du Système Nerveux, INSERM/Unité 161, 2 rue d'Alésia, 75014 Paris, France; TEL: 33-1-45-89-36-62; FAX: 33-1-45-88-13-04.

METHODS

The young (3–4 months, n = 15) and aged (25–32 months, n = 25) male Sprague-Dawley rats (SD) and the young and aged male Fisher 344 (F344) rats (3–4 months, n = 10 and 25 months, n = 9) were purchased from IFFA-CREDO (France). Young and aged male Wistar (WIS) rats (respectively 3–4 months, n = 15 and 25–27 months n = 15) were obtained from Troponwerke Gmbh (Germany). One young or one aged rat was studied alternatively each day. Standard intracellular recordings techniques in the current-clamp mode were used to record membrane potential and resistance, sodium and calcium action potential amplitudes and durations, afterhyperpolarization amplitude and duration, and various synaptic events (slow cholinergic excitatory postsynaptic potential, excitatory and inhibitory postsynaptic potentials due to the release of respectively excitatory amino-acids and GABA) from CA1 pyramidal neurons, in the *in vitro* hippocampal slice preparation.[1]

RESULTS

Sprague-Dawley Rats

No age-related differences were observed in resting membrane potential, input resistance, amplitude of the action potential or amplitude of the calcium spike. In contrast, the neuronal excitability (defined as the amplitude of the depolarizing current pulse necessary for the occurrence of one spike) was significantly decreased and the spike duration significantly increased in the aged rats as compared to the young rats. No consistent increase in AHP duration was observed. The depolarizing effect of bath-applied carbachol, as well as the associated increase in membrane resistance were reduced in neurons from the aged rats. In contrast, the effects of carbachol on the depression of synaptic events and the blockade of the AHP were similar in young and aged rats. The amplitude of the slow cholinergic excitatory postsynaptic potential induced by stimulation of the cholinergic afferents was also decreased in aged rats. The amplitude and duration of the excitatory postsynaptic potential (EPSP) following electrical stimulation of stratum radiatum were increased in the aged rats, but the difference did not reach statistical significance. The amplitude and duration of the fast inhibitory postsynaptic potential (IPSP) were not significantly modified in the aged rats. In contrast, the duration of the slow IPSP was significantly decreased. Since the hyperpolarization induced by baclofen was only slightly reduced in the aged rats, the most likely explanation is a decrease in the release of GABA, rather than an alteration of the postsynaptic response mediated by the GABA$_B$ receptors.

Wistar Rats

No age-related changes were observed in resting membrane potential, membrane input resistance, shape of the action potential or calcium spike. In contrast, the excitability was significantly decreased in aged rats. The duration of the AHP was significantly decreased. No significant differences were observed between young and aged animals in the amplitude or the duration of the EPSP, but the amplitude as well as the duration of the IPSP were decreased. The amplitude of the depolarization induced by carbachol was strongly and significantly depressed.

Fisher 344 Rats

No age-related differences were observed in resting membrane potential, membrane input resistance or in the shape of the action potential. As for SD and WIS, the excitability was decreased in the aged F 344 rats, but the difference was not statistically significant. No significant age-related change was observed in the amplitude of the AHP. Amplitude and duration of the EPSP did not differ between young and aged animals. In contrast, the duration of the IPSP was significantly decreased. The mean carbachol-induced depolarization was significantly decreased in aged rats, whereas the mean balofen-induced hyperpolarization was not significantly altered.

Comparison between Rat Strains

Several electrophysiological parameters such as resting membrane potential, membrane resistance, amplitude of the sodium spike, calcium spike, and EPSP are not significantly modified by aging in the three strains studied. In contrast, the excitability of the neurons is consistently decreased in the aged rats. The results concerning the AHPs are more complex: the duration of the AHP is decreased in the aged WIS rat while it tends to be slightly (but not significantly) increased in the other two strains. The age-related changes in the pharmacological properties of CA1 pyramidal neurons were similar in the three strains: the carbachol-induced depolarization was significantly smaller in aged animals, whereas no change in the baclofen-induced hyperpolarization was observed. Similarly, the amplitude and duration of the IPSP (which reflect the effect of GABA released from CA1 afferents) are significantly smaller in the aged rats.

DISCUSSION

The decrease in neuronal excitability in the aged rats observed in the present study was not associated with a change in membrane potential or membrane resistance. Our results suggest an age-related alteration in the mechanism of the sodium spike generation (see, however, refs. 2 and 3). The age-related changes in the duration of the AHP (which is driven by activation of a calcium-dependent potassium conductance) are not consistent among strains of rats. Therefore, the hypothesis of an increased calcium influx following the action potential in the neurons of the aged rat does not seem to be tenable for all strains (see refs. 4 and 5). Clearly, the age-related changes observed in the AHP duration in the three strains are different and cannot be explained by a single mechanism. Therefore, the AHP duration is not a reliable marker of neuronal aging in the rat brain.

Age-related changes in the pharmacology of CA1 hippocampal neurons were similar in the strains studied. Carbachol-induced depolarizations were decreased in aged WIS and F344 rats to the same extent as in aged SD rats. The reduced effect of carbachol suggests that the density and/or the affinity of the muscarinic receptors is decreased in the aged rat.[6,7] The data available in the literature on muscarinic receptors in the aged rat are inconsistent. It is thus difficult to know if the age-related change takes place at the receptor level, at the transduction mechanism level, or at the presynaptic level.

The size of the EPSP was not significantly altered in the aged rats, suggesting that the efficacy of the excitatory transmission is preserved during senescence. In contrast, there is an age-related decrease in IPSP duration in the three strains, due to a decrease in the duration of the slow phase of the IPSP. The slow IPSP is due to the action of GABA acting on $GABA_B$ receptors. The decreased duration of the IPSP strongly suggests an alteration of the $GABA_B$ response or a decrease in GABA release. However, we failed to observe any significant difference in the postsynaptic response to baclofen. This result suggests that the main alteration is probably a decrease in GABA release.

REFERENCES

1. POTIER, B., O. RASCOL, F. JAZAT, Y. LAMOUR & P. DUTAR. 1992. Alterations in the properties of hippocampal pyramidal neurons in the aged rat. Neuroscience **48:**793–806.
2. BARNES, C. A. & B. L. MCNAUGHTON. 1980. Physiological compensation for loss of afferent synapses in rat hippocampal granule cells during senescence. J. Physiol. **309:**473–485.
3. BARNES, C. A., G. RAO & B. L. MCNAUGHTON. 1987. Increased electrotonic

coupling in aged rat hippocampus: A possible mechanism for cellular excitability changes. J. Comp. Neurol. **259:**549–558.

4. LANDFIELD, P. W. & T. A. PITLER. 1984. Prolonged Ca^{2+}-dependent after-hyperpolarizations in hippocampal neurons of aged rats. Science **226:** 1089–1092.

5. REYNOLDS, J. N. & P. L. CARLEN. 1989. Diminished calcium currents in aged hippocampal dentate gyrus granule neurones. Brain Res. **479:**384–390.

6. LIPPA, A. S., D. J. CRITCHET, F. EHLERT, H. I. YAMAMURA, S. J. ENNA & R. T. BARTUS. 1981. Age-related alterations in neurotransmitter receptors. An electrophysiological and biochemical analysis. Neurobiol. Aging **2:**3–8.

7. SEGAL, M. 1982. Changes in neurotransmitter actions in the aged rat hippocampus. Neurobiol. Aging **3:**121–124.

Phospholipid and Phospholipid Metabolites in Rat Frontal Cortex Are Decreased following Nucleus Basalis Lesions[a]

TODD C. HOLMES, ROGER M. NITSCH, ANDREAS ERFURTH, AND RICHARD J. WURTMAN

Department of Brain and Cognitive Sciences, Massachusetts Institute of Technology, Cambridge, Massachusetts 02139 USA

ABSTRACT: Membrane phospholipid metabolism is abnormal in Alzheimer's disease (AD) brain. Phosphatidylcholine and phosphatidylethanolamine levels are decreased as are choline and ethanolamine, while glycerophosphocholine (GPC) and glycerophosphoethanolamine are increased.[1] To develop a rat model for these changes, we examined the effects of unilateral lesion of the cholinergic nucleus basalis (nBM) with ibotenic acid (10 mg/ml in PBS, 0.5 μl) and sham lesion on frontocortical phospholipid, choline and GPC. After one week, choline acetyltransferase activity in frontal cortex was decreased (26%, $p<0.005$, n=14) on the nBM ibotenate-lesion side relative to the contralateral side, while there were no differences following the nBM sham-lesion. Levels of membrane phospholipids (nmol/mg protein) in adjacent frontal cortex sections exhibited concomitant decreases (13%, $p<0.05$, n=14) on the nBM ibotenate-lesion side, while there were no differences following the nBM sham-lesion. Tissue nBM ibotenate-lesion frontocortical choline and GPC levels were also decreased relative to those in control tissues (choline: 21%, $p<0.05$, n=14; GPC:10%, $p<0.05$, n=14), while nBM sham-lesion showed no effect. Muscarinic receptor sensitivity in frontal cortex following nBM ibotenate-lesion was increased, as measured by carbachol-stimulated inositol phosphate production ($p<0.001$, n=12), indicating that increased receptor mediated phospholipid hydrolysis in cortex may occur following nBM ibotenate-lesion. These data suggest that impaired cholinergic transmission alters phospholipid metabolism in cholinergic target regions.

INTRODUCTION

The cerebral cortex receives major ascending inputs from neurotransmitter-specific subcortical nuclei, including cholinergic projections from the basal

[a] This research is supported by the National Institutes of Health, the NIA, and the Center for Brain Sciences and Metabolism Charitable Trust.

[b] *Send correspondence to:* T. Holmes, Department of Brain and Cognitive Sciences, E25-604/ M.I.T., Cambridge, MA 02139 USA; TEL: (617) 253-6706; FAX: (617) 253-6882.

forebrain nucleus basalis (nBM). There is evidence that this projection is compromised in the aging process and in neurodegenerative disorders such as Alzheimer's disease (AD).[2]

To determine whether abnormal phospholipid metabolism may occur as a consequence of impaired cholinergic transmission in the frontal cortex, we measured tissue phospholipid and phospholipid metabolites in cortical projection areas in rats one week after unilateral ibotenic acid lesions and sham lesion of the nBM. As phospholipid hydrolysis by phospholipases can be mediated by extracellular receptors, carbachol-stimulated inositol phosphate levels were also measured in frontal cortex one week following nBM lesion as an index of muscarinic receptor sensitivity.[3]

RESULTS AND DISCUSSION

ChAT activity in frontal cortex sections adjacent to tissue processed for phospholipids and phospholipid metabolites was significantly decreased ($p<0.005$, n = 14, Newman-Keuls test) by 26% on the nBM ibotenate-lesion side relative to the contralateral side one week following the lesion. The nBM sham-lesion did not effect ChAT activity in frontal cortex.

Tissue frontocortical phospholipid levels were decreased on the nBM ibotenate-lesion side relative to the non-lesioned contralateral control side by 13% one week following the lesion ($p<0.05$, n = 14, Newman-Keuls test), while nBM sham-lesion showed no effect. Tissue phospholipid water soluble metabolites were also decreased in nBM ibotenate-lesion side cortex relative to contralateral non-lesioned cortex. Choline levels were decreased by 21% ($p<0.05$, n = 14, Newman-Keuls test). In contrast to AD brain tissue, GPC levels were 10% lower in nBM ibotenate-lesion frontal cortex ($p<0.05$, n = 14, Newman-Keuls test). Tissues from nBM sham ibotenate-lesioned rats showed no difference in their levels of these metabolites.

Cortical muscarinic receptor sensitivity to agonist stimulation following nBM ibotenate-lesion was determined by comparing the ratio of lesion side carbachol response to control side carbachol response on inositol phosphate accumulation, using the method of Berridge.[3] Muscarinic receptor sensitivity linearly increased relative to the severity of the nBM lesion as measured by ChAT activity ($p<0.01$, n = 12, linear regression test). Further studies are underway to determine whether similar post-lesion increases occur in muscarinic-coupled phospholipase D activation and/or changes in phospholipid biosynthesis. The transmitter-specific lesion approach shows promise for examining phospholipid and acetylcholine metabolic interactions *in vivo* and may be useful for elucidating compensatory mechanisms for supporting neurotransmission following brain lesions.

ACKNOWLEDGMENTS

We would like to thank Drs. Barbara Slack and Arthur Lander for helpful discussions.

REFERENCES

1. NITSCH, R. N., J. K. BLUSZTAJN, A. G. PITTAS, B. E. SLACK, J. H. GROWDON & R. J. WURTMAN. 1992. Evidence for a membrane defect in Alzheimer's disease brain. Proc. Natl. Acad. Sci. USA **89:**1671–1675.
2. WURTMAN, R. J. 1992. Choline metabolism as a basis for the selective vulnerability of cholinergic neurons. TINS **15:**117–122.
3. BERRIDGE, M. J., C. P. DOWNES & M. R. HANLEY. 1982. Lithium amplified agonist-dependent phosphatidylinositol responses in brain and salivary glands. Biochem. J. **206:**587–595.

Decreased Density of Forebrain Cholinergic Neurons and Disintegration of the Spatial Organization of Behavior in Experimental Autoimmune Dementia (EAD)[a]

DANIEL M. MICHAELSON,[b] VLADIMIR DUBOVIK,
MARIA FAIGON, DAVID EILAM, AND JORAM FELDON

Tel Aviv University, Ramat Aviv 69978 Israel

ABSTRACT: Experimental autoimmune dementia (EAD) is a rat model designed to examine the potential role of anti-cholinergic neurons antibodies (Abs) in the neuropathology of Alzheimer's disease (AD) and dementia. We have previously shown that sera of AD and Down's syndrome patients contain Abs which bind specifically to the high molecular weight neurofilament protein (NF-H) of the purely cholinergic electromotor neurons of Torpedo. Production of such Abs in EAD rats by prolonged immunization with Torpedo cholinergic NF-H results in the accumulation of IgG in the septum and hippocampus of the immunized rats and in memory deficits.

In the present study, we examined immunohistochemically whether the anti-cholinergic NF-H immune response of the EAD rats affects their brain cholinergic neurons. In addition, since dementia is associated with severe deterioration in the spatio-temporal organization of behavior, we examined whether EAD rats also mimic this important feature of dementia. The results obtained show that production in EAD rats of anti-cholinergic NF-H Abs similar to those found in AD patients results in a marked decrease in the density of forebrain cholinergic neurons and in derangements in the spatio-temporal organization of their behavior. These findings may replicate pathogenic processes in AD and support a role for anti-cholinergic NF-H Abs in the degeneration of cholinergic neurons in the disease.

[a] This work was supported in part by grants to D.M.M. from the United States-Israel Binational Science Foundation (grant 89/86) and from The Harold Hyam Wingate Foundation Ltd., and by a grant to D.E. from the Israel Institute for Psychobiology.
[b] *Send correspondence to:* Daniel M. Michaelson, Department of Biochemistry, Tel Aviv University, Ramat Aviv 69978, Israel; TEL: (972)-3-6409624; FAX: (972)-3-6415053.

INTRODUCTION

We have previously shown that the heavy neurofilament protein NF-H of cholinergic neurons differs antigenically from that of chemically heterogeneous NF-H and that the degeneration of brain cholinergic neurons in Alzheimer's disease (AD) and in Down's syndrome is associated with serum IgG directed specifically against Torpedo and mammalian cholinergic NF-H.[1–3] In order to examine whether these antibodies (Abs) could play a role in neuronal degeneration in AD, we developed a rat model in which the cellular and behavioral effects of anti-cholinergic NF-H Abs are being examined. This model is termed Experimental Autoimmune Dementia (EAD).

Production of anti-cholinergic NF-H Abs in EAD rats by prolonged immunization with Torpedo cholinergic NF-H results in accumulation of IgG in the septum and hippocampus of the immunized rats and in memory deficits.[4,5] In the present study, we examined immunohistochemically whether the anti-cholinergic NF-H immune response of the EAD rats affects their brain cholinergic neurons. In addition, since dementia is associated with severe deterioration of the spatio-temporal organization of behavior,[6] we examined whether EAD rats also mimic this important feature of dementia. To enable an examination of the specificity of the neuronal and behavioral changes to the anti-cholinergic NF-H immune response of the EAD rats, three groups of rats were studied. They are: rats immunized with Torpedo cholinergic NF-H (EAD rats), rats immunized with the chemically heterogeneous Torpedo spinal cord NF-H (NFHC rats), and sham-injected controls.

RESULTS

Immunohistochemical Studies

The densities of forebrain cholinergic neurons in four EAD brains, four brains of NFHC rats and four brains of sham-injected controls were quantitated immunohistochemically utilizing an anti–low affinity nerve growth factor receptor monoclonal antibody.[7] TABLE 1 represents the results thus obtained in the medial septum and the vertical limb of the diagonal band (MS + DBv); in the horizontal limb of the diagonal band (DBh), and in the nucleus magnocellularis preoptic (MaPo). As can be seen, the average density of cholinergic neurons in the MS + DBv, in the DBh, and in the MaPo of the NFHC and sham-injected controls were virtually identical and were markedly higher than the corresponding values of the EAD rats. Maximal effect was observed in the MS + DBv where the density of cholinergic neurons of the

TABLE 1. Density of Forebrain Cholinergic Neurons

Brain Area	Control Rats	EAD Rats	NFHC Rats
MS + DBv	34.0 ± 1.2	26.3 ± 2.1[a]	33.4 ± 2.0
DBh	51.9 ± 3.6	44.6 ± 3.2	51.0 ± 4.2
MaPo	53.7 ± 2.9	46.8 ± 2.1	51.7 ± 1.5

The number of cholinergic neurons per mm^2 in the medial septum and the vertical limb of the diagonal band (MS + DBv), in the horizontal limb of the diagonal band (DBh) and in the magnocellular preoptic nucleus (MaPo), were measured immunohistochemically utilizing a monoclonal antibody against low affinity nerve growth factor receptors.[6] Results presented are the mean ± SEM of four rats in each group.

[a] $p < 0.05$.

EAD rats decreased by about 25%, whereas in the DBh and MaPo the decrease was only about 15%. Statistical analysis by ANOVA revealed a significant main effect of rat group and that the decreased density of cholinergic neurons in the EAD group was significant (F = 4.22, df 2/9, $p < 0.05$).

Behavioral Studies

Behavior of freely moving normal rats in the open field is spatio-temporally organized: they rapidly establish a home base from which they perform round trips of exploration of the open field. These round trips encompass most of the available area and are executed mainly along the walls of the open field.[8–10] In the present study, we analyzed the open field behavior of the EAD rats and employed it to examine whether the spatio-temporal organization of their behavior is impaired. The following results were obtained:

The Amount and Speed of Locomotion

The distance traveled by the EAD rats in the open field during the 30 minute observation period was 6 times lower than that of the control and NFHC rats. However, the speed of locomotion of the EAD rats was similar to that of the two groups. Furthermore, the activity of the EAD rats as measured in a small "activity monitor" was indistinguishable from that of the NFHC and sham-injected controls. This suggests that the reduced amount of locomotion of EAD rats is not due to motor disability but is linked to the specific testing conditions in the open field.

Spatial and Temporal Distribution of Locomotion

In addition to reduced locomotion, the organization of the behavior of the EAD rats differed from those of the NFHC and control rats in that: 1)

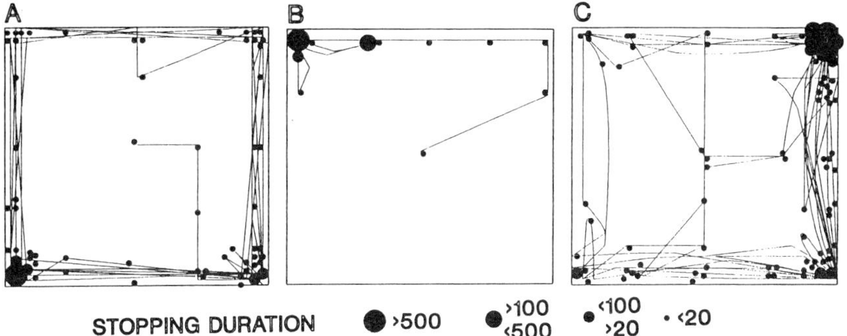

FIGURE 1. Representative trajectories of locomotion in the open field of a control rat (**A**), an EAD rat (**B**), and an NFHC rat (**C**). The squared enclosures correspond to the open field. Each circle represents a single stop and its diameter represents the duration of the stop as indicated in the figure. Lines represent the path of locomotion between successive stops.

They explored a smaller portion of the open field (~25% vs. 80% explored by both the NFHC and control rats); 2) they performed fewer round trips out of the location in which they spent the longest stopping time, namely the home base (2.1 ± 0.5 round trips vs. 8.4 ± 1.4 and 10.2 ± 2 round trips performed by the NFHC and control rats). These differences are illustrated in FIGURE 1, which depicts the trajectories of locomotion of a representative rat from each group. The decrease in explored space and number of round trips of the EAD rats was also apparent when the spatial and temporal distribution of locomotion of the three rat groups were compared for the same amount of locomotion and number of stops. This implies that the shrinkage of the explored space and the decrease in number of round trips of the EAD rats are independent of the level of locomotion and stem from a more general change in the spatio-temporal organization of open field behavior.

CONCLUSION

The present results show that production in EAD rats of anti-cholinergic NF-H Abs similar to those found in AD patients results in a marked decrease in the density of forebrain cholinergic neurons and in derangements in the spatio-temporal organization of their behavior. These changes are specific to the anti-cholinergic NF-H immune response of the EAD rats and are not observed in NFHC rats, which were immunized with chemically heterogeneous NF-H. These findings may replicate pathogenic processes in AD and support a role for anti-cholinergic NF-H Abs in the degeneration of cholinergic neurons in the disease.

REFERENCES

1. CHAPMAN, J., O. BACHAR, A. D. KORCZYN, E. WERTMAN & D. M. MICHAELSON. 1989. Alzheimer's disease antibodies bind specifically to a neurofilament protein in Torpedo cholinergic neurons. J. Neurosci. **9:**2710–2717.
2. HASSIN-BAER, S., E. WERTMAN, M. RAPHAEL, V. STARK, J. CHAPMAN & D. M. MICHAELSON. 1992. Antibodies from Down syndrome patients bind to the same cholinergic neurofilament protein recognized by Alzheimer's disease antibodies. Neurology **42:**551–555.
3. TCHERNAKOV, K., L. SOUSSAN, S. HASSIN-BAER, E. WERTMAN & D. M. MICHAELSON. 1992. Alzheimer's disease and Down's syndrome antibodies bind to the heavy neurofilament protein of cholinergic neurons. Res. Immunol. **143:** 671–675.
4. CHAPMAN, J., G. ALROY, Z. WEISS, M. FAIGON, J. FELDON & D. M. MICHAELSON. 1991. Anti-neuronal antibodies similar to those found in Alzheimer's disease induce memory dysfunction in rats. Neuroscience **40:**297–305.
5. MICHAELSON, D. M., G. ALROY, L. SOUSSAN, J. CHAPMAN & J. FELDON. 1991. Experimental autoimmune dementia (EAD): An immunological model of memory dysfunction and Alzheimer's disease. *In* Pharmacological Basis of Cholinergic Therapy in Alzheimer's Disease. R. E. Becker & E. Giacobini, Eds. 126–133. Birkhauser Inc. Boston.
6. ADAMS, R. D. & M. VICTOR. 1989. Principles of Neurology. McGraw-Hill. New York.
7. KORSCHING, S. & H. THOENEN. 1983. Nerve growth factor in sympathetic ganglia and corresponding target organs of the rat: Correlation with density of sympathetic innervation. Proc. Natl. Acad. Sci. USA **80:**3513–3516.
8. EILAM, D. & I. GOLANI. 1989. Home base of tame wild rats *(Rattus norvegicus)* in a novel laboratory environment. Behav. Brain Res. **34:**199–211.
9. GEYER, M. A. 1982. Variational and probabilistic aspects of exploratory behavior in space: Four stimulant styles. Psychopharmacol. Bull. **18:**48–51.
10. GOLANI, I., Y. BENJAMINI & D. EILAM. 1993. Stopping behavior: Constraints on exploration in rats *(Rattus norvegicus)*. Behav. Brain Res. **53:**21–33.

Age-related Increase in Galanin-binding Sites in the Rat Brain: Correlation with Behavioral Impairment[a]

P. KRZYWKOWSKI,[b] I. LAGNY-POURMIR,[c] F. JAZAT,[b]
Y. LAMOUR,[b,d] AND J. EPELBAUM[c]

[b] INSERM Unité 161, 2 rue d'Alésia, 75014 Paris, France
[c] INSERM Unité 159, 2 ter rue d'Alésia, 75014 Paris, France

ABSTRACT: The regional distribution of ^{125}I-galanin specific binding sites was determined by radioautography on brain sections in young (3- to 4-month-old) and aged (26- to 27-month-old) male Sprague-Dawley rats, previously tested for their performances in the Morris water maze task. In aged rats, a significant increase in specific binding was observed in piriform, perirhinal and entorhinal cortex, the CA1 field of the ventral hippocampus, ventral subiculum, and dorsal dentate gyrus, whereas no significant change was observed in the ventral dentate gyrus, the dorsal subiculum, the CA3 field of the hippocampus, the amygdala or the septal area. The area-specific regional increase in specific binding density in aged rats was significantly correlated with the impairment of their behavioral performances in the Morris water maze task. The change in ^{125}I-galanin specific binding in the aged rats was a result of an increase in the number of galanin-binding sites, without change in affinity.

INTRODUCTION

Galanin (Gal) is a 29 amino acid peptide, originally isolated from the small intestine of the pig.[1] Several immunocytochemical, *in situ* hybridization, and radioimmunoassay studies have shown its wide distribution in the peripheral and central nervous system.[2] The action of Gal in the brain involves the binding of the peptide to a high affinity and specific membrane recognition site that is sensitive to guanyl nucleotides. Gal-binding sites are widely distributed in the central nervous system and their regional localization generally fits with that of Gal-containing neuronal somata and fibers. The inhibitory action of Gal on ACh and histamine release in the hippocampus probably

[a] This work was supported in part by a grant from MGEN.
[d] *Send correspondence to:* Dr. Y. Lamour, INSERM/Unité 161, 2 rue d'Alésia, 75014 Paris, France; TEL: 33-1-45-893662; FAX: 33-1-45-881304.

involves presynaptic hippocampal Gal receptors. In turn, post-synaptic Gal receptors in the ventral hippocampus mediate the inhibitory effect of Gal on carbachol-stimulated phosphoinositide breakdown. In patients with Alzheimer's- and Parkinson-type dementias, a hypertrophy of Gal-immunoreactive fibers has been observed in the NBM.[3] Since no data were so far available on Gal receptors in the aged rat, we determined: 1) the distribution of Gal-binding sites in the brain of aged rats as compared to young rats, and 2) whether an impaired performance in the Morris water maze task correlates with a change in Gal receptors.

RESULTS

Five young (3- to 4-month-old, 250–300 g) and seven aged (26- to 27-month-old, 650–800 g) male Sprague-Dawley rats were used for behavioral and autoradiographic experiments. The behavioral[4] and autoradiographic[5] procedures have been previously described.

Behavioral Tests

The mean latency to find the platform in the water maze ranged from 10.1 to 16.9 seconds in the young rats (invisible platform paradigm) and from 28.9 to 60 seconds for the aged rats. Therefore, all aged rats had impaired performances as compared to the young rats. An arbitrary cut-off of 45 seconds was chosen, resulting in two groups of aged rats: the least impaired ($n = 3$), and the most impaired ($n = 4$). Although the performances of the aged rats were not as good as those of the young rats, there was an improvement in performance over the trials for the least impaired rats. In contrast, no improvement was observed for the most impaired aged rats.

Distribution of Gal-binding Sites in Young and Aged Rat Brains

The most intensely labeled structures in the young rat brain are telencephalic areas, *i.e.* piriform and entorhinal cortices, ventral portion of the hippocampal formation (ventral subiculum) and amygdaloid complex. Dense labeling is also seen in the ventral part of the dentate gyrus and in sub-cortical regions: dorsal and lateral septum, bed nucleus of the stria terminalis and some hypothalamic nuclei. Some labeling is also observed in the septo-hippocampal and septo-fimbrial nuclei, in the ventral field CA1 of the hippocampus and in the dorsal part of the dentate gyrus. Little binding is observed in medial septum, diagonal band of Broca, field CA3 of the hippocampus and dorsal subiculum.

The regional pattern of ^{125}I-Gal binding is qualitatively similar in aged and young rats. The quantitative analysis of the radioautograms along the rostro-caudal axis shows that ^{125}I-Gal-specific binding is enhanced in aged rats as compared to young rats in selective areas such as piriform, perirhinal and entorhinal cortices, ventral CA1 field of the hippocampus, dorsal dentate gyrus and ventral subiculum. Moreover, when the aged rats are divided into two groups on the basis of their performances in the Morris water maze test, the increase of the ^{125}I-Gal-specific binding is consistently larger in the most impaired rats than in the least impaired rats. No age-dependent change in binding is observed in ventral dentate gyrus, dorsal subiculum, field CA3 of hippocampus, amygdala, or in the septal area.

There is a positive correlation between the latencies in the Morris water maze and the amount of ^{125}I-Gal-specific binding in the piriform cortex, the entorhinal cortex ($r = 0.6$, $p = 0.04$), the dorsal dentate gyrus ($p = 0.04$), the ventral subiculum ($p = 0.05$) (but not in the CA1 area), *i.e.,* the rats with the best behavioral performances have the lowest Gal-binding density in these structures.

Competition Experiment

The difference in ^{125}I-Gal-specific binding between the young and the most impaired rats is dependent on an increase in maximal specific binding (Bmax), without significant change in affinity. The values of maximal specific binding are 1666 ± 57 and 2227 ± 91 cpm/surface unit respectively for young and most impaired rats in the piriform cortex. The difference is statistically significant ($p < 0.01$). The values of the IC50 determined from these curves (0.16 ± 0.04 and 0.25 ± 0.07 nM, respectively for young and most impaired rats) did not differ significantly.

DISCUSSION

Our results in the young adult rat brain are in close agreement with previous reports of the regional distribution of Gal-binding sites as visualized by radioautographic techniques. The present study shows that there is no qualitative change in regional distribution in the aged rat brain. However, there is a significant increase in the amount of ^{125}I-Gal-specific binding in the aged rats in piriform, perirhinal and entorhinal cortex, field CA1 of the ventral hippocampus, ventral subiculum and dorsal dentate gyrus. This increase is due to an increased receptor number rather than to a change in affinity. No significant changes in binding sites density were observed in other structures such as the amygdala, the septal area, the dorsal subiculum, the field CA3 of the hippocampus or the ventral dentate gyrus. Thus, the increase in binding density in the aged rats is not a general increase but is area-specific. It is therefore likely that it is not due to a generalized and unspecific modification of neuronal membranes with age, but rather that it has a functional significance in relation with its topography. In this context, it is specially interesting to note that the largest increase in specific binding level is observed in animals with the worst performances in the Morris water maze task.

The relationships between Gal and behavioral performances are unclear. A few studies suggest that Gal could impair performances in the Morris water maze, or in a T-maze after icv injection.[2] In our own experiments,[6] a loss of Gal immunoreactive cells was found in the medial septa area,[7] though no clear relationship was found between the number of Gal positive neurons in the medial septum-diagonal band of Broca (MS-DBB) complex and behavioral performances in the aged rats. The present results suggest a correlation between behavioral performances and the density of Gal binding sites in specific brain regions in aged rats.

It is necessary to put our results in the context of the changes in neurotransmitter systems which occur in aged rodents and primates, and more specifically the changes in the cholinergic systems, since Gal and ACh are colocalized in the septo-hippocampal pathway. Alterations in the functions of the central cholinergic systems occur in physiological aging.[8,9] In patients with Alzheimer's disease, a significant decrease of cholinergic markers in the hippocampal formation and neocortex and a loss of cholinergic neurons in the basal forebrain are observed. The "Gal component" of the cholinergic system, located in the MS-DBB complex, seems to be specially vulnerable to aging. We found an age-related decrease in the number of Galanin immunoreactive cells in the MS-DBB, but not in locus coeruleus or hypothalamus.[7] Taken together, our results show that there is not only a loss of Gal immunoreactive cells in the MS-DBB, but also an increased density of the Gal binding sites in some of the projection areas of the Gal-ACh system in the hippocampal formation. This is new evidence that complex changes occur in the septo-hippocampal system with aging.

REFERENCES

1. TATEMOTO, K., A. RÖKAEUS, H. JÖRNVALL, T. J. MCDONALD & V. MUTT. 1983. Galanin, a novel biologically active peptide from porcine intestine. FEBS Lett. **164:**124–128.
2. CRAWLEY, J. N. & G. L. WENK. 1989. Co-existence of galanin and acetylcholine: Is galanin involved in memory processes and dementia? TINS **12:**278–282.

3. CHAN-PALAY, V. 1988. Galanin hyperinnervates surviving neurons of the human basal nucleus of Meynert in dementias of Alzheimer's and Parkinson's disease: A hypothesis for the role of galanin in accentuating cholinergic dysfunction in dementia. J. Comp Neurol. **273**:543–557.

4. POTIER, B., O. RASCOL, F. JAZAT, Y. LAMOUR & P. DUTAR. 1992. Alterations in the properties of hippocampal pyramidal neurons in the aged rat. Neuroscience **48**:793–806.

5. LAGNY-POURMIR, I. & J. EPELBAUM. 1992. Regional stimulatory and inhibitory effects of guanine nucleotides on [^{125}I] galanin binding in rat brain: Relationship with the rate of occupancy of galanin receptors by endogenous galanin. Neuroscience **49**:829–847.

6. DE BILBAO, F., M. C. SENUT, J. SWEENEY, F. JAZAT & Y. LAMOUR. 1991. Etude comparative chez le rat âgé des déficits comportementaux et des modifications morphométriques des neurones contenant de la galanine dans la région septale médiane. C. R. Acad. Sci. Paris **312**(III):503–509.

7. DE BILBAO, F., F. JAZAT, Y. LAMOUR & M. C. SENUT. 1991. Age-related changes in galanin-immunoreactive cells of the rat medial septal area. J. Comp. Neurol. **313**:613–624.

8. DECKER, M. W. 1987. The effects of aging on hippocampal and cortical projections of the forebrain cholinergic systems. Brain Res. Rev. **12**:423–438.

9. LAMOUR Y., P. DUTAR, M. H. BASSANT & M. C. SENUT. 1989. Brain aging, Alzheimer's disease and neurotransmitters. *In* Neurotransmission and Cerebrovascular Function. Vol. 1:3–28. J. Seylaz & E. T. MacKenzie, Eds. Elsevier Science Publisher. Amsterdam.

Age-related Cognitive Deficits in Rats Are Associated with a Combined Loss of Cholinergic and Serotonergic Functions[a]

GAL RICHTER-LEVIN AND MENAHEM SEGAL[b]

Department of Neurobiology, The Weizmann Institute, Rehovot 76100 Israel

ABSTRACT: The cholinergic hypothesis of senile dementia proposes that an age-dependent reduction of central cholinergic functions accounts for the severe cognitive deficits seen in aged rats. A careful examination of the experimental evidence cited in support of this hypothesis reveals that it cannot account for some behavioral observations. We have modified this hypothesis and wish to propose that serotonin and acetylcholine interact to allow normal cognitive functions in the brain. Thus, a partial reduction in both cholinergic and serotonergic functions will cause severe memory impairment in young as well as in aged rats. We found that restoration of the serotonergic innervation in the hippocampus of serotonin depleted rats, using tissue transplants, can restore impaired behavior. We have localized a memory-related interaction between serotonin and acetylcholine in the hippocampus and are in the process of identifying a physiological function which may underly this interaction.

The cholinergic hypothesis of senile dementia, formulated over a decade ago[1] proposes that aging is associated with a loss of cholinergic neurotransmission, which is essential for some cognitive functions of the brain. This hypothesis is supported by several lines of evidence including a marked degeneration of cholinergic neurons found in aged brains,[2] the loss of cognitive functions following lesion of the forebrain cholinergic system,[3] and the effect of cholinergic drugs on cognitive functions. However, the cholinergic hypothesis does not provide a sufficient explanation for all of age-related cognitive deterioration. First, aging is associated with only a partial reduction of cholinergic functions,[4] reaching, at most, 50% of young adult values. Production of equivalent cholinergic damage in the young does not produce cognitive deficits.[5] Second, cholinergic drugs which are supposed to overcome the reduced

[a] Supported by a research grant from the Henry S. and Anne S. Reich Research Fund in Mental Health.

[b] *Send correspondence to:* M. Segal, Department of Neurobiology, The Weizmann Institute, Rehovot 76100 Israel; TEL: 972 8 342 553; FAX: 972 8 344 140.

cholinergic transmission (*e.g.*, anticholinesterases) do not ameliorate cognitive deficits in humans. On the basis of our results and others, we would like to modify the cholinergic hypothesis of senile dementia and propose that it is an interaction between the cholinergic and serotonergic systems in the forebrain that is crucial for the normal operation of cognitive functions of the brain. This hypothesis is based on results obtained with both young and aged rats in the following experiments:

Behavioral Studies

Spatial Performance Is Severely Impaired in Rats with a Combined Reduction of Cholinergic/Serotonergic Transmission[6]

We found that rats that were depleted of serotonin, using *p*-chlorophenylalanine (PCPA), and had a blockade of cholinergic neurotransmission, with atropine, were markedly impaired in water maze performance, unlike rats that were injected with only one drug, which were not different from controls. Similar results were obtained when the septo-hippocampal system was damaged, with either electolytic lesion[5] or septal injection of colchicine (unpublished), and the serotonergic system destroyed with the selective neurotoxin, 5,7-dihydroxytryptamine.

The Double Lesion-induced Behavioral Deficits Could Be Ameliorated by a Serotonin-containing Raphe Graft Implanted into the Hippocampus[7]

The graft grows in the host brain and sends fibers to innervate the hippocampus. Upon proper chemical stimulation, it can release serotonin which affects the electrical activity of the host. In serotonin-containing, raphe-grafted rats, the behavioral deficit associated with the double lesion, is no longer apparent. This restoration of behavioral functions was not seen when the graft was located in the host entorhinal cortex or hypothalamus. Non-serotonergic grafts were also unable to restore the impaired behavior.

Aged Rats Are Impaired in the Water Maze Spatial Memory Task, Like Young, Double-Lesioned Rats

The behavioral deficits are seen already in adult, non-aged, 14-month-old rats, but a severe deficit is clear in 2-year-old rats.

The Behavioral Deficits Seen in Aged Rats Could Be Ameliorated by Treatment with a Serotonergic Precursor, 5-Hydroxytryptophane (5-HTP)

While this precursor did not affect the behavior of young, normal rats, it did enhance water maze performance in the old rats. It did not affect other, non-cognitive performances. The treatment with 5-HTP enhances basal and evoked serotonin levels in the brain, as seen in experiments where serotonin effects on hippocampal activity were measured.

Physiological Studies

A series of physiological tests were conducted with the perforant path, the major excitatory afferent to the hippocampus, in an attempt to identify a parameter, or a series of parameters most affected by the double lesion of the serotonergic/cholinergic afferents to the hippocampus. Further attempts were made to determine if these changes can be restored by a serotonergic transplant. Once such parameters were identified, we searched for similar changes in aged rats. Among the parameters examined were input/output relationships, frequency responses (potentiation and depression), long-term potentiation, feed-back and feed-forward inhibition, and excitation. Several changes could be observed when single lesions were made, but the most striking effect of double lesions is on feed-forward inhibition, produced by priming stimulation of the commissural afferents to the hippocampal dentate gyrus. The reduced efficacy of the commissural inhibition is restored by a raphe graft in the hippocampus. Interestingly, aged rats are also impaired in commissure-evoked feed-forward inhibition.

These results suggest that the commissural connection is most relevant to the normal operation of the hippocampus, and that its disruption may be associated with impaired functions of the hippocampus. It is not clear at the present time, what might be the functional significance of this pathway, and further experiments are designed to test this.

The present experiments indicate that an interaction between the cholinergic and serotonergic systems is crucial for the normal operation of the hippocampus. It is not clear if the two neurotransmitters act independently on target neurons in the hippocampus or if they indeed interact. Indirect evidence exists in favor of the second possibility; serotonin can affect release of acetylcholine—and vice versa—and serotonin can serve to enable the action of acetylcholine on target neurons in the hippocampus. These possibilities are being examined now in *in vitro* preparations.

REFERENCES

1. BARTUS, R. T., R. L. DEAN, G. BEER & A. S. LIPPA. 1982. The cholinergic hypothesis of geriatric memory dysfunction. Science **217:**408–412.

2. FISCHER, W., K. S. CHEN, F. H. GAGE & A. BJORKLUND. 1991. Progressive decline in spatial learning and integrity of forebrain cholinergic neurons in rats during aging. Neurobiol. Aging **13**:9–24.

3. KELSEY, J. E. & B. A. LANDRY. 1988. Medial septal lesions disrupt spatial mapping ability in rats. Behav. Neurosci. **102**:289–293.

4. BIEGON, A., M. HANAU, V. GREENBERGER & M. SEGAL. 1989. Aging and brain cholinergic muscarinic subtypes: An autoradiographic study in the rat. Neurobiol. Aging **10**:305–310.

5. RICHTER-LEVIN, G. & M. SEGAL. 1991. The effects of serotonin depletion and raphe grafts on hippocampal electrophysiology and behavior. J. Neurosci. **11**:1585–1596.

6. RICHTER-LEVIN, G. & M. SEGAL. 1989. Spatial performance is severely impaired in rats with combined reduction of serotonergic and cholinergic transmission. Brain Res. **477**:404–407.

7. RICHTER-LEVIN, G. & M. SEGAL. 1990. Grafting of midbrain neurons into the hippocampus restores serotonin modulation of hippocampal activity in the rat. Brain Res. **521**:1–6.

Neural Transplantation for Neurodegenerative Diseases: Past, Present, and Future[a]

D. EUGENE REDMOND, JR.,[b,c,e] ROBERT H. ROTH,[b,c]
DENNIS D. SPENCER,[b] FREDERICK NAFTOLIN,[b]
CSABA LERANTH, RICHARD J. ROBBINS,[b]
KENNETH L. MAREK,[b] JOHN D. ELSWORTH,[b,c]
JANE R. TAYLOR,[b,c] KIMBERLEE J. SASS,[b]
JOHN R. SLADEK, JR.[c,d]

[b] *The Neural Transplant Program, Yale University School of Medicine,
New Haven, Connecticut 06510 USA*
[c] *The St. Kitts Biomedical Research Foundation, P.O. Box 47, Basseterre,
St. Kitts, West Indies*
[d] *The Chicago Medical School, Neuroscience Institute, 3333 Green Bay Road,
North Chicago, Illinois 60064-3095 USA*

ABSTRACT: After almost 100 years of sporadic, and marginally successful, studies of neural transplantation in animals, we are now on the threshold of a clinical treatment of the damaged brain. The initial studies of neural transplantation have focused on Parkinson's disease, primarily as a model for a more general strategy of "repair by cellular replacement." Parkinson's is known to result from the loss of a small population of cells that produce the essential neuromodulator, dopamine, for much of the brain. Further, the disease is improved significantly, during the early part of its course, by chemical augmentation of dopamine activity through drug therapies, such as L-dopa. Finally, the disease is often fatal in spite of the best medical treatments, therefore justifying more radical therapeutic experiments. If transplantation of brain cells can be accomplished successfully in humans, as it has been in animals, then replacement of a small population of dopamine-producing cells in Parkinson's disease should have important functional effects and possibly reverse the course and symptoms of the disease. Other useful applications will surely follow for conditions affecting millions of people for whom medicine now has only palliative and ineffective treatments.

Just as Parkinson's disease is a model clinical condition for testing cellular replacements, fetal neural tissue transplants are also a first step for a broader strategy of molecular and cellular therapies. Fetal cells are, in many respects, the

[a] Supported in part by PO1-NS24032 and KO1-MH00643 (to D.E.R.). Studies using human fetal tissue were supported entirely by private funds from Yale University, the Axion Research Foundation, and others.
[e] *Send correspondence to:* Dr. Eugene Redmond, Jr., The Neural Transplant Program, Yale University School of Medicine, P.O. Box 3333, New Haven, CT USA 06510; TEL: 203-785-4432; FAX: 203-776-2893.

best replacements one could imagine, since precursor cells have the capacity to develop into every cell found in the adult. So, the best replacement for a dopamine neuron would likely be a precursor dopamine neuron or "neuroblast." Animal research through 1985 had demonstrated the unique properties of such fetal cells, but survivability after transplantation had not been attained with primate or human neural tissue. Our programs developed techniques to transplant monkey fetal neural tissue, to cryopreserve it, and to reverse functional effects of the neurotoxin, MPTP, in monkeys. This technique was applied to the collection and preservation of human tissue, and preliminary successful results have been obtained in patients with idiopathic Parkinson's disease. Others have reported success with different techniques in two MPTP-Parkinsonian patients and a small number of patients with idiopathic disease. If the most dramatic improvements can be replicated consistently and the benefits last for a reasonable period without complications, a clinical treatment might develop using "random-source" fetal cadaver cells.

THE FIRST NINETY YEARS OF NEURAL TRANSPLANTATION

The idea that the brain could be repaired by transplanting tissue from another individual is not new. The first reported efforts were made in 1890 by W. Gilman Thompson.[1] Although he was clearly unsuccessful, the idea persisted and eventually led to the discovery of interesting phenomena which now underlie its present-day feasibility. The presence of neurotropic factors was observed early in the century,[2,3] and it is still not clear whether "circuit reconstruction" with synaptic connections or released factors will be the most useful in the future. The relative absence of immune response in the brain was also noted,[4] a fact which makes neural transplantation much easier than transplants of peripheral cells and organs. The most critical discovery was the fact that fetal tissue uniquely survives transplantation,[5] probably due to its capacity to migrate and organize in complex ways in the developing brain, and the fact that its removal in early stages does not destroy axonal and dendritic extensions from the perikarya. During this phase of research, neural transplantation was generally undertaken as a means to study neural plasticity and development rather than a means to produce functional effects in the new host.

More optimism followed a new phase of research in the late 1970s which documented functional effects, first with hormonal replacements,[6] and then with changes in the 6-hydroxydopamine model in rodents reported by Perlow *et al.*[7] and Björklund *et al.*[8] These and a whole series of subsequent studies demonstrating aspects of neural function in the recipient of grafted cells and tissues supported the possibility that clinical applications might someday be possible. But the failure to achieve survival with primate neurons[9] led to a detour using adrenal tissue, which had political and immune advantages if it worked.[10]

SUCCESS WITH TRANSPLANTATION OF PRIMATE FETAL MESENCEPHALIC TISSUE

Our studies began with the effort to document a better model of Parkinson's disease than the old rodent models, using MPTP. Quite accidentally, the African green monkey, appears to model the human idiopathic disease more completely than other monkeys after the administration of the neurotoxin (MPTP), with remarkable neurological, physiological, biochemical, pharmacological, and neuropathological parallels. The two major differences from the human disease appear to be a dramatically accelerated course and the absence of progression after the initial toxic substances are cleared. Using the model, we were able to demonstrate graft survival and functional reversal of parkinsonism that were highly correlated[11] and to reverse functional deficits that were extremely dramatic.[12] Several other groups also reported some success with transplants in monkeys.

For logistical and safety reasons, we next developed a cryopreservation technique in monkeys[13] that would allow tissue eventually to be obtained from routine, unmodified, elective abortions in humans,[14] and demonstrated its use in monkeys with fetal tissue from monkeys and from elective human abortions.[15] As a part of this process, we had to work out procedures which could withstand strict ethical scrutiny and political opposition which were likely in the United States when clinical studies began. Similar to ethical guidelines developed elsewhere, these were based upon entirely separating decisions about pregnancy termination from any possible research use of fetal tissue and eliminating conceivable inducements such as directed donations or payments.

FIRST CLINICAL FETAL NEURAL TRANSPLANTS

The first fetal neural transplants for Parkinson's disease were reported by Madrazo et al.,[16] following previous reports of success with adrenal tissue which had not been satisfactorily replicated by other investigators. Hitchcock et al.[17] and Lindvall et al.[18] reported that studies had begun in England and in Sweden, but the outcome was not convincing or encouraging. Lindvall et al. reported that their two patients had essentially failed to improve. Lindvall et al. were more optimistic in a case report with a 5-month outcome,[19] although a second patient transplanted about the same time apparently did not improve until later, according to a later report.[20] Many of the patients reported in these early studies have been difficult for outside investigators to evaluate due to differences in techniques and assessment methods between the studies, with the result that there remained a significant basis for skepticism as to the actual benefits which are derived from surviving implanted cells.[21]

THE YALE STUDIES

Our group was determined to address a number of problems in these earliest reports: 1) the absence of control data in a condition that is associated with significant daily variability; 2) the effects of medication as a confounding variable; and 3) the reliance on self-report measures such as "on-off" records rather than blind and objectively assessed standard tests as a basis for determining improvement. Finally, we agreed not to report individual and impressionistic results on any patient nor to report any data until a reasonable time had elapsed for all of the patients after transplantation. This time was selected as 18 months, since it was clear that adrenal autografts had failed by this time even if earlier improvement had been seen. We have now reported data on our four initial patients transplanted unilaterally into the caudate nucleus, with the group limited to the first four, since our next seven patients were transplanted bilaterally into the caudate.[22]

The study methods were detailed previously.[21,22] The second patient died four months after transplantation, of disease progression and without demonstrable benefit; his brain was recovered and showed evidence of graft and neuronal survival,[22] but no tyrosine hydroxylase activity, along with a pathological finding that his correct diagnosis was striatonigral degeneration. Although he met standard criteria for Parkinson's disease and the CAPIT criteria for L-dopa response,[24] either his continued high medication doses or the pathology of his disease may have been responsible for the absence of tyrosine hydroxylase activity which is routinely demonstrated to be present in tissue prepared for grafting as well as in comparably aged grafts in monkeys. The remaining three patients showed convincing improvements, which were statistically detectable by 6 months after grafting, and which also showed significant improvement slopes until the end of the 18-month follow-up reported.

Improvement in the ability to perform standard motor function tests, scored quantitatively (rather than qualitatively) from videotaped records, was seen across all tasks and on both sides of the body, although only some of these were statistically significant (FIG. 1). Neither the patients studied before transplantation, nor the control subjects, identically selected but randomly delayed a year before surgery, showed improvement. These quantitative motor improvements were consistent with neurologist-rated and patient self-report data on reductions in parkinsonian symptoms and ability to perform activities of daily living rated from standard scales, such as the Unified Parkinson Disease Rating Scale (FIG. 2). There was no increase in psychiatric symptoms or decline of cognitive ability; surprisingly, two patients showed a 9–10 point increase in full-scale I.Q.; one showed a 14 point increase in performance IQ. All of these changes occurred in spite of the complete elimination of dopamine agonist drugs and a mean reduction of 38% of presurgical L-dopa doses; the controls required increasing doses throughout a one-year

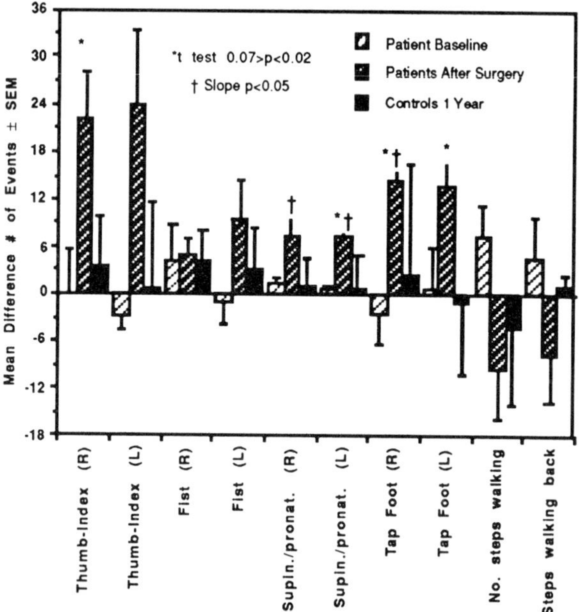

FIGURE 1. After transplantation patients significantly improved their performance on standard neurological evaluation tasks, whereas controls showed no changes. The mean difference in number of events, performed in a fixed time interval, is plotted for each task on the right (R) or the left (L). Improvement appears to occur equally on both sides. For the walking task, the number of steps required to walk 15 feet in each direction is plotted (fewer steps to walk the entire distance indicates improvement). The statistical significance of changes was determined by paired *t*-test between initial and final values for each period and by slope analyses which utilized all of the data points for each patient. (FIGURES 1 and 2 reproduced with the kind permission of Raven Press from Redmond *et al.*[21])

period (slope $p<0.01$) and a mean increase of 34%, which was significantly different from the patients ($p<0.03$).

Positive effects of grafts could be inferred from the fact that patients were also better during drug holiday periods when all anti-Parkinson medications were withheld for 40 hours (FIG. 3), as well as during optimum functional periods after medication. This analysis showed significant differences after surgery in the off-drug as well as the on-drug periods. Furthermore, the scores after surgery, off all drugs, were lower than the optimum on-drug periods before surgery, suggesting that in these severe patients, transplantation was more efficacious than their drug treatment. Nonetheless, this group of patients, while showing some significant and beneficial individual effects, remained significantly impaired by their disease and improved less than severely parkinsonian, MPTP-treated monkeys which were transplanted bilaterally into the caudate.

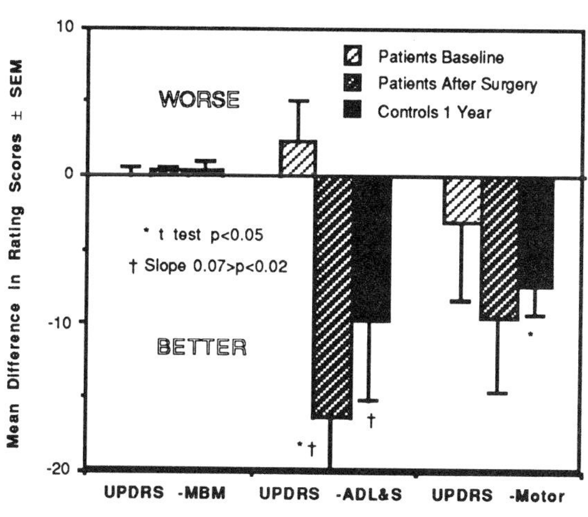

FIGURE 2. Three patients showed significant improvements in Unified Parkinson's Disease Rating Scale (UPDRS) activities of daily living and symptoms scale after transplantation. Control patients also showed improvement on this measure, as well as on the UPDRS Motor scale. There were no changes in the UPDRS Mood, Behavior, and Mentation scale in either group. Mean differences between the first and last measurement within the baseline and post-surgical periods are plotted for the patients, and between the entry to the study and approximately one year later for the control patients. The statistical significance of slopes, which used all data for each patient, is indicated, but not plotted on the graph.

PRESENT STATE OF KNOWLEDGE ABOUT NEURAL TRANSPLANTS

Two other reports, just published, support functional effects of fetal neural grafts in humans. Two patients with MPTP-induced Parkinsonism were reported to be improved by Widner *et al.*[25] for 22 and 24 months after extensive bilateral grafting into the caudate and putamen. These patients were primarily medication-intolerant; the benefits of transplantations were most clear as a

FIGURE 3. Neurological UPDRS ratings—effects of drugs vs. transplants. The possible effects of transplantation on UPDRS Subscale scores are compared with the effects of medication treatment as indicated by the comparison of the data from optimal drug treatment "On Drugs" with 40 hour drug holidays ("Off Drugs"). Each of these comparisons is shown during baseline and at the end of the evaluation period after surgery. This figure provides comparisons of the magnitude of drug vs. transplant effects in this group of severely affected, but L-dopa responsive patients.

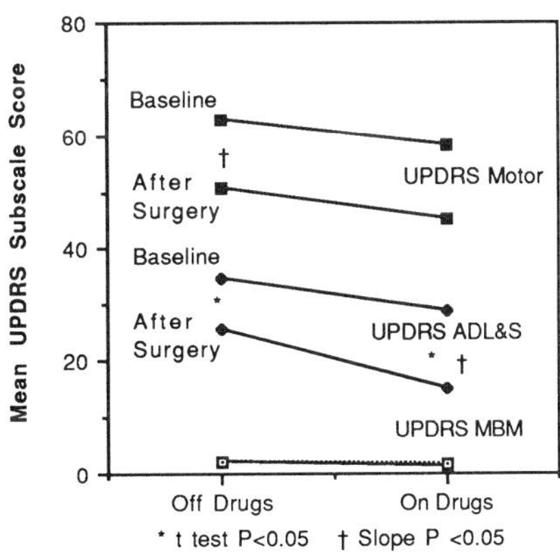

means of reducing L-dopa doses and attendant side effects. Freed *et al.*[26] reported that one patient implanted into caudate and putamen on one side had improved at 46 months, one had not at 33 months, and five patients implanted bilaterally only into the putamen had improved at 11 to 13 months. Although the total number of patients in any of these reports, studied in the same fashion, is still quite small, the overall positive results are encouraging. In spite of sensationalistic case reports and media coverage, all investigators agree that important research questions must be answered before fetal neural tissue transplants are offered as a therapeutic choice.

THE FUTURE OF NEURAL TRANSPLANTATION

Obviously, there is significant research remaining to develop and evaluate a transplant "treatment" for Parkinson's disease using dopamine neuroblasts.[27] Data are inadequate to determine the necessity or advantages of multiple fetal source grafts, immune suppression treatment, and implantation sites, which differed among these studies. What is the best method of tissue preparation and preservation? Are the changes seen on some PET studies due to release of dopamine from functioning grafts or from stimulated host mechanisms? Why are bilateral effects seen after unilateral grafts in most studies? Can all patients be restored to normal by increasing the quantitative replacement of dopamine deficits by implanting cells in dopamine target areas, or will more physiologic circuit restoration be necessary through implantation into the substantia nigra, where afferent connections may be necessary? Can long-term tissue survival be improved? Clearly, larger studies must be carried out and evaluated using standard and comparable methodology and replicated by different groups of investigators. Animal studies must also be continued and may continue to provide technological advances that will further improve human clinical outcomes.

Since fetal cells may eventually produce cellular rejection or introduce infectious disease, can alternative sources of tissue be developed? Although the supply of fetal tissue through elective abortions seems more than adequate at present, increased uses for fetal cells may eventually outpace the supply of tissue while changes in the law or in medical practice could drastically decrease the supply of usable fetal tissue. Techniques are being explored which would increase the supply of replacement cells through propagated cell lines, address problems such as infection and rejection, or provide more specific repair of cellular defects where these are understood, using molecular techniques or gene therapy. The Parkinson's model should also encourage studies of other neural conditions which might benefit from regulated replacement of neurotransmitters, neuromodulators, or growth factors, such as Alzheimer's or Huntington diseases.

REFERENCES

1. THOMPSON, W. G. 1890. Successful brain grafting. N. Y. Med. J. **51:**701–702.
2. GASH, D. M. 1984. Neural transplants in mammals: A historical overview. *In* Neural Transplants: Development and Function. J. R. Sladek & D. M. Gash, Eds. 1–12. Plenum Press. New York and London.
3. BJÖRKLUND, A. & U. STENEVI. 1985. Intracerebral neural grafting: A historical perspective. *In* Neural Grafting in the Mammalian CNS. A. Björklund & U. Stenevi, Eds. 3–14. Elsevier Science Publishers. Amsterdam, New York, Oxford.
4. SHIRAI, Y. 1921. Transplantation of rat sarcoma in adult heterogeneous animals. Jap. Med. World **1:**14–15.
5. LE GROS CLARK, W. E. 1940. Neuronal differentiation in implanted foetal cortical tissue. J. Neurol. Psychiatry **3:**263–284.
6. HALÁSZ, B., L. PUPP, S. UHLARIK & L. TIMA. 1963. Growth of hypophysectomized rats bearing pituitary transplants in the hypothalamus. Acta Physiol Acad. Sci. Hung. **23:**287–292.
7. PERLOW, M. J., W. J. FREED, B. J. HOFFER, A. SEIGER, L. OLSON & R. J. WYATT. 1979. Brain grafts reduce motor abnormalities produced by destruction of nigrostriatal dopamine system. Science **204:**643–653.
8. BJÖRKLUND, A. & U. STENEVI. 1979. Reconstruction of the nigrostriatal dopamine pathway by intracerebral nigral transplants. Brain Res. **177:**555–560.
9. MORIHISA, J. M., R. K. NAKAMURA, W. J. FREED, M. MISHKIN & R. J. WYATT. 1984. Adrenal medulla grafts survive and exhibit catecholamine-specific fluorescence in the primate brain. Exp. Neurol. **84:**643–653.
10. LEWIN, R. 1988. Cloud over Parkinson's therapy. Science **240:**390–392.
11. REDMOND, D. E. JR., J. R. SLADEK JR., R. H. ROTH, T. J. COLLIER, J. D. ELSWORTH, A. Y. DEUTCH, *et al.* 1986. Fetal neuronal grafts in monkeys given methylphenyltetrahydro-pyridine. Lancet **1:**125–127.
12. TAYLOR, J. R., J. D. ELSWORTH, R. H. ROTH, J. R. SLADEK, JR., T. J. COLLIER & D. E. REDMOND, JR. 1991. Grafting of fetal substantia nigra to striatum reverses behavioral deficits induced by MPTP in primates: A comparison with other types of grafts as controls. Exp. Brain Res. **85:**335–348.
13. COLLIER, T. J., D. E. REDMOND, JR., C. SLADEK, M. J. GALLAGHER & J. R. SLADEK, JR. 1987. Intracerebral grafting and culture of cryopreserved primate dopamine neurons. Brain Res. **436:**363–366.
14. ROBBINS, R., I. TORRES-ALEMAN, C. LERANTH, C. BRADBURY, A. DEUTCH, S. WELSH, *et al.* 1990. Cryopreservation of human brain tissue. Exp. Neurol. **107:**208–213.
15. REDMOND, D. E., JR., F. NAFTOLIN, T. J. COLLIER, C. LERANTH, R. J. ROBBINS, C. D. SLADEK, *et al.* 1988. Cryopreservation, culture, and transplantation of human fetal mesencephalic tissue into monkeys. Science **242:**768–771.
16. MADRAZO, I., V. LEÓN, C. TORRES, M. AGUILERA, G. VARELA, F. ALVAREZ, *et al.* 1988. Transplantation of fetal substantia nigra and adrenal medulla to the caudate nucleus in two patients with Parkinson's disease. N. Engl. J. Med. **318:**51.

17. HITCHCOCK, E. R., C. CLOUGH, R. C. HUGHES & B. G. KENNY. 1988. Embryos and Parkinson's disease. Lancet i:1274.

18. LINDVALL, O., S. REHNCRONA, P. BRUNDIN, B. GUSTAVII, B. ASTEDT, H. WIDNER, et al. 1989. Human fetal dopamine neurons grafted into the striatum in two patients with severe Parkinson's disease: A detailed account of methodology and a 6-month follow-up. Arch. Neurol. 46:615–631.

19. LINDVALL, O., P. BRUNDIN, H. WIDNER, S. REHNCRONA, B. GUSTAVII, R. FRACKOWIAK, et al. 1990. Grafts of fetal dopamine neurons survive and improve motor function in Parkinson's disease. Science 247:574–577.

20. LINDVALL, O., H. WIDNER, S. REHNCRONA, P. BRUNDIN, P. ODIN, B. GUSTAVI, R. FRACKOWIAK, K. L. LEENDERS, G. SAWLE, J. C. ROTHWELL, A. BJÖRKLUND & C. D. MARSDEN. 1992. Transplantation of fetal dopamine neurons in Parkinson's disease: One-year clinical and neurophysiological observations in two patients with putaminal implants. Ann. Neurol. 31:155–165.

21. REDMOND, D. E., R. J. ROBBINS, F. NAFTOLIN, K. L. MAREK, T. VOLLMER, C. LERANTH, et al. 1992. Cellular replacement of dopamine deficit in Parkinson's disease using human fetal mesencephalic tissue: Preliminary results in four patients. In Molecular and Cellular Approaches to the Treatment of Brain Disease. S. G. Waxman, Ed.: 325–359. Raven Press. New York.

22. SPENCER, D. D., R. J. ROBBINS, F. NAFTOLIN, K. L. MAREK, T. VOLLMER, C. LERANTH, R. H. ROTH, L. H. PRICE, A. GJEDDE, B. S. BUNNEY, K. J. SASS, J. B. ELSWORTH, E. KIER, R. MAKUCH, P. B. HOFFER & D. REDMOND, JR. 1992. Unilateral transplantation of human fetal mesencephalic tissue into the caudate nucleus of patients with Parkinson's disease. New Engl. J. Med. 327:1541–1548.

23. REDMOND, D. E., JR., C. LERANTH, D. D. SPENCER, R. ROBBINS, T. VOLLMER, J. H. KIM et al. 1990. Fetal neural graft survival. Lancet, ii:820–822.

24. CAPIT COMMITTEE: J. W. LANGSTON, H. WIDNER, C. G. GOETZ, D. BROOKS, S. FAHN, T. FREEMAN & R. WATTS. 1992. Core assessment program for intracerebral transplantations (CAPIT). Movement Disorders. 7:2–13.

25. WIDNER, H., J. TETRUD, S. REHNCRONA, B. SNOW, P. BRUNDIN, B. GUSTAVII, A. BJÖRKLUND, O. LINDVALL & J. W. LANGSTON. 1992. Bilateral fetal mesencephalic grafting in two patients with parkinsonism induced by 1-methyl-4-phenyl-1,2,3,6-tetrahydropyridine (MPTP). New Engl. J. Med. 327:1556–1563.

26. FREED, C., R. E. BREEZE, N. L. ROSENBERG, S. A. SCHNECK, E. KRIEK, J-X. QI, T. LONE, Y-B. ZHANG, J. A. SNYDER, T. H. WELLS, L. O. RAMIG, L. THOMPSON, J. C. MAZZIOTTA, S. C. HUANG, S. T. GRAFTON, D. BROOKS, G. SAWLE, G. SCHROTER & A. A. ANSARI. 1992. Survival of implanted fetal dopamine cells and neurologic improvement 12 to 46 months after transplantation for Parkinson's disease. New Engl. J. Med. 327:1549–1555.

27. FAHN, S. 1992. Fetal-tissue transplants in Parkinson's disease. New Engl. J. Med. 327:1589–1590.

Basal Forebrain Grafts in the Hippocampus and Neocortex: Regulation of Acetylcholine Release[a]

OLA G. NILSSON,[b] GIAMPIERO LEANZA,[c] CARL ROSENBLAD, AND ANDERS BJÖRKLUND

Department of Medical Cell Research, Section of Neurobiology, University of Lund, S-223 62 Lund, Sweden

ABSTRACT: The regulation of acetylcholine (ACh) release from cholinergic neurons transplanted to the hippocampus or neocortex was studied by microdialysis in awake rats. Fetal basal forebrain tissue was implanted as a cell suspension or solid graft into the fimbria-fornix—lesioned hippocampus, or as a cell suspension into the frontal cortex after excitotoxic lesion of the nucleus basalis. Several months after transplantation, microdialysis probes were implanted in areas of the hippocampus or frontal cortex reinnervated by the grafts. The grafts restored lesion-induced deficits in steady-state ACh release up to normal or above normal levels in both hippocampus and frontal cortex. The responses to KCl and tetrodotoxin suggested that the ACh release exhibited normal firing-dependent properties. By applying various behaviorally arousing stimuli that normally activate the basal forebrain projection systems, we wished to investigate the functional integration of the grafts in the host brain. In the hippocampus, sensory stimulation, immobilization stress and motor activity all resulted in increased release of graft-derived ACh amounting to 25–65% of the normal response. Variations in ACh levels during the day-night cycle was, however, not observed in the grafted rats. In the frontal cortex, immobilization enhanced the graft-derived ACh release (60% of normal response), whereas the response to sensory stimulation did not reach significance. Since the activity of the normal basal forebrain projection systems is under influence of monoaminergic brainstem afferents, we investigated the effects of systemic administration of amphetamine or apomorphine on ACh release in the hippocampus. Both drugs produced increases in graft-derived ACh release although the response was variable and less pronounced than normal. In conclusion, the graft-derived ACh release was affected by behavioral manipulations and catecholaminergic drugs that normally modify cholinergic septo-hippocampal and basalo-cortical activity. This strongly suggests a high degree of functional integration of the graft in the host brain allowing for a regulated release of transmitter that can be adjusted during ongoing behavior.

[a] The studies were supported by grants from the Swedish Medical Research Council (04X-3874), the National Institutes of Health (NS06701), the Greta and Johan Kock Foundation, and the Gun and Bertil Stohnes Foundation.

[b] *Send correspondence to:* Ola G. Nilsson, Department of Medical Cell Research, Section of Neurobiology, University of Lund, Biskopsgatan 5, S-223 62 Lund, Sweden; TEL: 46-46-107915; FAX: 46-46-107927.

[c] *Present address:* Institute of Human Physiology, University of Catania, Catania, Italy.

INTRODUCTION

Grafts of fetal basal forebrain (BF) tissue rich in developing cholinergic neurons implanted in the hippocampus or neocortex have previously been shown to ameliorate lesion-induced or age-dependent impairments in a range of conditioned behaviors.[1,2] Improved performance has, thus, been reported in active or passive avoidance learning, delayed match-to-sample or attentional tasks, and spatial navigation memory in rats with neurotoxin or surgical lesions to the septo-hippocampal or basalo-cortical cholinergic projection systems. Similar effects of intrahippocampal cholinergic grafts on learning impairments have been demonstrated in fornix-lesioned monkeys.[3] Several lines of evidence indicate that the graft-derived functional recovery is dependent on a cholinergic reinnervation of host target areas.[2] First, functional synaptic connections between grafted choline acetyltransferase-positive neurons and the denervated neurons of the host has been observed. Second, restoration of lesion-induced 2-deoxyglucose utilization in the hippocampus was correlated with the degree of acetylcholinesterase-positive reinnervation produced by the graft. Third, functional effects similar to those obtained with cholinergic-rich BF tissue has not been obtained with control grafts of non-cholinergic tissue or when a cholinergic graft is placed in an inappropriate location. Fourth, it has been possible to block the graft-induced behavioral recovery by muscarinic receptor antagonists.

The activity of the normal septo-hippocampal and basalo-cortical cholinergic systems has been shown to be intimately related to the behavioral state of the animal,[4] and arousing, stressful or otherwise behaviorally activating stimuli increase cholinergic firing rate or transmitter release in the target areas.[5-11] Electrophysiological and transmitter release studies suggest that important regulatory inputs to the BF cholinergic neurons comes from the brainstem.[4,12-16] Thus, electrical stimulation of brainstem nuclei and administration of drugs that affect ascending brainstem monoaminergic systems modulate ACh release and electroencephalographic activity in the hippocampus and neocortex.

In the present series of experiments we wished to study the *in vivo* ACh release from BF grafts in the hippocampus or frontal cortex of awake freely moving animals by using the microdialysis technique. In particular, we were interested in whether ACh released from the grafts would show any variations with the behavior of the animal and, therefore, a range of behavioral manipulations were applied that are known to activate the intact BF cholinergic projection systems.

METHODS

A unilateral aspirative lesion of the fimbria-fornix (FF) and the overlying cortex (including the supracallosal striae) was made in order to produce a complete and permanent cholinergic denervation of the dorsal two-thirds of the hippocampal formation. The frontal cortex was unilaterally depleted of its BF input by stereotaxic injections of quisqualic acid in the vicinity of the nucleus basalis magnocellularis (NBM).[17] One to two weeks later, the BF was dissected out from 14- to 16-day-old rat fetuses (crown-rump length = 12–16 mm) of the same outbred strain. Rats with FF lesions received either solid BF grafts into the lesion cavity (one bilateral BF region per recipient) or stereotaxic injections of cell suspension grafts into the hippocampal parenchyma. The cell suspension was prepared by incubating BF tissue pieces in 0.1% trypsine followed by mechanical dissociation. Rats with NBM lesions received only suspension grafts. Details on grafting procedures can be found in Nilsson and Björklund[10] and Rosenblad and Nilsson.[17]

Microdialysis of ACh was carried out several months after lesion and transplantation surgery in graft-reinnervated areas of the dorsal hippocampus or frontal cortex.[10,14,17,18] The dialysis probes consisted of a loop of semi-permeable tubing with a molecular weight cut-off of about 10,000 and an outer diameter of 0.30 mm in the wet state. They were implanted stereotaxically, and kept in place by scull screws and dental acrylic. Four millimeters of probe membrane (dorso-ventral distance 2 mm) was exposed to the brain tissue. *In vitro* tests performed with dialysis probes immersed in Ringer containing different amounts of ACh revealed that the recovery across the probe membrane was $10.8 \pm 0.1\%$. One day after probe implantation (*i.e.*, at least 15 hours after implantation surgery), the probe inlet cannula was connected to a microinfusion system and perfused continuously at a rate of 2 or 4 μl/min with Ringer's solution containing 5 μM neostigmine bromide in order to inhibit degradation of ACh. Samples were collected every 7.5 or 15 minutes during: 1) baseline conditions, 2) infusion of KCl (100 mM) or tetrodotoxin (TTX; 1 μM); 3) a range of behaviorally activating stimuli (see RESULTS section); and 4) systemic treatment with amphetamine (2.5 mg/kg) or apomorphine (2 mg/kg). Samples were assayed for ACh using high-performance liquid chromatography with enzyme reaction and electrochemical detection.[11,19] The detection limit for ACh was approximately 0.2 pmol.

After dialysis, the brains were perfusion fixed and a histological evaluation, using AChE histochemistry, was performed in order to confirm the location of the probes, the completeness of the lesions, and the survival and fiber outgrowth of the grafts. Immunohistochemical identification of host monoaminergic fibers in the intrahippocampal grafts was made using antibodies directed against 5-hydroxytryptamine (5-HT) and tyrosine hydroxylase (TH).[10,18]

RESULTS

ACh Release from Grafts in the Hippocampus

Steady-state Release

Baseline levels of ACh sampled in the normal hippocampus was typically around 2 pmol/30 μl during standard day-time dialysis (not corrected for recovery). The FF lesion reduced the ACh overflow by approximately 70–90%. In both suspension and solid grafted rats, baseline hippocampal ACh overflow was significantly increased compared to the lesion-only controls. Suspension grafts restored baseline hippocampal ACh release up to the level seen in the normal rats or higher, and the levels were significantly higher than those recorded from rats with solid grafts.

Effects of KCl or TTX

A depolarizing concentration of KCl (100 mM) increased ACh release by 340% in the intact hippocampi, whereas no response was detected in the rats with FF lesions. All grafted rats responded significantly to the KCl with average increases of 140% in the suspension graft group and 210% in the solid graft group. Addition of TTX to the perfusion fluid reduced ACh release in both the intact and the grafted hippocampi to levels seen in the FF-lesioned hippocampi. The reductions amounted to about 75–80%. No effect of the TTX was seen in the FF-lesioned rats.

Effects of Behavioral Manipulation

Sensory stimulation by handling (gentle stroking of the fur and tail), immobilization stress or motor activity by swimming during one sampling period each produced a marked twofold increase in hippocampal ACh release in the normal hippocampus. These stimulus-induced changes were entirely absent in the FF-lesioned control rats. Both in rats with solid and suspension grafts, ACh release responded to the various stimuli although the magnitude of the response was generally lower and more variable than in normal rats. The response amounted to 25–65% of that seen in the intact hippocampus with no obvious difference between the two types of grafts. The difference in ACh release between day and night time as monitored in the normal rats (100% higher levels during night) was not seen in any of the grafted groups.

Effects of Catecholaminergic Drugs

In normal rats, systemic administration of apomorphine or amphetamine caused a 168% or 250% increase in ACh overflow compared to the previous baseline level, respectively. The drug-induced increases in ACh levels in the FF-lesioned controls was substantially lower than normal. Rats with solid septal grafts responded significantly more strongly than FF lesion controls to the amphetamine with twofold increased ACh levels, whereas the response to apomorphine was less clear. Both apomorphine and amphetamine resulted in increased ACh release in rats with suspension grafts (an approximately twofold increase), a significantly stronger response as compared to rats with FF lesions only.

Immunohistochemical Analysis

TH- and 5-HT-positive fibers from the host brain were seen to cross the host-graft border and grow into the depth of both solid grafts placed in the FF lesion cavity and cell suspension grafts in the hippocampus. The crossing of fibers was particularly conspicuous in animals with solid grafts where the transected fibers of the host lateral septum provided a dense innervation TH- or 5-HT-positive fibers in parts of the grafts.

ACh Release from Grafts in the Frontal Cortex

Steady-state Release

Baseline levels of ACh in the frontal cortex of intact rats averaged 2 pmol/ 15 minute sample. The quisqualic acid lesion of the NBM caused a 65% decrease in ACh overflow. Cell suspension implants of BF tissue restored the steady-state ACh release to 70% above normal levels.

Effects of KCl or TTX

Addition of 100 mM KCl to the perfusion fluid resulted in increased ACh levels in all groups, although to different extents. Normal and grafted animals thus responded significantly stronger (2- and 3-fold increase, respectively) than did animals with lesions only. When TTX was added to the perfusion-medium (1 μM), a pronounced reduction in ACh release was evident in all animals amounting to 80–90%.

Effects of Behavioral Manipulations

Sensory stimulation by handling or immobilization stress each produced a marked twofold increase in hippocampal ACh release in the intact frontal cortex. These effects were also evident in NBM-lesioned control rats, although the responses were considerably weaker. In rats with BF grafts, ACh overflow increased after immobilization to an extent significantly larger than the lesioned-only controls amounting to 60% of the response seen in the normal controls. The grafted rats' responses to handling did not differ significantly from any of the other groups.

CONCLUSION

The graft-induced restoration of near normal steady-state levels of ACh in the hippocampus and frontal cortex shows that grafted fetal BF tissue maintain its ability to spontaneously synthesize and release ACh despite the ectopic location. The graft-derived increases in ACh release after potassium-evoked depolarization and the reduction in release after blockade of sodium channels by TTX provide further evidence that the ACh levels recovered in the grafted animals depend on normal neuronal activity and axonal impulse flow in the graft-derived cholinergic fibers.

The main finding was that the graft-derived ACh overflow in the hippocampus increased in response to behavioral activation by sensory stimulation, immobilization stress, and motor activity. In the frontal cortex, the same effect was seen after immobilization stress. These responses were similar to those observed in normal rats, although smaller in magnitude, and strongly suggest a high-degree of functional integration of the graft in the host brain. The present results suggest that monoaminergic host afferents may play a role in the control of graft activity. Direct or indirect brainstem afferents, allowing for the host brain to modulate the activity of the grafted cholinergic neurons during ongoing behavior, may play a role in the lesion-induced recovery of function seen with these types of transplants.

REFERENCES

1. DUNNETT, S. B. 1990. Neural transplants in animal models of dementia. Eur. J. Neurosci. **2:**567–587.
2. BJÖRKLUND, A., O. G. NILSSON & P. KALEN. 1990. Reafferentation of the subcortically denervated hippocampus as a model for transplant-induced functional recovery in the CNS. Progr. Brain Res. **83:**411–426.
3. RIDLEY, R. M., H. D. THORNLEY, H. F. BAKER & A. FINE. 1991. Cholinergic neural transplants into hippocampus restore learning ability in monkeys with fornix transections. Exp. Brain Res. **83:**533–538.

4. VANDERWOLF, C. H. 1988. Cerebral activity and behavior: Control by central cholinergic and serotonergic systems. Int. Rev. Neurobiol. **30:**225–340.

5. AKAISHI, T., A. KIMURA, A. SATO & A. SUZUKI. 1990. Responses of neurons in the nucleus basalis of Meynert to various afferent stimuli in rats. Neuroreport **1:**37–39.

6. DAY, J., G. DAMSMA & H. C. FIBIGER. 1991. Cholinergic activity in the rat hippocampus, cortex and striatum correlates with locomotor activity: An in vivo microdialysis study. Pharmacol Biochem Behav **38:**723–729.

7. DUTAR, P., Y. LAMOUR & A. JOBERT. 1985. Activation of identified septo-hippocampal neurons by noxious peripheral stimulation. Brain Res **328:**15–21.

8. IMPERATO, A., S. PUGLISI-ALLEGRA, P. CASOLINI & L. ANGELUCCI. 1991. Changes in brain dopamine and acetylcholine release during and following stress are independent of the pituitary-adrenocortical axis. Brain Res. **538:**111–117.

9. MIZUNO, T., J. ENDO, J. ARITA & F. KIMURA. 1991. Acetylcholine release in the rat hippocampus as measured by the microdialysis method correlates with motor activity and exhibits a diurnal variation. Neuroscience **44:**607–612.

10. NILSSON, O. G., & A. BJÖRKLUND. 1992. Behavior-dependent changes in acetylcholine release in normal and graft-reinnervated hippocampus: Evidence for host regulation of grafted cholinergic neurons. Neuroscience **49:**33–44.

11. NILSSON, O. G., P. KALÉN, E. ROSENGREN & A. BJÖRKLUND. 1990. Acetylcholine release in the rat hippocampus as studied by microdialysis is dependent on axonal impulse flow and increases during behavioral activation. Neuroscience **36:**325–338.

12. CASAMENTI, F., G. DEFFENU, A. L. ABBAMONDI & G. PEPEU. 1986. Changes in cortical acetylcholine output induced by modulation of the nucleus basalis. Brain Res. Bull. **16:**689–695.

13. COSTA, E., P. PANULA, H. K. THOMSON & D. L. CHENEY. 1983. The transsynaptic regulation of the septal hippocampal cholinergic neurons. Life Sci. **32:** 165–179.

14. NILSSON, O. G., G. LEANZA & A. BJÖRKLUND. 1992. Acetylcholine release in the hippocampus: Regulation by monoaminergic afferents as assessed by in vivo microdialysis. Brain Res **584:**132–140.

15. ROBINSON, S. E. 1986. 6-Hydroxydopamine lesion of the ventral noradrenergic bundle blocks the effect of amphetamine on hippocampal acetylcholine. Brain Res. **397:**181–184.

16. VERTES, R. P. 1985. Brainstem-septohippocampal circuits controlling the hippocampal EEG. *In* Electrical Activity of the Archicortex. G. Buzsáki & C. H. Vanderwolf, Eds. 33–45. Akadémia Kiadó. Budapest.

17. ROSENBLAD, C. & O. G. NILSSON. Basal forebrain grafts in the rat neocortex restore in vivo acetylcholine release and respond to behavioral activation. In press.

18. NILSSON, O. G., P. KALÉN, E. ROSENGREN & A. BJÖRKLUND. 1990. Acetylcholine release from intrahippocampal septal grafts is under control of the host brain. Proc. Natl. Acad. Sci. USA **87:**2647–2651.

19. POTTER, P. E., J. L. MEEK & N. H. NEFF. 1983. Acetylcholine and choline in neuronal tissue measured by HPLC with electrochemical detection. J. Neurochem. **41:**188–194.

Behavioral Effects of Cholinergic Grafts[a]

R. M. RIDLEY[b] AND H. F. BAKER

Division of Psychiatry, MRC Clinical Research Centre, Harrow
Middlesex HA1 3UJ United Kingdom

ABSTRACT: Experimental work in animals and, to a more limited extent, in humans, has demonstrated that the cholinergic system is involved in mechanisms which control learning and memory. Since there is cholinergic loss in a variety of dementing illnesses, any treatment designed to alleviate the mental symptoms of these diseases must address the issue of cholinergic dysfunction even if other treatments are also required to overcome other neurotransmitter imbalances. Work in rodents has demonstrated that cholinergic-rich fetal neural tissue transplants can, under certain circumstances, alleviate the behavioral effects of cholinergic lesions or of cholinergic decline associated with aging. More complex cognitive testing can be achieved using primates and, in this case, the common marmoset is a suitable species to use because its rapid and reliable reproductive rate aids the provision of appropriate transplant tissue. Marmosets with transection of the fornix are deprived of a cholinergic input into the dentate gyrus, posterior hippocampus and entorhinal cortex and are specifically impaired on learning tasks which require remembering a rule of responding (non-evaluative memory). Transplantation of cholinergic-rich fetal septal tissue into the hippocampus of such animals completely restores their ability to learn this type of task, whereas transplantation of cholinergic-poor fetal hippocampal tissue into the same area produces no such improvements. These results demonstrate that where a learning impairment is produced by a relatively simple procedure which has a major effect on one neurotransmitter, that function can be restored by transplantation of tissue containing that neurotransmitter even where the impairment consists of a very "high level" cognitive dysfunction.

Degeneration of the central rising cholinergic projections occurs in many neurodegenerative diseases. Although decline in the cholinergic system is unlikely to be the primary pathological event in neurodegenerative disease, the correlation between the decrease in markers of cholinergic activity and mental deterioration in disease and the wealth of experimental evidence detailing learning impairments following disruption of the cholinergic system indicate that therapeutic strategies aimed at ameliorating the symptoms of dementia and amnesia will have to address the issue of cholinergic dysfunction.

[a] This work was supported by the Medical Research Council, U.K.
[b] *Send correspondence to:* Dr. R. M. Ridley, Division of Psychiatry, MRC Clinical Research Centre, Watford Road, Harrow, Middlesex HA1 3UJ United Kingdom; TEL: 44-081-869-3518; FAX: 44-081-869-3511.

The cholinergic neurons of the basal forebrain project to many areas of the telencephalon. If it is supposed that these projections contribute to and sustain the functions of those areas to which they project, then it is to be expected that they will have a role in learning and memory as well as other higher cognitive functions. In order to demonstrate this experimentally, however, it is necessary to test animals on those tasks which are appropriate for those target areas which it can be demonstrated have been affected by the lesions. This in turn requires precise neuropsychological localization studies. This area of animal psychology is more advanced in primates than rats since primatologists have always aligned themselves with clinical psychologists who have been concerned mainly with cortical localization, whereas rodentologists are, to some extent, still laboring under the influence of Lashley's "Law of Mass Action." Nonetheless, important advances in understanding the cholinergic system and pioneering work demonstrating the behavioral effects of cholinergic grafts have been made using rats. Cholinergic-rich fetal septal grafts in the hippocampus and/or neocortex can produce improvement in a variety of behavioral tasks in rats with either circumscribed or widespread cholinergic lesions.

The marmoset is a small New World primate which is particularly suitable for use in behavioral transplantation studies using fetal tissue because it breeds rapidly in captivity, producing 4–6 offspring in two pregnancies per year and its learning ability can be assessed in the Wisconsin General Test Apparatus. In this apparatus, the monkey is presented with a series of discrete trials on which it must choose one of two objects in order to find a piece of food reward. Tasks on which the reward is always hidden under the same object require evaluative memory[1] because one object has greater reward value than the other. Tasks on which the reward can only be found according to a specific rule (*e.g.*, go to the left object if one pair of identical objects is presented; go to the right object if an alternative pair of identical objects is presented) require non-evaluative memory[1] because neither pair of objects has greater reward value than the other. Transection of the fornix, which interrupts the cholinergic projection to the hippocampus and entorhinal cortex, produces very specific impairments on acquisition and retention of tasks requiring non-evaluative memory. This model has been used to assess the effect on acquisition of non-evaluative tasks of cholinergic-rich (septal) and cholinergic-poor (hippocampal) tissue grafts taken from the ~80 day marmoset fetus and transplanted into the hippocampus of adult marmosets whose cholinergic projection to the hippocampus had been destroyed by fornix transection (see Fig. 1 and refs. 2 and 3).

Several different tasks were assessed before and after transplantation. These tasks have been grouped into those which required evaluative memory (termed "control" tasks because impairment was not expected after fornix transection) and those requiring non-evaluative memory (termed "experimen-

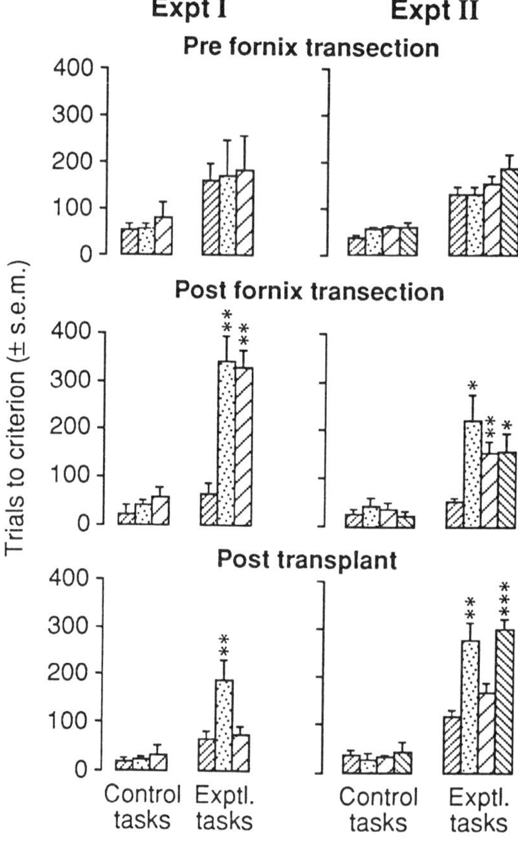

FIGURE 1. Mean number of trials required to reach criterion (usually 27/30 for each task) on "control" (evaluative) tasks and "experimental" (non-evaluative) tasks before and after fornix transection and after transplantation in experiments I[2] and experiments II.[3] ▨ = fornix-intact marmosets; ▧ = marmosets with fornix transections alone; ▨ = marmosets with fornix transection and cholinergic-rich grafts into hippocampus; ▨ = marmosets with fornix transection and cholinergic-poor grafts into hippocampus. *$p < 0.05$; **$p < 0.01$; ***$p < 0.001$, compared to control (fornix-intact) marmosets.

tal" tasks because impairment was predicted after fornix transection). FIGURE 1 shows that transplantation of cholinergic-rich tissue into the hippocampus produced complete restitution of learning ability on tasks requiring non-evaluative memory systems, whereas animals with fornix transection alone or with intra-hippocampal grafts of cholinergic-poor tissue remained impaired on these tasks throughout the post-transplant test period which lasted about 8 months. The lack of effect of the grafts on the control tasks indicates that the grafts, though space occupying, did not impair the function of the surrounding temporal neocortex or amygdala (which is required for performance of these "control" tasks).

At the end of behavioral testing all animals were killed and the lesions and grafts were examined using acetylcholinesterase histochemistry.

These results are consistent with the idea that the cholinergic projection to the hippocampus sustains the function of the hippocampus by providing an appropriate level of cholinergic tone without carrying the information to be remembered encoded in impulse activity. This is comparable to the role of the rising dopaminergic pathway in sustaining the function of the basal ganglia. Good restitution of function can be achieved in Parkinson's disease by replacing the level of dopaminergic tone either with L-dopa or with dopamine-rich fetal neural tissue transplants. Hippocampal function in fornix transected marmosets can be restored by treatment with cholinergic agonist drugs such as pilocarpine[2] as well as, as is shown in this paper, by transplantation of cholinergic tissue.

In the case of these rising neurotransmitter projection systems, it would seem that where the lesion is relatively simple, the behavioral deficit can be overcome by a transplant which restores neurotransmitter levels to the target area irrespective of the complexity of the behavioral or cognitive function in question. In the normal, and therefore optimal, condition the activity in the rising pathways may be modulated to cope with varying demands. This may be possible to only a limited extent for transplant-produced neurotransmitter, but the production of reasonable amounts of such transmitter may be sufficient to produce substantial improvements in performance.

REFERENCES

1. RIDLEY, R. M. & H. F. BAKER. 1991. A critical evaluation of monkey models of amnesia and dementia. Brain Res. Rev. **16**:15–37.
2. RIDLEY, R. M., H. D. THORNLEY, H. F. BAKER & A. FINE. 1991. Cholinergic neural transplants into hippocampus restore learning ability in monkeys with fornix transections. Exp. Brain Res. **83**:533–538.
3. RIDLEY, R. M., S. GRIBBLE, B. A. CLARK, H. F. BAKER & A. FINE. 1992. Restoration of learning ability in fornix-transected monkeys after fetal basal forebrain but not fetal hippocampal tissue transplantation. Neuroscience **48:** 779–792.

Cells Engineered to Produce Acetylcholine: Therapeutic Potential for Alzheimer's Disease[a]

LISA J. FISHER[b], HEATHER K. RAYMON, AND FRED H. GAGE

Department of Neurosciences, University of California, San Diego,
La Jolla, California USA

ABSTRACT: Alzheimer's disease (AD) is a debilitating disorder of the central nervous system which may affect up to 50% of the population over the age of 85 years. The etiology of AD is unknown and there is currently no cure for the disease. Well-documented losses in cholinergic and other neurotransmitter systems have provided a focal point for attempting pharmacological interventions in AD to ameliorate some of the cognitive deficits that occur. However, current systemic strategies have met with limited success. An alternative strategy, that has been pursued in animal models of neurodegenerative disease, is to augment neurotransmitter function within the brain through tissue transplantation. Such implants have an advantage over conventional drug therapies in that the cells can be precisely placed within compromised areas of the brain. We have pursued a strategy of designing cells, through the use of molecular biology techniques, to produce neurotrophic factors and neurotransmitters. Recently, we developed a primary fibroblast cell line that was genetically modified to express choline acetyltransferase (ChAT). *In vitro*, these cells produced and released acetylcholine at levels that varied with the amount of choline in the culture media. When implanted into the hippocampus of rats, the *in vivo* microdialysis technique revealed that the ChAT-expressing fibroblasts continued to produce and release acetylcholine after grafting. Most importantly, the levels of acetylcholine synthesized by the cells could be regulated by the localized infusion of choline in the vicinity of the grafts. These results confirmed previous work which indicated that engineered fibroblasts provide an effective delivery vehicle of different substances to the brain. While the intracerebral implantation of genetically modified cells will not cure AD, the continuing development of this strategy may ultimately provide a powerful approach for ameliorating the devastating cognitive impairments which are a hallmark of this disease.

Alzheimer's disease (AD) is clinically characterized by a gradual deterioration of intellectual functioning. Neuropathological examination of AD brains re-

[a] These studies were supported by grants from the National Institutes of Health (AG 104 35-02) and the Broad Foundation.

[b] *Send correspondence to:* Dr. Lisa J. Fisher, Department of Neurosciences, University of California San Diego, Clinical Sciences Building, La Jolla, CA 92093-0627; TEL: (619) 534-7186; FAX: (619) 534-5748.

veals neuronal loss, senile plaques, a reduction in synaptic density, β-amyloid protein deposition, and neurofibrillary tangles throughout the association areas of the parietal-temporal cortex, the hippocampus, the entorhinal cortex, and the amygdala.[1] In addition to these anatomical changes, several neurotransmitter systems in subcortical areas which project to the cortex and hippocampus are affected in AD brains, such as the cholinergic neurons in the nucleus basalis of Meynert, serotonergic cells in the dorsal raphe and noradrenergic neurons in the locus ceruleus. Of these ascending projection pathways, changes in cholinergic systems in AD have been the focus of most research, forming the foundation for a "cholinergic hypothesis of geriatric memory dysfunction."[2] There is a dramatic loss of cholinergic cells within both the nucleus basalis and the medial septum of the AD brain as compared to aged matched controls.[3] Choline acetyltransferase (ChAT), the synthetic enzyme for acetylcholine (ACh), has been reported to be decreased 60–90% in the cerebral cortex and hippocampus of AD brains,[4,5] and there is a correlation between the extent to which cholinergic markers are decreased in cortical areas of the AD brain and the degree of cognitive impairments observed.[5]

Therapeutic strategies for AD which have targeted the replacement or replenishment of deficient neurotransmitters have met with limited success. To date, most neurotransmitter augmentation strategies for AD have involved cholinergic agents. Overall, ACh precursor administration does not seem to effectively ameliorate cognitive deficits of AD patients.[2] Somewhat moderate improvements in cognitive performances have been reported following the administration of cholinesterase inhibitors.[6] The reasons for the limited effectiveness of cholinergic and non-cholinergic treatments are probably varied, but may include sub- or supra-optimal dosing, non-specific target stimulation, and short durations of action of the different compounds. Further, achieving optimal improvements in cognition in AD may require the pharmacological manipulation of multiple neurotransmitter systems, potential therapies which have not yet been explored.

An alternative technique for enhancing deficient neurotransmitters within the brain, which has been the focus of much research over the past decade, is the intracerebral implantation of fetal neurons. The aged rat has been used as a model of cognitive decline to examine the ability of neuronal grafts to improve deficits on learning and memory tasks. While aged rats do not generally show pathological changes within the brain which are typical of AD, such as plaques and tangles, they do have marked reductions in both cholinergic and non-cholinergic systems and show impairments on a variety of cognitive tasks.[7] Fetal neurons grafted to the brain of aged rats have been found to survive well and extend processes into the host parenchyma.[7] In a population of aged rats with marked deficits in spatial learning and memory in the Morris water maze, cholinergic-rich tissue has been reported to induce a significant improvement in the performance of this task.[8] Further, this graft-induced amelioration of spatial deficits was shown to be abolished by the cholinergic antagonist atropine, demonstrating the crucial role of ACh in mediating the cognitive improvement.[9]

GENETICALLY MODIFIED CELLS

Intracerebral grafting of fetal neurons is a powerful technique for achieving site-specific enhancement of neurotransmitters. However, in considering neural grafting as a therapeutic intervention in human disease, there are concerns about the procurement of fetal tissue and with achieving histocompatibility between host and donor tissues. Genetically modifying cells obtained from a patient would significantly facilitate tissue acquisition and, when implanted into the brain, such autologous transduced cells would be protected from immunological attack. Further, gene transfer techniques would allow for the possibility that cells may be customized to synthesize and release one or more desired compounds. One population of primary cells that may be easily obtained from a patient are fibroblasts from a skin biopsy. Therefore, we have explored the possibility that primary fibroblasts may provide an effective donor cell for genetic manipulation and intracerebral grafting.[10] In our work with fibroblasts derived from an inbred strain of rats, the primary skin cells have been found to survive well within the rodent brain for over 1 year. These grafts are readily vascularized by cerebral blood vessels and are characterized by a compact and stable size.[11,12] To date, we have genetically modified primary rat fibroblasts to produce a variety of molecules, including nerve growth factor, L-dopa and γ-aminobutyric acid. Work with fibroblasts engineered to produce L-dopa, the precursor of the neurotransmitter dopamine, revealed good survival of the cells for 10 weeks after implantation into the brain of rats with experimental Parkinson's disease.[13] Further, the implanted fibroblasts significantly ameliorated some of the behavioral abnormalities of the rats, suggesting that the genetically modified cells continued to release L-dopa *in vivo* and affect the functioning of the host brain.

ACETYLCHOLINE-PRODUCING FIBROBLASTS

In considering genetically modified cells that would be appropriate for the neurodegenerative changes observed in Alzheimer's disease, we recently developed a primary fibroblast line that produces ACh.[14] These cells were obtained by infecting cultured fibroblasts with a retroviral vector that expressed *Drosophila* ChAT (dChAT) from the 5′ long terminal repeat. *In vitro*, these cells were found to contain ChAT protein that was biologically active, as assessed through immunohistochemical staining and biochemical assays.

Consistent with these observations, the dChAT-expressing fibroblasts were found to produce and release ACh into the culture media.

The ability of the engineered fibroblasts to take in choline from the culture media, which was then converted into ACh, was found to be at least partly mediated through high affinity choline uptake mechanisms. In brain synaptosomes, high affinity choline uptake is defined by three properties: a K_m less than 5 μM; sensitivity to hemicholinium-3 (HC-3); and Na+ dependence.[15] Both human and avian skin fibroblasts exhibit all of these properties,[16,17] suggesting that fibroblasts in general display high affinity accumulation of choline. However, such mechanisms have not been explored in rat fibroblasts. Using a protocol described by Riker and colleagues for exploring choline uptake in human fibroblasts,[16] rat fibroblasts were found to display a K_m of 3.2 μM (mean of two experiments). An example of a Lineweaver-Burk plot of choline accumulation in rat fibroblasts is shown in FIGURE 1. The K_m observed for the rat fibroblasts was similar to those obtained for human (5 μM) and avian fibroblasts (3 μM).[16,17] In addition to the low K_m value, rat fibroblasts also showed inhibition of choline uptake in the presence of HC-3 (IC_{50} = 50 μM) and in the absence of Na+. Therefore, consistent with results obtained with other fibroblast populations, rat fibroblasts contain a high affinity choline uptake system.

The choline uptake system in the rat fibroblasts appears to provide an avenue for manipulating ACh production within the engineered cells. When dChAT-expressing fibroblasts were exposed to increasing concentrations of

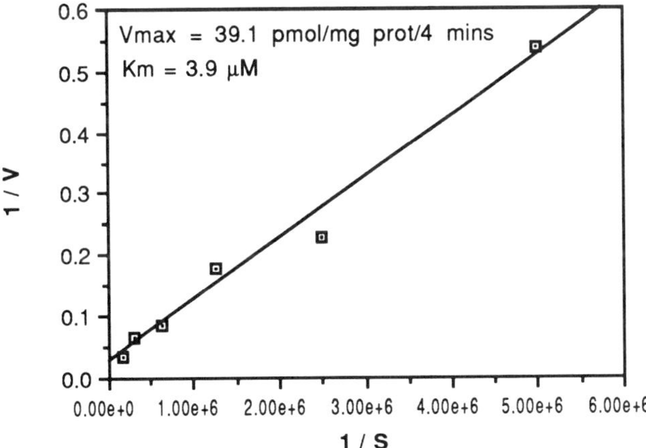

FIGURE 1. Representative Lineweaver-Burk plot of [³H]choline accumulation in primary rat fibroblasts. The 4 minute assay was performed at 37°C on cultures that were 1- to 2-days post-confluent. Choline concentrations were varied from 0.2 μM to 6.4 μM. The uptake observed at 37°C was typically 3- to 8-fold higher than that observed in cultures kept at 1°C. The mean V_{max} for 2 experiments was 27.5 pmol/mg prot/4 min assay.

choline *in vitro* (0.25–500 μM), the cells showed up to a threefold increase in the levels of ACh produced.[14] This choline-induced increase in ACh synthesis was consistent with results obtained with immortalized fibroblasts that were genetically modified to express dChAT[18] and has also been described in other cells lines that express a ChAT transgene.[19]

In considering the primary dChAT-expressing fibroblasts as a source of ACh for grafting, it was important to establish that the cells continued to produce and release ACh after implantation into the brain. The cells were therefore grafted into the hippocampus of adult rats and the *in vivo* microdialysis technique was used to measure ACh levels in the vicinity of the grafts. Samples collected from anesthetized rats 7–10 days after grafting revealed ACh levels around the dChAT-fibroblast grafts that averaged 20.9 ± 2.9 pmol/30 μl (FIG. 2). This was in marked contrast to the fourfold lower levels of ACh that were typical in both the non-grafted hippocampus (5.2 ± 1.8 pmol/30 μl) and adjacent to control grafts containing β-galactosidase-expressing fibroblasts (5.0 ± 1.2 pmol/30 μl). Following the collection of baseline samples from the grafted rats, choline chloride was infused through the indwelling microdialysis probe. This localized choline administration was found to induce a significant increase in ACh levels around the dChAT-fibroblast grafts (FIG. 2). While there was a profound effect of the choline on the dChAT grafts, there was no change in ACh overflow within the control

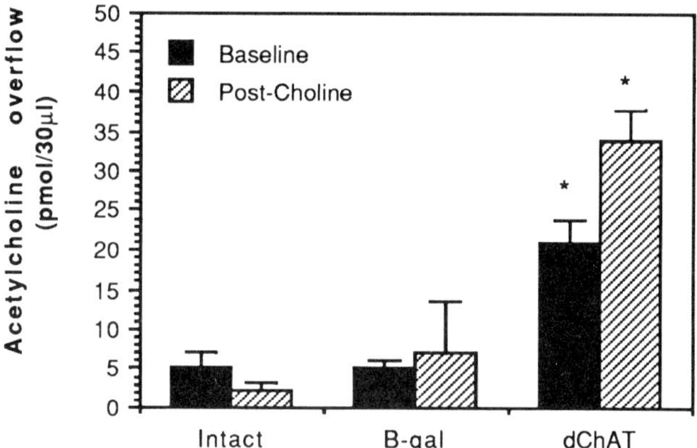

FIGURE 2. Acetylcholine levels measured within the intact and grafted hippocampi. *In vivo* microdialysis samples were collected in the presence of 15 μM neostigmine bromide from anesthetized rats. Grafted rats were implanted with primary fibroblasts that expressed either β-galactosidase (B-gal) or *Drosophila* ChAT (dChAT). Baseline samples were obtained 60–90 minutes after probes were positioned within the hippocampus. After the baseline samples were collected, choline chloride (200 μM) was infused through the indwelling probe for 20 minutes. The post-choline samples were then obtained immediately after the choline was removed from the perfusate. Data represent mean ± standard error of the mean. Statistical comparisons between groups were performed using a one-way analysis of variance (*$p < 0.05$).

hippocampi. These results indicated that dChAT-expressing fibroblasts continue to synthesize and release ACh for at least one week after grafting. Further, the increase in ACh levels after choline infusion indicates that the cells are amenable to exogenous manipulations.

CONCLUSION

The results obtained with the ACh-producing fibroblasts confirmed previous work which indicated that engineered cells provide an effective method for achieving localized delivery of discrete molecules to the brain. However, there are issues that remain to be addressed to optimize the functioning of genetically modified cells after grafting. In particular, it has been reported that transgenes driven from a retroviral promoter may not display stable activity for prolonged periods *in vivo*.[20] Since stable transgene production is essential for long term therapeutic applications, we have initiated studies to explore alternative approaches for obtaining sustained transgene expression in fibroblasts and other cellular populations. In addition, we are particularly interested in developing genetically modified cells that can be easily regulated exogenously. Finally, while fibroblasts are an excellent vehicle for achieving passive delivery of substances to the brain, they will always lack the ability to functionally incorporate into the host system. Thus, continued developments in gene delivery to the brain will show an increased emphasis on using neurons for genetic manipulation and in refining techniques that allow the direct injection of therapeutic genes into cells *in vivo*.

ACKNOWLEDGMENTS

We would like to thank Malcolm Schinstine, Paul Salvaterra, Ad Dekker, and Jasodhara Ray for collaborative interactions and helpful discussions. We would also like to acknowledge the technical assistance of Henry Grajeda, Barbara Miller, Stephen Forbes, Regina Wu, and Jennifer Hablewitz in conducting some of the work described.

REFERENCES

1. KATZMAN, R. 1986. Alzheimer's disease. N. Engl. J. Med. **314:**964–973.
2. BARTUS, R. T., R. L. DEAN, B. BEER & A. S. LIPPA. 1982. The cholinergic hypothesis of geriatric memory dysfunction. Science 7:408–417.
3. WHITEHOUSE, P. J., D. L. PRICE, R. G. STRUBLE, A. W. CLARK, J. T. COYLE & M. R. DeLONG. 1982. Alzheimer's disease and senile dementia: Loss of neurons in the basal forebrain. Science **215:**1237–1239.

4. DAVIES, P. & A. J. F. MALONEY 1976. Selective loss of central cholinergic neurons in Alzheimer's disease. Lancet **2:**1403.

5. PERRY, E. K., B. E. TOMLINSON, G. BLESSED, K. BERGMANN, P. H. GIBSON & P. H. PERRY. 1978. Correlation of cholinergic abnormalities with senile plaques and mental test scores in senile dementia. Br. Med. J. **2:**1457–1459.

6. SCHWARTZ, R. D., R. E. DAVIS, S. GRACON, T. HOOVER, W. H. MOOS & R. PAVIA. 1991. Next generation tacrine. Neurobiol. Aging **12:**185–187.

7. DUNNETT, S. B. 1990. Neural transplantation in animal models of dementia. Eur. J. Neurosci. **2:**567–587.

8. GAGE, F. H., A. BJORKLUND, U. STENEVI, S. B. DUNNETT & P. A. T. KELLY. 1984. Intrahippocampal septal grafts ameliorate learning impairments in aged rats. Science **225:**533–536.

9. GAGE, F. H. & A. BJORKLUND. 1986. Cholinergic septal grafts into the hippocampal formation improve spatial learning and memory in aged rats by an atropine-sensitive mechanism. J. Neurosci. **6:**2837–2847.

10. GAGE, F. H., M. D. KAWAJA & L. J. FISHER. 1991. Genetically modified cells: Applications for intracerebral grafting. Trends Neurosci. **14:**328–333.

11. KAWAJA, M. D., A. M. FAGAN, B. L. FIRESTEIN & F. H. GAGE. 1991. Intracerebral grafting of cultured autologous skin fibroblasts into the rat striatum: An assessment of graft size and ultrastructure. J. Comp. Neurol. **307:**695–706.

12. KAWAJA, M. J. & F. H. GAGE. 1992. Morphological and neurochemical features of cultured primary skin fibroblasts of Fischer 344 rats following striatal implantation. J. Neurochem. **317:**102–116.

13. FISHER, L. J., H. A. JINNAH, L. C. KALE, G. A. HIGGINS & F. H. GAGE. 1991. Survival and function of intrastriatally grafted primary fibroblasts genetically modified to produce L-dopa. Neuron, **6:**371–380.

14. FISHER, L. J., M. SCHINSTINE, P. SALVATERRA, A. J. DEKKER, L. THAL & F. H. GAGE. 1993. In vivo production and release of acetylcholine from primary fibroblasts genetically modified to express choline acetyltransferase. J. Neurochem. In press.

15. KUHAR, M. J. & L. C. MURRIN. 1978. Sodium-dependent, high affinity choline uptake. J. Neurochem. **30:**15–21.

16. RIKER, D. K., R. H. ROTH & X. O. BREAKEFIELD. 1981. High-affinity [³H]choline accumulation in cultured human skin fibroblasts. J Neurochem **36:**746–752.

17. BARALD, K. F. & D. K. BERG. 1978. High affinity choline uptake by spinal cord neurons in dissociated cell culture. Dev. Biol. **65:**90–99.

18. SCHINSTINE, M., M. B. ROSENBERG, C. ROUTLEDGE-WARD, T. FRIEDMANN & F. H. GAGE. 1992. Effects of choline and quiescence on Drosophila choline acetyltransferase expression and acetylcholine production by transduced rat fibroblasts. J. Neurochem. **58:**2019–2029.

19. HABERT, E., S. BIRMAN & J. MALLET. 1992. High-level synthesis and fate of acetylcholine in baculovirus-infected cells: Characterization and purfication of recombinant rat choline acetyltransferase. J. Neurochem. **58:**1447–1453.

20. PALMER, T. D., G. J. ROSMAN, R. A. OSBORNE & A. D. MILLER. 1991. Genetically modified skin fibroblasts persist long after transplantation but gradually inactivate introduced genes. Proc. Natl. Acad. Sci. USA **88:**1330–1334.

Neural Stem Cells for CNS Transplantation

E. EDWARD BAETGE[a]

CytoTherapeutics, Inc., Providence, Rhode Island USA 02906

ABSTRACT: Neurodegenerative disorders such as Parkinson's, Alzheimer's, and Huntington's disease are becoming ever more prominent in our society. A direct approach towards therapeutic treatment of these diseases is through replacement therapy where normal tissue is transplanted back to the nervous system. Recently, significant progress has been achieved with transplants in Parkinson's disease, but the process is heavily dependent on an unstable and problematic source of fetal tissue. Neural stem cells may become the tissue/cell source necessary for developing the therapeutic potential of neural transplantation. Stem cells are self-renewing, multipotent and could provide a well-characterized and clean source of transplantable material. A number of new *in vitro* approaches have led to the development of continuously propagated stem cells that are potential candidates for nervous system transplantation. These include oncogene-induced immortalization and growth-factor stimulation of naturally occurring central and peripheral nervous system stem cells. The nature of these cells and their suitability for transplantation into the CNS will be evaluated.

Transplantation into the mammalian nervous system has long been a dream of neurobiologists. Until the 1970s only a few such experiments had been attempted and with little success. Over the last two decades a large number of rodent transplantation paradigms have been successfully employed to investigate both the survival of implanted tissue and its ability to repair damaged CNS structures.

The success of the rodent studies has led to the application of these procedures to human transplantation, particularly in Parkinson's disease. Recently some of the most promising transplantation successes have been observed in patients with MPTP-induced and idiopathic Parkinsonism.[1-3] At present, these procedures are dependent on the availability of suitable fetal mesencephalic tissue obtained from 6- to 8-week-old aborted fetuses. Currently, the state of the art technique generates fetal cells that are 70–80% viable with 10–15% of these cells immunoreactive for tyrosine hydroxylase. In the majority of cases it is estimated that only 5–10% of the engrafted tissue survives long-term at the implant site.[1]

Although these fetal tissue isolation and transplantation procedures are

[a] *Send correspondence to:* E. Edward Baetge, Ph.D., CytoTherapeutics, Inc., 2 Richmond Square, Providence, RI 02906; TEL: 401-272-3310; FAX: 401-421-8587.

likely to improve with time, there are many obvious disadvantages for its use in brain transplantation. Serious questions arise as to whether the supply of fetal tissue will be an adequate or consistent source of safe, transplantable material for the ever increasing patient population afflicted with neurodegenerative disorders. In addition, the moral and ethical debate over the use of fetal tissue continues to be one of the most serious obstacles to this form of transplantation.

If one could choose the ideal source of cells or tissue for nervous system transplantation, it might have the following qualities: 1) the cells or tissue to be transplanted would be produced in large quantities in a reproducible fashion like a cell line; 2) the material would be well-characterized, free of adventitious agents, and would be non-transformed and non-tumorigenic when implanted into the host; 3) the transplanted tissue would be capable of differentiating into both neurons and glial cells (pluripotential), and be capable of integrating into the host brain in a relevant functional/regenerative manner, and; 4) the transplanted material would not require long-term immunosuppression for survival. All of this may be possible if homogeneous, allogenic or even xenogenic neuronal populations are transplanted which have been demonstrated to lack or express very low levels of the major histocompatibility antigens (MHC) necessary for antigen presentation.[4,5] Neural-derived stem cells possess many of the characteristics listed above as they are self-renewing and under the proper conditions capable of producing differentiated progeny,[6,7] and as such they may prove to be widely applicable for CNS transplantation.

Recently, a rodent neural cell line with a number of these characteristics has been derived from the embryonic hippocampal anlagen. These cells, termed HiB5, were derived by infection of the embryonic (E16) rat hippocampus with a retrovirus expressing a temperature-sensitive SV40 large T-antigen.[8] The cells express an intermediate filament protein called nestin[9] which is expressed *in vivo*[10] and *in vitro*[11] by neuroepithelial-derived stem cells. This intermediate filament protein appears to be specifically expressed by early stem/progenitor cells in both the peripheral and central nervous systems and upon terminal differentiation is replaced by either glial (glial fibrillary acidic protein - GFAP) or neuronal- (neurofilaments) specific intermediate filament proteins. Although the HiB5 cell line does not assume highly differentiated phenotypes *in vitro*, it can be transplanted back into the postnatally developing hippocampal dentate gyrus or cerebellum and assume differentiated morphologies and some antigenic markers associated with both neurons and glia.[8] In this respect, the HiB5 cells have been demonstrated to be multipotential after transplantation into either the developing hippocampal dentate gyrus or cerebellar granule layer. These experiments indicate that the developmental fate of at least some transplanted neural precursor cells is influenced by the CNS environment.

With respect to the ideal cell source for neural transplantation, the HiB5 line satisfies the requirement for large numbers of transplantable cells. The HiB5 line is conditionally immortalized with a temperature-sensitive SV40 T-antigen, which is inactivated at the non-permissive temperature of 37–39°C. As the rodent core temperature is believed to be in this range, the transplanted HiB5 cells appear to become non-immunoreactive for T-antigen, cease cell division, and terminally differentiate. It is reported that no tumors form anywhere in the recipient CNS after implantation of the HiB5 cells. The HiB5 cells can be transplanted allogenically into rats, but it is not clear what percentage of the cells survive and become appropriately differentiated and integrated *in vivo* and whether these cells are functionally active. These cells represent an excellent system for studying the interaction of neuronal stem cells with the normal or lesioned nervous system and satisfy many of the characteristics of a renewable source of transplantable neuronal stem-like cells. It remains to be determined how multipotenital these cells are and whether a similar version of this cell might be obtained from the human nervous system.

A number of other precursor cell lines with some of the features of the HiB5 cells have also been established from the embryonic nervous system using retrovirally mediated oncogene transfer. However, further characterization is necessary in order to demonstrate that these cells possess at least some features of true CNS stem cells.[12–15] The application of a large number of oncogenes for the derivation of continuous or immortalized neuronal and glial cell lines has yielded a vast array of these lines. Many of these immortalized cell lines have greatly contributed to our understanding of some of the complex processes and interactions within the nervous system. It is worth noting however, that the continuous nature of these lines and their capacity for producing large quantities of material is a direct result of the presence of the oncogene. Even though the expression of some of these oncogenes is conditional in nature, and some of the cell lines apparently do not readily form tumors in the rodent brain, they raise serious safety issues in the context of human transplantation.

The ideal neural stem cell would be continuous in culture, with growth and differentiation properties under normal epigenetic control and preferably not modified with transforming or immortalizing genes. In attempts to develop culture conditions for the propagation of endogenous neural stem cells *in vitro*, a number of investigators have demonstrated growth factor[11,16,17] and conditioning cell requirements[18,19] for stimulation of neuronal stem cell proliferation. However, these culture methods have not enabled the continuous propagation of cells possessing true stem cell characteristics *in vitro*. Recently, Ray *et al.*[27] have demonstrated that primary embryonic hippocampal progenitor cells can be propagated long-term in the presence of 10–20 ng/ml bFGF. This growth factor–stimulated progenitor cell population appears restricted to the generation of nerve cells as determined by immuno-cytochemical and ultrastructural analysis.

Reynolds and Weiss,[20,21] have discovered a novel striatal progenitor cell that can be continuously propagated *in vitro*. The EGF-responsive progenitor cells can be isolated from embryonic[21] and adult mouse brain,[20] and can be continuously propagated in EGF-containing culture medium. Removal of EGF prevents proliferation. A single cell from one of these EGF-generated clusters can be plated by limiting dilution giving rise to an "identical" cell cluster within 10 days. Both EGF and TGFα can stimulate the propagation of similar clusters of cells while NGF, PDGF or TGFβ are not capable of stimulating cell proliferation. The majority of cells in the EGF-generated clusters also express the intermediate filament nestin. When these cell clusters are allowed to proliferate for 25 days *in vitro* (DIV), a variety of neuronal and glial phenotypes appear. These include, NSE, neurofilament, substance P, GABA, and met-enkephalin immunoreactive cells, in addition to GFAP immunoreactive astrocytes. BrdU-labeling of EGF-generated clusters between 14 and 21 DIV results in NSE and GFAP double-labeled cells at 25 DIV. These results indicate that the EGF-generated cell clusters are capable of differentiating into the majority of cell types that exist within the striatum. Furthermore, the production of differentiated BrdU-labeled neurons and glia indicate that the progenitor cells are actively dividing before terminal differentiation.

It remains to be determined whether these progenitor cells are limited to producing only cells present in the striatum or whether they are capable of generating neurons and glia found in other regions of the CNS. It is suggested from the work by Reynolds and Weiss that the EGF-responsive cells have self-renewing properties in that isolated cell clusters can be split into single cells which can reproducibly give rise to a multipotential cluster of cells containing an unknown number of the original "stem" cells. It is suggested that these stem-like cells can continue to be self-renewing and divide in an asymmetric fashion (divide to produce an identical stem cell and a more differentiated daughter cell) and are capable of giving rise to neuronal and glial cells throughout the life span of the organism. In support of this idea, apparently identical, multipotent EGF-dependent cells can be isolated from both E14 and adult mouse brain. Currently, these cells remain pluripotential up to 30 passages *in vitro*. It is very likely that the true potential of these cells will be discovered using a combination of *in vitro* (growth factor, co-culture) and in vivo differentiation paradigms similar to those used for the HiB5 cells.

It will also be important to relate the Weiss/Reynolds EGF-dependent progenitor cells to the O_2A precursor cell which gives rise to the oligodendrocyte and type II astrocyte described by Raff and collaborators[22,23] and to the recently identified NO precursor cell[24] that gives rise to both neurons and oligodendrocytes.

Interestingly, it has been previously reported that EGF and TGFα also stimulate retinal neuroepithelial cell mitosis in primary cultures.[25] This work clearly shows that a variety of retinal neuronal and glial phenotypes can be generated in these cultures in the presence of EGF and low serum conditions. Under these culture conditions these cells were not demonstrated to be capable of continuous propagation.

Finally, recently published experiments indicate that a multipotent neural crest stem cell can be identified and cultured *in vitro*.[26] It is of interest to mention here that the initial culturing medium contains 100 ng/ml EGF together with βFGF and 2.5S NGF. The neural crest stem/progenitor cell can be isolated by FACS sorting of surface labeled crest cells or through replating and cell surface labeling using antibodies to low affinity nerve growth factor receptor (LNGFR). In this work, Stemple and Anderson have demonstrated that all of the LNGFR positive neural crest cell progenitors express high levels of the intermediate filament protein, nestin. Primary clones cultured for 9–14 days generated neuronal morphologies reacting with antibodies to neurofilament 160KD, N-CAM, and peripherin. Peripherin is an intermediate filament protein expressed almost exclusively within the peripheral nervous system. These differentiated cells no longer express nestin or LNGFR. Furthermore, addition of forskolin (5μm) and 10% FBS to the culture medium results in the expression of Schwann cell markers, GFAP, P_0 and sulfatide-0_4 in many of the non-neuronal cells remaining in these cultures.

If 6 day-old LNGFR receptor positive clones are dispersed into single cells and replated, 50% of those cells survive and grow into colonies that produce peripherin positive neurons and GFAP-positive Schwann cells. These experiments suggest that the neural crest progenitor/stem cell is multipotent and can reproduce both asymmetrically and symmetrically giving rise to itself and a differentiated daughter cell.

Although the neuronal phenotype(s) produced by these cells are not known, it is clear that both neurons and Schwann cells can be generated from a single neural crest "stem" cell and that these cells appear to be both self-renewing and pluripotential. It now remains to be demonstrated whether these cells can be continuously propagated and employed for *in vivo* transplantation paradigms.

In summary, a number of neuroepithelial derived "stem" cell populations have been adapted to the culture environment. This is a significant advance towards developing a reproducible and highly manipulatable source of uniform cells for application to transplantation in the nervous system. Whether these cells can be continuously cultured with no loss of renewing potential remains to be shown. Furthermore, it is not clear whether any of the cells described are pluripotential for all CNS and PNS cell types or have a more limited potential. Finally, there is little evidence for the ability of these "stem"-like cells to be successfully transplanted into the nervous system. Much work remains to determine the true potential of these putative nervous system stem cell populations, but the prospects are incredibly exciting.

REFERENCES

1. WIDNER, H., J. TETRUD, S. REHNCRONA, B. SNOW, P. BRUNDIN, B. GUSTAVII, A. BJORKLUND, O. LINDVALL & J. W. LANGSTON. 1992. Bilateral fetal mesencephalic grafts in two patients with Parkinsonism induced by 1-methyl-4-phenyl-1,2,3,6-tetrahydropyridine (MPTP). N. Engl. J. Med. **327:**1556–1563.

2. FREED, C. R., R. E. BREEZE, N. L. ROSENBERG, S. A. SCHNECK, E. KRIEK, J. QI, T. LONE, Y. ZHANG, J. A. SNYDER, T. H. WELLS, L. O. RAMIG, L. THOMPSON, J. C. MAZZIOTTA, S. C. HUANG, S. T. GRAFTON, D. BROOKS, G. SAWLE, G. SCHROTER & A. A. ANSARI. 1992. Survival of implanted fetal dopamine cells and neurologic improvement 12 to 46 months after transplantation for Parkinson's disease. N. Engl. J. Med. **327:**1549–1555.

3. SPENCER, D. D., R. J. ROBBINS, F. NAFTOLIN, K. L. MAREK, T. VOLLMER, C. LERANTH, R. H. ROTH, L. H. PRICE, A. GJEDDE, B. S. BUNNEY, K. J. SASS, J. D. ELSWORTH, L. KIER, R. MAKUCH, P. B. HOFFER & E. REDMOND, JR. 1992. Unilateral transplantation of human fetal mesencephalic tissue into the caudate nucleus of patients with Parkinson's disease. N. Engl. J. Med. **327:**1541–1548.

4. LAMPSON, L. A. 1987. Molecular bases of the immune response to neural antigens. Trends Neurosci. **10:**211–216.

5. SLOAN, D. J., M. J. WOOD & H. M. CHARLTON. 1991. The immune response to intracerebral neural grafts. Trends Neurosci. **14:**341–346.

6. HALL, P. A. & F. M. WATT. 1989. Stem cells: The generation and maintenance of cellular diversity. Development **106:**619–633.

7. POTTEN, C. S. & M. LOEFFLER. 1990. Stem cells: Attributes, cycles, spirals, pitfalls and uncertainties. Lessons for and from the crypt. Development **110:**1001–1020.

8. RENFRANZ, P. J., M. G. CUNNINGHAM & R. D. G. MCKAY. 1991. Region-specific differentiation of the hippocampal stem cell line HiB5 upon implantation into the developing mammalarian brain. Cell **66:**713–729.

9. LENDAHL, U., L. B. ZIMMERMAN & R. D. G. MCKAY. 1990. CNS stem cells express a new class of intermediate filament protein. Cell **60:**585–595.

10. FREDERIKSEN, K. & R. MCKAY. 1988. Proliferation and differentiation of rat neuroepithelial precursor cells in vivo. J. Neurosci. **8:**1144–1151.

11. CATTANEO, E. & R. D. G. MCKAY. 1990. Proliferation and differentiation of neuronal stem cells regulated by nerve growth factor. Nature **347:**762–765.

12. BARTLETT, P. F., H. H. REID, K. A. BAILEY & O. BERNARD. 1988. Immortalization of mouse neural precursor cells by the c-myc oncogene. Proc. Natl. Acad. Sci. USA **85:**3255–3259.

13. GELLER, H. M. & M. DUBOIS-DALCQ. 1988. Antigenic and functional characterization of a rat central nervous system-derived cell line immortalized by a retroviral vector. J. Cell Biol. **107:**1977–1986.

14. EVRARD, C., I. BORDE, P. MARIN, B. E. GALIANA, J. PREMONT, F. GROS & P. ROUGET. 1990. Immortalization of bipotential and plastic glio-neuronal precursor cells. Proc. Natl. Acad. Sci. USA **87:**3062–3066.

15. SNYDER, E. Y., D. L. DEITCHER, C. WALSH, S. ARNOLD-ALDEA, E. A. HARTWIG & C. L. CEPKO. 1992. Multipotent neural cell lines can engraft and participate in development of mouse cerebellum. Cell **68:**33–51.

16. GENSBURGER, C., G. LABOURDETTE & M. SENSENBRENNER. 1987. Brain basic fibroblast growth factor stimulates the proliferation of rat neuronal precursor cells in vitro. FEBS Lett. **217:**1–5.

17. MURPHY, M., J. DRAGO & P. F. BARTLETT. 1990. Fibroblast growth factor stimulates the proliferation and differentiation of neural precursor cells in vitro. J. Neurosci. Res. **25:**463–475.

18. TEMPLE, S. 1989. Division and differentiation of isolated CNS in microculture. Nature **340:**471–473.

19. RICHARDS L. J., T. J. KILPATRICK & P. F. BARTLETT. 1992. De novo generation of neuronal cells from the adult mouse brain. Proc. Natl. Acad. Sci. USA **89:** 8591–8595.

20. REYNOLDS, B. A. & S. WEISS. 1992. Generation of Neurons and astrocytes from isolated cells of the adult mammalian central nervous system. Science **255:** 1707–1710.

21. REYNOLDS, B. A., W. TETZLAFF & S. WEISS. 1992. A multipotent EGF-responsive striatal embryonic progenitor cell produces neurons and astrocytes. J. Neurosci **12:**4565–4574.

22. RAFF, M. C. 1989. Glial cells diversification in the rat optic nerve. Science **243:** 1450–1455.

23. RAFF, M. C., L. E. LILLIEN, W. D. RICHARDSON, J. F. BURNE & M. NOBLE. 1988. Platelet-derived growth factor from astocytes drives the clock that times oligodendrocyte development in culture. Nature **333:**562–565.

24. WILLIAMS, B. P., J. READ & J. PRICE. 1991. The generation of neurons and oligodendrocytes from a common precursor cell. Neuron **7:**685–693.

25. ANCHAN, R. M., T. A. REH, J. ANGELLO, A. BALLIET & M. WALKER. 1991. EFG and TGF-α stimulate retinal neuroepithelial cell proliferation in vitro. Neuron **6:**923–936.

26. STEMPLE. D. K. & D. J. ANDERSON. 1992. Isolation of a stem cell for neurons and glia from the mammalian neural crest. Cell **71:**973–985.

27. RAY, J., D. A. PETERSON, M. SCHINSTINE & F. H. GAGE. 1993. Proliferation, differentiation, and long-term culture of primary hippocampal neurons. Proc. Natl. Acad. Sci. USA **90:**3602–3606.

Neurotrophic Strategies for Treating Alzheimer's Disease: Lessons from Basic Neurobiology and Animal Models[a]

VASSILIS E. KOLIATSOS[b], DONALD L. PRICE, RICHARD E. CLATTERBUCK, ALICJA L. MARKOWSKA, DAVID S. OLTON, AND BARBARA J. WILCOX

The Johns Hopkins University School of Medicine, Neuropathology Laboratory, Baltimore, Maryland USA 21205

ABSTRACT: Because neurotrophic factors can prevent natural and experimental cases of neural cell death and induce and maintain differentiation, they are especially attractive agents for the treatment of neurodegenerative diseases, such as Alzheimer's disease (AD). The present report argues for the specific role of particular families of trophic factors, such as neurotrophins (*e.g.,* nerve growth factor [NGF]) and neurokines (*e.g.,* ciliary neurotrophic factor [CNTF]), for the promotion of the survival and phenotype of subsets of central nervous system (CNS) neurons vulnerable in AD, such as basal forebrain cholinergic neurons and cortical projection neurons. Although there is ample evidence for the therapeutic role of NGF in experimental or natural injury of cholinergic neurons, not enough progress has been made on trophic models involving cortical neurons. Further understanding of the mechanisms of cell death in AD and elucidation of the transduction cascades of trophic factors will undoubtedly refine our current concepts of a neurotrophic treatment for AD.

THE PLACE OF TROPHIC FACTORS IN THE TREATMENT OF ALZHEIMER'S DISEASE

Alzheimer's disease (AD) is a chronic neurodegenerative disorder that accounts for the majority of cases of senile dementia. During the course of AD, selective populations of neurons manifest progressive abnormalities,

[a] This work was supported by grants from the U.S. Public Health Service (NS 20471, AG 05146, NS 07179) as well as the American Health Assistance Foundation and the Metropolitan Life Foundation. Drs. Koliatsos and Price are the recipients of a Leadership and Excellence in Alzheimer's Disease (LEAD) award (AG 07914). Dr. Price is also the recipient of a Javits Neuroscience Investigator Award (NS 10580).

[b] *Send correspondence to:* Dr. Vassilis Koliatsos, The Johns Hopkins University School of Medicine, Neuropathology Laboratory, 558 Ross Research Building, 720 Rutland Avenue, Baltimore, MD 21205-2196; USA TEL: (410) 955-5632; FAX: (410) 955-9777.

including alterations in neurotransmitter metabolism and in the neuronal cytoskeleton. These changes lead to effective denervation of target systems in the brain and, ultimately, to the clinical manifestations of dementia, including disorders of memory, verbal skills and visuospatial orientation, ideomotor apraxia, and behavior abnormalities. The mechanisms of dysfunction and death of neurons in AD are not well understood; therefore, for the sake of this discussion, AD will be viewed as a complement of pathologies in the cell bodies and neuropil (the latter term including synapses and the extracellular space). Although it is likely that all the above pathologies are linked via direct or third-party associations, for the sake of simplicity, they will be considered as independent targets for treatment (FIG. 1). For instance, to inhibit the progression of amyloid deposition, the use of competitive protease substrates could be implemented.[1] To stimulate the remaining functional synapses (*e.g.*, cholinergic synapses), acetylcholinesterase (AChE) inhibitors could be used that could address the molecular forms of AChE resistant to the degenerative process[2] or directly stimulate the disconnected postsynaptic site with cholinergic agonists. Obviously, a very important target for therapy is the cell body of the afflicted neuron, which is losing its signaling capabilities and gradually degenerating via multiple mechanisms that involve membrane failure, displacement and/or entanglement of cell organelles by abnormal cytoskeletal constituents, calcium overload, free radicals, or even the transcription of new and, as yet, unidentified genes mediating cell death.[3] A variety of agents could be used theoretically for the above changes, including calcium-binding proteins, free-radical scavengers, *etc.* Trophic factors are particularly relevant to the treatment of the degenerative process at the perikaryal level. Certain classes of trophic factors (*i.e.*, neurotrophins, exemplified by NGF) are defined by their prevention of developmental cell death in peripheral neurons and their sustenance of the survival of peripheral and central neurons in the adult under various conditions of injury, ranging from traumatic and neurotoxic insults to age-associated degenerative processes.[4]

Another interesting effect of neurotrophins is the induction of differentiation of peripheral and central neurons and the maintenance of the mature phenotype of responsive populations of neurons.[5] Because neurons in AD degenerate through a protracted course during which they show alterations in neurotransmitter and cytoskeletal markers as well as changes in their shape and size, the differentiating effects of neurotrophins are particularly attractive. In the present summary, we will deal with two broad classes of neurotrophic factors, the neurotrophins (see above) and the neurokines. As mentioned above, the former, a family with high amino acid homology, includes peptides such as NGF, BDNF, NT-3, and NT-4/5.[6] The latter represent a group of heterogeneous pleiotropic peptides, many of which are known for their effects on nonneural cells; neurokines include the fibroblast growth factors (FGF), interleukins, transforming growth factors β, leukemia inhibitory factor, and

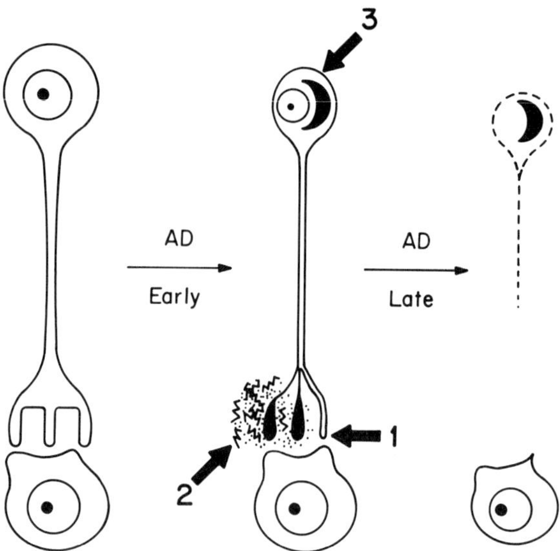

FIGURE 1. A schematic representation of an idealized progression of pathology in the brain of an individual with AD. The diagram is based on the basic circuit of two neurons, one of which *(top)* is synapsing on the other *(bottom)*. The putative targets for treatment are indicated by arrows. 1 represents remaining functional synapses. 2 represents abnormal terminals (neurites) in an area of an amyloid deposition (plaque). Abnormalities in nerve terminals are manifested by gross alterations in shape and size and loss of apparent contacts with postsynaptic structures; according to some investigators, synaptic destruction contributes more significantly to dementia than any other pathological change associated with the disease.[21] Amyloid deposits are made up of a 4-kD peptide termed β-amyloid or Aβ; this peptide polymerizes into 4–8 nm filaments with β-pleated conformation. Amyloid forms the core of the senile plaque, the periphery of which recruits abnormal neuronal processes (neurites) (in this schema, abnormal nerve terminals). Perikaryal abnormalities **(3)** affect all major domains of neuronal function, but the most representative changes are the disappearance of differentiated neuronal phenotypes (including breakdown in neurotransmitter synthesis and alterations in perikaryal morphology) and a wide range of complex and interdependent alterations of the cytoskeleton.[22] The most characteristic cytoskeletal alteration is the neurofibrillary tangle (NFT) (black semilune in the diagram). The NFT is composed primarily of paired helical filaments (that contain phosphorylated tau) but also contains other abnormal constituents, such as phosphorylated neurofilament proteins. Sequestration of these cytoskeletal alterations is incompatible with normal cell function and may be a major cause of death of the afflicted neurons (late AD, *right panel*).

CNTF.[7] We will examine the effects of the previous classes of factors on CNS neurons, focusing on basal forebrain cholinergic neurons and projection neurons in neocortex and hippocampus, two populations of neurons implicated in complex CNS functions at risk in AD.

NEUROTROPHINS AND BASAL FOREBRAIN CHOLINERGIC NEURONS

Cholinergic neurons of the basal forebrain express p75[NGFR] and trkA,[8] whereas their targets in the hippocampus and neocortex are the main sites of NGF expression in the CNS.[9] During development as well as in the adult, NGF up-regulates the expression of ChAT and p75[NGFR] in these neurons and increases their size.[10] Although there is no direct evidence that changes in levels of NGF play a primary role in the degeneration of these cholinergic neurons in AD, it is possible that the administration of NGF could prevent cell death and restore some functions of these neurons in AD patients.[11] Among other neurotrophins, BDNF and NT-3 are also enriched in hippo-campus.[12] However, neither BDNF nor NT-3 appears to influence intact cholinergic neurons of the basal forebrain *in vivo*. Transection of the axons of cholinergic neurons in the fimbria-fornix leads to rapid loss of the transmitter phenotype of these neurons and cytoskeletal and morphological alterations. This model has been very useful in assessing the effects of various preparations of NGF in reversing the phenotypic injury in basal forebrain cholinergic neurons. In all of these experiments, mouse and at least two preparations of human recombinant NGF have proven to afford full protection in axotomized cholinergic neurons of the medial septum. The specificity of the NGF effect can be assessed using ChAT biochemistry in medial septal tissue punches and constructing dose-response curves. Using this approach, it becomes apparent that the stimulatory effect of NGF on axotomized cholinergic neurons is dose dependent and saturates at a dose of 10 μg/week. Other neurotrophins enriched in targets of basal forebrain cholinergic neurons (*i.e.*, hippocampus) do not have any significant protective effect on these cholinergic neurons (measured by p75[NGFR]/ChAT immunocytochemistry *in situ* hybridization, or ChAT biochemistry in tissue punches). In view of the comparable efficacies of NGF and BDNF on basal forebrain cholinergic neurons *in vitro*,[13] the previous findings suggest an important discrepancy between the *in vitro* and *in vivo* effects of BDNF on cholinergic neurons, which merits further investigation. The same degree of NGF protection of cholinergic phenotype is seen in macaques with lesions of the fornix, followed by 2–4 weeks of treatment with either mouse or human NGF.[14,15]

Based on prelabeling studies with fluorescent dyes prior to axotomy, retrograde cell death settles in the complete fimbria-fornix model in the third week postaxotomy. Because, for the most part, treatment of rats with complete fimbria-fornix lesions has been limited to two weeks, it is unknown whether NGF merely reduces the phenotypic injury or, more importantly, prevents retrograde cell death in this system. More recently, we have extended the treatment of fimbria-fornix lesioned rats to four weeks postaxotomy, using sequential implantation of Alzet 2002 minipumps. We have found that NGF affords full protection of the phenotype and viability of cholinergic neurons up to four weeks postaxotomy. These results indicate that NGF not only protects basal forebrain cholinergic neurons from phenotypic injury, but also prevents retrograde cell death in this system.

Another set of experiments has focused on the efficacy of NGF on memory impairments that occur in aged rodents. The pioneering studies of Fisher *et al.*[16] indicated that NGF has effects on acetycholine-dependent mnemonic functions, as exemplified by the improved performance of aged rats on a place discrimination task that was manipulated to primarily assess retention. More recently, we were able to assess the behavioral effects of NGF in Fisher 344 rats in three tests: recent memory in a T-maze; place learning in water maze; and sensorimotor skills. Each rat was trained in all tasks, treated with NGF or vehicle, and retested following three weeks of continued infusion. Both high (40 μg/week) and low (10 μg/week) doses of NGF were used, and two age groups were tested: 4 months old and 23 months old. In 23-month-old rats, both doses of NGF improved performance in the place learning and recent memory tasks but did not improve sensorimotor skills. In young rats, performance on the T-maze deteriorated even with low doses of NGF. NGF increased ChAT activity in hippocampus and neocortex and sizes of cholinergic neurons in all sectors of the basal forebrain cholinergic system.

The next phase in the investigations of the behavioral effects of NGF will be to assess its effects on memory disorders that occur in aged-nonhuman primates and appear to be, at least in part, sensitive to cholinergic agents.[17] The behaviorally impaired aged monkeys comprise the most appropriate model of AD, and the efficacy of NGF treatment in this setting would likely precipitate carefully designed trials of NGF in a small group of patients with AD.[18]

NEUROKINES AND DEGENERATING CNS NEURONS

CNTF was described originally as an activity that supports the survival of neurons of the chick ciliary ganglia *in vitro*. The widespread expression of CNTF in the CNS and PNS suggests a broader trophic role for this peptide. CNTF prevents axotomy-induced cell death of neurons in the anteroventral and anterodorsal thalamic nuclei of the adult rat following transections of the cingulum bundle.[19] In the anteroventral nucleus of vehicle-treated animals there is a 75% reduction in the number of cells; additional evidence of retrograde degeneration is also present, including marked gliosis and the thalamic retrograde dust, a particulate deposit characteristic of degenerating thalamic neurons. In CNTF-treated animals, the magnitude of cell loss is decreased to 34% and other evidence of degeneration is either ameliorated (gliosis) or abolished (retrograde dust). In the anterodorsal nucleus, there is a 56% reduction in the number of cells in untreated lesioned animals but only a 20% reduction in CNTF-treated rats. Using the polymerase chain reaction, we have also demonstrated the presence of CNTFR (the CNTF binding protein) and gp130 (the principal CNTF/LIF/IL-6 transducing protein) mRNA in the anteroventral and anterodorsal thalamic nuclei. The coincidence of CNTF and two of its receptor proteins in a population of neurons responding to the factor suggests a paracrine function for CNTF. The thalamic axotomy paradigm should be viewed as a classical example of retrograde degeneration in the CNS and not as a model to demonstrate the selective effects of CNTF. The rescue of degenerating thalamic neurons by CNTF implies more broadly that neurokines have significant effects on CNS neurons in vivo and that they can prevent cell death in the adult CNS. Therefore, they should be tested in models involving CNS neurons more closely associated with AD, such as basal forebrain cholinergic neurons and cortical projection neurons (see below).

TROPHIC FACTORS FOR CORTICAL NEURONS

Except for sporadic reports, very little is known about the effects of different factors on cortical neurons. BDNF, NT-3, and NGF are all expressed in pyramidal cortical neurons (an expression pattern consistent with the utilization of these factors in corticocortical pathways). Cortical neurons also express trkB and trkC, although it is presently unknown whether these receptors represent the full-length receptor isoforms, which contain the tyrosine kinase domain or truncated isoforms, representing nonfunctional receptors. A major obstacle in the effective pursuit of trophic factors for cortical neurons has been the lack of a reliable model of experimental degeneration of cortical neurons. However, there is recent evidence that transection of the axons of entorhinal projection neurons in the perforant pathway results in 30% reduction of large layer II-III entorhinal neurons one month posttransection.[20] We have recently performed similar lesions including perforant pathway transections as well as subtotal hippocampectomies; by applying stereological methods of quantitation of the retrograde changes in entorhinal cortex, we found that the above lesions result in shrinkage of large layer II-III entorhinal neurons (20–30%) but not in cell death. Whatever the case, it appears that lesions similar to those used in basal forebrain and thalamic degeneration models can be applied in the case of cortical neurons and can lead to measurable retrograde changes. In the same report, Cummings *et al.*[20] have found that the neurokine basic FGF can prevent retrograde pathology in entorhinal neurons. Although this finding is very interesting, the generally recognized local and systemic complications associated with this neurokine limit its application in patients with AD. In summary, the limited but encouraging information from novel models of cortical degeneration and the use of FGF should stimulate efforts to assess the efficacy of other neurotrophic factors (*i.e.*, neurotrophins) for different populations of cortical neurons.

CONCLUSIONS AND FUTURE DIRECTIONS

In the present account, we discuss the status of trophic factors as potential therapeutic agents for AD and we use examples of animal models to illustrate the relevance of particular neurotrophic factors for AD. We focus on basal forebrain cholinergic neurons and cortical projection neurons and show that neutrophins can prevent both the phenotypic injury and retrograde cell death in cholinergic neurons and that the neurokine CNTF can prevent retrograde cell death in the CNS, using axotomized thalamic neurons as a model. It is still unknown whether the beneficial effects of trophic factors in the above animal models can be maintained over time under sustained infusion; this issue is very relevant for a chronic degenerative disorder, such as AD. Another issue is the precise mechanisms of cell death in AD. Further insights into these mechanisms can provide additional arguments for the use of trophic factors in this disease or can place certain limitations. Finally, the elucidation of trophic factor transduction pathways may lead to the use of smaller molecules which could act on second messenger substrates, thereby mimicking the neurotrophic effects by bypassing the receptor site; such molecules may easily cross the blood-brain barrier and, therefore, present clear clinical advantages. Progress along the frontiers outlined above will lead to a comprehensive trophic approach to treat AD and may simplify methods of treatment via the delivery of drugs that influence trophic cascades; the latter developments may not be less important than the former.

REFERENCES

1. CAPUTO, C. B. & A. I. SALAMA. 1989. The amyloid proteins of Alzheimer's disease as potential targets for drug therapy. Neurobiol. Aging **10:**451–461.
2. GIACOBINI, E., D. LINVILLE, E. MESSAMORE & N. OGANE. 1991. Toward a third generation of cholinesterase inhibitors. *In* Cholinergic Basis for Alzheimer Therapy. R. Becker & E. Giacobini, Eds. 477–490. Birkhäuser. Boston.
3. CHOI, D. W., Y. BARDE, M. CHALFIE, U. HEINEMANN, H. R. HORVITZ, K. S. KOSIK, H. W. MÜLLER, R. SCHWARCZ, M. SCHWARZ, E. M. SHOOTER, B. K. SIESJÖ & K. UNSICKER. 1991. Group report: Neuronal death and survival. *In* Neurodegenerative Disorders. Mechanisms and Prospects for Therapy. D. L. Price, H. Thoenen & A. J. Aguayo, Eds. 233–248. John Wiley & Sons. New York.
4. HAMBURGER, V., J. K. BRUNSO-BECHTOLD & J. W. YIP. 1988. Neuronal death in the spinal ganglia of the chick embryo and its reduction by nerve growth factor. J. Neurosci. **1:**60–71.
5. HAYASHI, Y. & N. MIKI. 1985. Purification and characterization of a neurite outgrowth factor from chicken gizzard smooth muscle. J. Biol. Chem. **260:** 14269–14278.
6. BERKEMEIER, L. R., J. W. WINSLOW, D. R. KAPLAN, K. NIKOLICS, D. V. GOEDDEL & A. ROSENTHAL. 1991. Neurotrophin-5: A novel neurotrophic factor that activates trk and trkB. Neuron **7:**857–866.
7. UNSICKER, K., C. GROTHE, R. WESTERMANN & K. WEWETZER. 1992. Cytokines in neural regeneration. Curr. Opin. Neurobiol. **2:**671–678.
8. HOLTZMAN, D. M., Y. LI, L. F. PARADA, S. KINSMAN, C-K. CHEN, J. S. VALLETTA, J. ZHOU, J. B. LONG & W. C. MOBLEY. 1992. p140[trk] mRNA

marks NGF-responsive forebrain neurons: Evidence that trk gene expression is induced by NGF. Neuron **9:**465–478.

9. KORSCHING, S., G. AUBURGER, R. HEUMANN, J. SCOTT & H. THOENEN. 1985. Levels of nerve growth factor and its mRNA in the central nervous system of the rat correlate with cholinergic innervation. EMBO J. **4:**1389–1393.

10. CAVICCHIOLI, L., T. P. FLANIGAN, J. G. DICKSON, G. VANTINI, R. D. TOSO, M. FUSCO, F. S. WALSH & A. LEON. 1991. Choline acetyltransferase messenger RNA expression in developing and adult rat brain: Regulation by nerve growth factor. Mol. Brain Res. **9:**319–325.

11. HEFTI, F. & W. J. WEINER. 1986. Nerve growth factor and Alzheimer's disease. Ann. Neurol. **20:**275–281.

12. MAISONPIERRE, P. C., L. BELLUSCIO, S. SQUINTO, N. Y. IP, M. E. FURTH, R. M. LINDSAY & G. D. YANCOPOULOS. 1990. Neurotrophin-3: A neurotrophic factor related to NGF and BDNF. Science **247:**1446–1451.

13. KNÜSEL, B., J. W. WINSLOW, A. ROSENTHAL, L. E. BURTON, D. P. SEID, K. NIKOLICS & F. HEFTI. 1991. Promotion of central cholinergic and dopaminergic neuron differentiation by brain-derived neurotrophic factor but not neurotrophin 3. Proc. Natl. Acad. Sci. USA **88:**961–965.

14. KOLIATSOS, V. E., R. E. CLATTERBUCK, H. J. W. NAUTA, B. KNÜSEL, L. E. BURTON, F. F. HEFTI, W. C. MOBLEY & D. L. PRICE. 1991. Human nerve growth factor prevents degeneration of basal forebrain cholinergic neurons in primates. Ann. Neurol. **30:**831–840.

15. TUSZYNSKI, M. H., H. SANG, K. YOSHIDA & F. H. GAGE. 1991. Recombinant human nerve growth factor infusions prevent cholinergic neuronal degeneration in the adult primate brain. Ann. Neurol. **30:**625–636.

16. FISCHER, W., K. Z. WICTORIN, A. BJÖRKLUND, L. R. WILLIAMS, S. VARON & F. H. GAGE. 1987. Amelioration of cholinergic neuron atrophy and spatial memory impairment in aged rats by nerve growth factor. Nature **329:**65–68.

17. BARTUS, R. T., R. L. DEAN & B. BEER. 1983. An evaluation of drugs for improving memory in aged monkeys: Implications for clinical trials in humans. Psychopharmacol. Bull. **19:**168–184.

18. PHELPS, C. H., F. H. GAGE, J. H. GROWDON, F. HEFTI, R. HARBAUGH, M. V. JOHNSON, Z. KHACHATURIAN, W. MOBLEY, D. PRICE, M. RASKIND, J. SIMPKINS, L. THAL & J. WOODCOCK. 1989. Potential use of nerve growth factor to treat Alzheimer's disease. Neurobiol. Aging **10:**205–207.

19. CLATTERBUCK, R. E., D. L. PRICE & V. E. KOLIATSOS. 1993. Ciliary neurotrophic factor prevents retrograde neuronal death in the adult central nervous system. Proc. Natl. Acad. Sci. USA. **90:**2222–2226.

20. CUMMINGS, B. J., G. J. YEE & C. W. COTMAN. 1993. bFGF promotes the survival of entorhinal layer II neurons after perforant path axotomy. Brain Res. In press.

21. TERRY, R. D., E. MASLIAH, D. P. SALMON, N. BUTTERS, R. DETERESA, R. HILL, L. A. HANSEN & R. KATZMAN. 1991. Physical basis of cognitive alterations in Alzheimer's disease: Synapse loss is the major correlate of cognitive impairment. Ann. Neurol. **30:**572–580.

22. PRICE, D. L., L. J. MARTIN, R. E. CLATTERBUCK, V. E. KOLIATSOS, S. S. SISODIA, L. C. WALKER & L. C. CORK. 1992. Neuronal degeneration in human diseases and animal models. J. Neurobiol. **23:**1277–1294.

Selective Signaling via Unique M1 Muscarinic Agonists[a]

ABRAHAM FISHER,[b,d] ELIAHU HELDMAN,[b] DAVID GURWITZ,[b] RACHEL HARING,[b] DOV BARAK,[b] HAIM MESHULAM,[b] DANIELE MARCIANO,[b] RACHEL BRANDEIS,[b] ZIPORA PITTEL,[b] MENAHEM SEGAL,[c] ZVI VOGEL,[c] AND YISHAI KARTON[b]

[b] *Israel Institute for Biological Research, Ness-Ziona, Israel*
[c] *The Weizmann Institute, Rehovot, Israel*

ABSTRACT: Rigid analogs of acetylcholine (ACh) were designed for selective actions at muscarinic receptor (mAChR) subtypes and distinct second messenger systems. AF102B, AF150, and AF151 are such rigid analogs of ACh. AF102B, AF150 and AF151 are centrally active M1 agonists. AF102B has a unique agonistic profile showing, inter alia: only part of the M1 electrophysiology of ACh and unusual binding parameters to mAChRs. AF150 and AF151 are more efficacious agonists than AF102B for M1 AChRS in rat cortex and in CHO cells stably transfected with the m1 AChR subtype. Notably, the selectivity of the new m1 agonists is reflected also by activation of select second messenger systems via distinct G-proteins. These compounds reflect a new pharmacological concept, tentatively defined as ligand-selective signaling. Thus, agonist/m1AChR complexes may activate different combinations of signaling pathways, depending on the ligand used. Rigid agonists may activate a limited repertoire of signaling systems. In various animal models for Alzheimer's disease (AD) the agonists AF102B, AF150 and AF151, exhibited positive effects on mnemomic processes and a wide safety margin. Such agonists, and especially AF102B, can be considered as a rational treatment strategy for AD.

INTRODUCTION

Five distinct human mAChR subtypes (m1–m5) have been cloned.[1] The mAChRs are G-protein coupled receptors having, in addition to the agonist-binding domain, a G-protein binding intracellular domain. This domain, by interaction with distinct G-proteins, controls second messenger systems. M1 or m1 agonists,[2–4] M2 or m2 antagonists, m3 agonists[2,3] or m3 antagonists,[e,4] or a combination of these in one compound were suggested as treatment

[a] Supported in part by Snow Brand Milk Products, Japan.
[d] *Send correspondence to:* Abraham Fisher, Ph.D., Israel Institute for Biological Research, P.O. Box 19, Ness-Ziona 70450, Israel; TEL: (972)-8-381-603; FAX: (972)-8-401-094.
[e] The terms m1–m5 and M1–M3 agonists (or antagonists) are used for agonists (or antagonists) defined using the cloned m1–m5 and M1–M3 pharmacologically characterized mAChRs, respectively.

strategies in AD. Yet, in AD a crucial abnormality may also occur along various signal transduction pathways.[5] Thus, m1 agonists selective both at the level of the ligand binding domain and at the level of second messengers are needed. We have shown that such selective m1 agonists can be designed via rigid analogs of ACh including: cis-2-methyl-spiro(1,3-oxathiolane-5,3′)quinuclidine (AF102B),[3,6–10] 2-methyl-spiro(1,3-oxazoline-5,4′)-*N*-methyl-piperidine (AF150) and 2-methyl-spiro (3,1-oxazoline-5,4′)-*N*-methyl-piperidine (AF151).[6,7,10] This presentation will survey new data on these compounds, which may be relevant for a rational treatment strategy in AD.

RESULTS AND DISCUSSION

The findings obtained to date indicate that AF102B is a selective M1 agonist.[3,6–10] Notably, AF102B can act as a full agonist, a partial agonist, or an antagonist depending on the tissue, the mAChR subtype and the functional assays studied. Thus, AF102B can best be considered as a selective M1 or m1 agonist when defined through functional assays. AF150 and AF151 are more efficacious agonists than AF102B for M1 AChRs in rat cerebral cortex (C T) vs. cerebellum (CER) {binding of [^{3}H]pirenzepine $\pm$ GppNHp (Gp) vs. [^{3}H]QNB, respectively; *e.g.*, for AF150 in CT: $K_{H-Gp} = 0.11$ μM (21%), $K_{L-Gp} = 11$ μM; $K_{L+Gp} = 19$ μM (100%); in CER: $K_H = 5.1$ μM (62%), $K_L = 81$ μM}. In Chinese hamster ovary (CHO) fibroblasts transfected with m1 AChR or m3 AChR and in SK-N-SH cells (expressing mostly m3 AChRs), AF102B shows partial m1 agonistic activity and m3 antagonistic activity, AF150 and AF151 are full m1 agonists and partial m3 agonists (cc 25% vs. CCh) (assayed by phosphoinositides [PI] hydrolysis and arachidonic acid [AA] release). Yet these compounds, unlike CCh, had no effect on either cAMP levels in intact m1AChR-transfected cells, or adenylyl cyclase activity in isolated membranes prepared from the same cells.[8] In CHO cells transfected with m1–m5 AChRs and assayed for changes of $[Ca^{2+}]_i$ (intracellular Ca^{2+}) levels, AF102B showed almost full m1 and partial m3 agonistic profiles, no effects on m4 and weak m2 and m5 agonistic effects; AF150 and AF151 showed for the transfected cells, almost full m1, m3 and m5 agonistic, yet only marginal agonistic profiles on m2 and m4 AChRs.[7] In CA1 neurons of rat hippocampal slices AF150 appears to be an M1>M2 agonist, but is more effective than AF102B (an M1 agonist). While AF102B induced only part of the M1 electrophysiological response to ACh, *e.g.*, reduction of the slow afterhyperpolarization (sAHP),[9] AF150 produced two effects mediated via M1 AChRs, a depolarization and a reduction of the sAHP, but had little effect on EPSPs or on input resistance.[10]

AF102B, AF150 and AF151 improved memory and learning deficits in a variety of animal models, which mimic cholinergic deficits reported in AD, without producing adverse central or peripheral side effects at the effective doses and showing a relatively wide safety margin.[3,6,10] AF102B is a promising candidate drug and is presently in Phase II clinical trials in AD patients. Notably, mRNA for $G_s\alpha$[11] were elevated in post-mortem brain tissues of AD patients, and an elevation of Gs and decrease of Gi were reported in aged human brains.[12] Taken together, these observations may imply increased sensitivity of m1AChR-mediated elevation in adenylyl cyclase in these situations. It is thus possible that the desired M1 or m1-selective agonists for the treatment of AD, should not stimulate adenylyl cyclase via m1AChR. These concepts of ligand-mediated selective signaling[6-8] might be tied with the recent findings that activation of m1 AChR resulted in a rapid increase in secretion of a soluble form of amyloid precursor protein.[13] In such a scenario, it can be implied that highly selective m1 agonists might have a more important role in the treatment of AD than originally envisaged.

REFERENCES

1. BONNER, T. I., N. J. BUCKLEY, A. C. YOUNG & M. R. BRANN. 1987. Identification of a family of muscarinic acetylcholine receptor genes. Science **237:** 527–532.

2. POTTER, L. T. 1992. Strategies for the treatment of Alzheimer's disease: Cholinergic agonist. *In* Alzheimer's Disease: New Treatment Strategies. Z. S. Khachaturian & J. P. Blass, Eds. 57–66. Marcel Dekker, New York.

3. FISHER, A., R. BRANDEIS, I. KARTON, Z. PITTEL, D. GURWITZ, R. HARING, M. SAPIR, A. LEVY & E. HELDMAN. 1991. Cis-2-methyl-spiro(1,3-oxathiolane-5,3')quinuclidine an M1 selective cholinergic agonist attenuates cognitive dysfunctions in an animal model of Alzheimer's disease. J. Pharmacol. Exp. Ther. **257:**392–403.

4. SUGITA, S., N. UCHIMURA, Z.-G. JIANG & R. A. NORTH. 1991. Distinct muscarinic receptors inhibit release of gama-aminobutyric acid and excitatory amino acids in mammalian brain. Proc. Natl. Acad. Sci. USA **88:**2608–2611.

5. FOWLER, C. J., C. O'NEILL, A. GARLIND & R. F. COWBURN. 1990. Alzheimer's disease: Is there a problem beyond recognition. TIPS **11:**183–184.

6. FISHER, A., Y. KARTON, E. HELDMAN, D. GURWITZ, R. HARING, H. MESHULAM, R. BRANDEIS, Z. PITTEL, Y. SEGALL, D. MARCIANO, I. MARKOVITCH, Z. SAMOCHA, E. SHIRIN, M. SAPIR, B. GREEN, G. SHOHAM & D. BARAK. 1993. Progress in medicinal chemistry of novel selective muscarinic agonists. Drug Design Disc. **9:**221–235.

7. FISHER, A., D. GURWITZ, D. BARAK, R. HARING, I. KARTON, R. BRANDEIS, Z. PITTEL, D. MARCIANO, H. MESHULAM, Z. VOGEL & E. HELDMAN. 1992. Rigid analogs of acetylcholine can be M1-selective agonists: Implications for a rational treatment strategy in Alzheimer's disease. Biorg. Med. Chem. Lett. **2:** 839–844.

8. GURWITZ, D., R. HARING, C. M. FRASER, E. HELDMAN & A. FISHER. 1991.

Selective signal transduction by the M1 agonist, AF102B. Soc. Neurosci. Abstr. **17:**388.

9. SEGAL, M. & A. FISHER. 1992. AF102B, an M1 muscarinic agonist, mimics some effects of acetylcholine on neurons of rat hippocampus slices. Eur. J. Pharmacol. 220:103–106.

10. FISHER, A., Y. SEGALL, H. MESHULAM, E. SHIRIN, D. GURWITZ, R. HARING, R. BRANDEIS, M. SEGAL, H. MARKRAM, Z. PITTEL, C. M. FRASER. E. HELDMAN & I. KARTON. 1991. AF150 and AF151: Novel efficacious M1 muscarinic agonists. Soc. Neurosci. Abstr. **17:**388.

11. HARRISON, P. J., A. J. L. BARTON, B. McDONALD & R. C. A. PEARSON. 1991. Alzheimer's disease: Specific increases in a G-protein subunit ($G_s\alpha$) mRNA in hippocampal and cortical neurons. Mol. Brain Res.**10:**71–81.

12. YOUNG, L. T., J. J. WARSH, P. P. LI, K. P. SIU, L. BECKER, J. GILBERT, O. HORNYKIEWICZ & S. J. KISH. 1991. Maturational and aging effects on guanine nucleotide binding protein immunoreactivity in human brain. *Dev. Brain Res.* **61:**243–248.

13. NITSCH, R. N., B. E. SLACK, R. J. WURTMAN & J. H. GROWDON. 1992. Release of Alzheimer amyloid precursor derivatives stimulated by activation of muscarinic acetylcholine receptors. Science **258:**304–307.

Natural and Synthetic Huperzine A: Effect on Cholinergic Function *in Vitro* and *in Vivo*[a]

ISRAEL HANIN,[b,e] XI-CAN TANG,[c] GISELA L. KINDEL,[b] AND
ALAN P. KOZIKOWSKI[d]

[b] *Department of Pharmacology and Experimental Therapeutics, Loyola University
Chicago, Stritch School of Medicine, Maywood, Illinois 60153 USA*
[c] *Shanghai Institute of Materia Medica, Academia Sinica, Shanghai, China*
[d] *Department of Chemical Research, Mayo Clinic, Jacksonville,
Jacksonville, Florida USA*

ABSTRACT: Huperzine A has been shown to be useful in the treatment of symptoms of dementia of the Alzheimer type. Our initial attempts to synthesize (−)Huperzine A resulted in the racemic mixture of (±)Huperzine A. We have therefore compared the *in vitro* and *in vivo* effects of (±)Huperzine A with those of (−)Huperzine A in rats. The results indicate a similar biological mechanism of action between the two, but that the racemic mixture of (±)Huperzine A has a weaker biological activity than the natural product (−)Huperzine A, presumably due to the presence in the mixture of (+)Huperzine A, which is considerably less potent than the (−)isomer.

The cholinergic hypothesis of Alzheimer's disease (AD) has provided the initiative for several clinical studies to test the efficacy of cholino-active agents (*e.g.*, cholinesterase inhibitors) in the alleviation of the symptoms of this disease state.[1–4] In 1968, reports in the Chinese literature indicated that the naturally occurring alkaloid, (−)Huperzine A, is an effective agent for the treatment of myasthenia gravis as well as for memory problems in patients with AD.[5–8] This was of particular interest to investigators in the field, since (−)Huperzine A was also shown to have a long duration of action (hours, rather than minutes as in the case of physostigmine[9]), and minimal side effects.[10] (−)Huperzine A, however, is scarce in nature; large quantities of the original clubmoss, *Huperzia serrata,* from which the alkaloid is extracted, are necessary in order to provide sufficient amounts of the pure material for clinical use.

[a] This work was partially supported by NIA Grant AG07591, and by the Retirement Research Foundation, Illinois.
[e] *Send correspondence to:* Dr. I. Hanin, Department of Pharmacology and Experimental Therapeutics, Loyola University Chicago, Stritch School of Medicine, Maywood, IL 60153 USA; TEL: (708) 216-3261; FAX: (708) 216-6596.

Our attempts to develop a synthetic approach which could enable the preparation of the product in quantity in the laboratory yielded the racemic $(\pm)$Huperzine A mixture,[11] rather than the $(-)$Huperzine isomer, which is the active component found in nature. In the absence of a chiral procedure for the synthesis of pure $(-)$Huperzine A, we sought to compare the *in vitro* and *in vivo* pharmacological profile of the $(\pm)$Huperzine A mixture with that of the natural $(-)$Huperzine A.

In vitro studies, seeking to determine the IC_{50} for inhibition of acetylcholinesterase obtained from rat hippocampal crude homogenates, indicated a threefold difference between the potency of $(\pm)$Huperzine A $(3 \times 10^{-7}M)$ and $(-)$Huperzine A $(10^{-7}M)$. Comparative studies in rats *in vivo*, demonstrated an inhibitory effect on acetylcholinesterase levels in hippocampus, striatum, hypothalamus and frontal cortex by both components, with $(-)$Huperzine A being slightly more potent than $(\pm)$Huperzine A. The same trend was noticed in the ability of both $(-)$Huperzine A and $(\pm)$Huperzine A to elevate acetylcholine levels in the cortex. Neither component affected brain choline acetyltransferase levels, and both exerted a duration of action exceeding 60 minutes in vivo. The reason for the comparatively reduced potency of $(\pm)$Huperzine A is inherent in the fact that the $(+)$Huperzine analog is considerably weaker as an inhibitor of acetylcholinesterase $(IC_{50}$ in vitro $= 7 \times 10^{-6}M)$; hence, its presence in the $(\pm)$Huperzine A racemic mixture dilutes the overall effect of this mixture.[12]

These studies indicate that synthetically obtained $(\pm)$Huperzine A compares in its biological effects with $(-)$Huperzine A, both *in vitro* and *in vivo*. If the ratio of enantiomers can be controlled, the mixture may conceivably serve as a viable substitute for the scarce natural product in future clinical studies.

REFERENCES

1. BECKER, R. E., P. MORIEARTY & L. UNNI. 1991. The second generation of cholinesterase inhibitors: Clinical and pharmacological effects. *In* Cholinergic Basis for Alzheimer Therapy. R. Becker & E. Giacobini, Eds. 263–296. Birkhauser. Boston.
2. GAUTHIER, S. & L. GAUTHIER. 1991. Status of THA as therapy for Alzheimer's disease. *In* Cholinergic Basis for Alzheimer Therapy. R. Becker & E. Giacobini, Eds. 224–230. Birkhauser. Boston.
3. THAL, L. 1991. Physostigmine in Alzheimer's disease. *In* Cholinergic Basis for Alzheimer Therapy. R. Becker & E. Giacobini, Eds. 209–215. Birkhauser. Boston.
4. WINBLAD, B., A. ADEM, L. BACKMAN, A. NORDBERG, F. ELINDER & P. ARHEM. 1991. Cholinesterase inhibitors in Alzheimer's disease: Evaluation of

clinical studies. *In* Cholinergic Basis for Alzheimer Therapy. R. Becker & E. Giacobini, Eds. 238–243. Birkhauser. Boston.

5. CHENG, Y. S., C. Z. LU, Z. L. YING, W. Y. NI, C. L. ZHANG & G. W. SANG. 1986. 128 cases of myasthenia gravis treated with Huperzine A. New Drugs Clin Rem **5:**197–199.

6. ZHANG, C. L. 1986. Therapeutic effects of Huperzine A on the aged with memory impairment. New Drugs Clin. Rem. **5:**260–262.

7. ZHANG, C. L. & G. Z. WANG. 1990. Effects of Huperzine A tablet on memory. New Drugs Clin. Rem. **9:**339–341.

8. ZHANG, R. W., X. C. TANG, Y. Y. HAN, G. W. SANG, Y. D. ZHANG, Y. X. MA, C. L. ZHANG & R. M. YANG. 1991. Drug evaluation of Huperzine A in the treatment of senile memory disorders. Acta Pharmacol. Sin. **12:**250–252.

9. TANG, X. C., P. DE SARNO, K. SUGAYA & E. GIACOBINI. 1989. Effect of Huperzine A, a new cholinesterase inhibitor, on the central cholinergic system of the rat. J. Neurosci. Res. **24:**276–285.

10. YAN, X. F., W. H. LU, W. J. LOU & X. C. TANG. 1987. Effects of Huperzine A and B on skeletal muscle and electroencephalogram. Acta Pharmacol. Sin. **8:**117–123.

11. KOZIKOWSKI, A. P., Y. XIA, E. R. REDDY, W. TUCKMANTEL, I. HANIN & X. C. TANG. 1991. Synthesis of Huperzine A and its analogues, and their anticholinesterase activity. J. Org. Chem. **56:**4636–4645.

12. TANG, X. C., G. H. KINDEL, A. P. KOZIKOWSKI & I. HANIN. Comparison of the effects of natural and synthetic Huperzine-A on rat brain cholinergic function in vitro and in vivo. Submitted.

PKC Translocation in Rat Brain Cortex Is Promoted *in Vivo* and *in Vitro* by α-Glycerylphosphorylcholine, a Cognition-enhancing Drug[a]

S. GOVONI[b], F. BATTAINI[c], L. LUCCHI[b], A. PASCALE[b], AND M. TRABUCCHI[c]

[b] *Institute of Pharmacological Sciences, University of Milan, Milan, Italy*
[c] *Department of Experimental Medicine and Biochemical Sciences, University of Roma–Tor Vergata, Rome, Italy*

ABSTRACT: Protein kinase C (PKC) activity was measured in soluble and particulate fractions of rat individual brain areas after treatment with α-glycerylphosphorylcholine (GPC), a cognition-enhancing drug which promotes acetylcholine synthesis and release. The drug induced both *in vivo* and *in vitro* PKC translocation. *In vivo*, an increase of particulate PKC activity was observed 1 hour following the acute oral administration of a behaviorally active dose (600 mg/kg); the effect was transient. *In vitro*, GPC promoted PKC translocation in cortical slices at concentrations as low as 50 nM; the concentration-response curve was bell shaped. The increased PKC activity may be related to the cortical effects of GPC.

INTRODUCTION

PKC is a family of diacylglycerol and phospholipid-dependent kinases that have been implicated in the control of neuronal plasticity. PKC is, in fact, involved in processes underlying memory trace formation in both invertebrates and vertebrates.[1] In rodent models spatial learning is facilitated by PKC activators and genetic differences in acquisition trials directly correlate with changes in brain PKC activity. PKC has also been involved in LTP and is modified in physiopathologic conditions known to be related to memory impairment.[2]

Cognition enhancers are a heterogeneous group of compounds belonging to diverse chemical classes facilitating memory and learning. These compounds may be grouped into three categories: cholinergic, nootropics, neuro-

[a] Supported in part by a grant by LPB Pharmaceutical Institute, Cinisello Balsamo, Milan, Italy.

[d] *Send correspondence to:* Dr. S. Govoni, Institute of Pharmacological Sciences, University of Milano, Via Balzaretti 9, 20133 Milano, Italy; TEL: 39-2-20488333; FAX: 39-2-29404961.

modulators.[3] In spite of a large body of behavioral studies, the molecular mechanisms by which cognition enhancers exert their action are not yet fully understood. Data have been reported on the possibility of interaction of nootropics with glutamatergic transmission, with cholinergic function and with synaptic facilitation as well.

The present study investigates the effect of the *in vivo* and *in vitro* administration of GPC, an acetylcholine synthesis precursor with documented effect on acetylcholine release and passive avoidance training facilitation,[4,5] on brain PKC activity.

METHODS

Male Wistar rats (Charles River, Calco, Italy) weighing 175–200 g were sacrificed by decapitation. Brain areas were quickly dissected, frozen on dry ice and kept at $-80°C$ until assayed. Areas from individual animals were prepared and PKC activity in soluble and particulate fractions assayed as detailed in.[6] For in vitro studies, pooled brain areas were cross-chopped (300 μm) with a McIlwain tissue chopper and re-suspended in oxygenated Krebs Ringer medium. Slices were exposed to the drug for 15 min, the slices sedimented, and fractions prepared as described above.

RESULTS

TABLE 1 shows that the *in vivo* administration of a behaviorally active dose of GPC induced the translocation of PKC, (detected as an increase in histone directed phosphorylating activity in the particulate fraction and a decrease in the soluble one) at 1 hour following the treatment. The effect was transient; 3 hours following the oral administration of the drug PKC activity in the particulate fraction returned to the control range and at a later time (5 hours) was decreased both in the soluble and in the particulate fraction. The treat-

TABLE 1. Effect of Acute GPC and Amphetamine Administration on PKC Activity in Rat Brain Cortex

Treatment	Time (h)	PKC Activity (nmoles/min/mg prot.) Particulate	Soluble
Saline		4.2 ± 0.3 (15)	$2.2 \pm 0.3*$ (15)
GPC (600 mg/kg, p.o.)	1	$6.3 \pm 0.8*$ (10)	$1.4 \pm 0.2*$ (10)
	3	4.6 ± 0.4 (7)	$1.5 \pm 0.1*$ (7)
	5	$2.7 \pm 0.6*$ (9)	$1.3 \pm 0.1*$ (9)
Amphetamine	1	3.9 ± 0.3 (5)	2.2 ± 0.4 (5)
(3 mg/kg, i.p.)	5	4.0 ± 0.4 (5)	2.1 ± 0.3 (5)

Values are means $\pm$ SD of (N) rats. $* p < 0.05$ vs. saline treated rats, Dunnett's *t*-test.

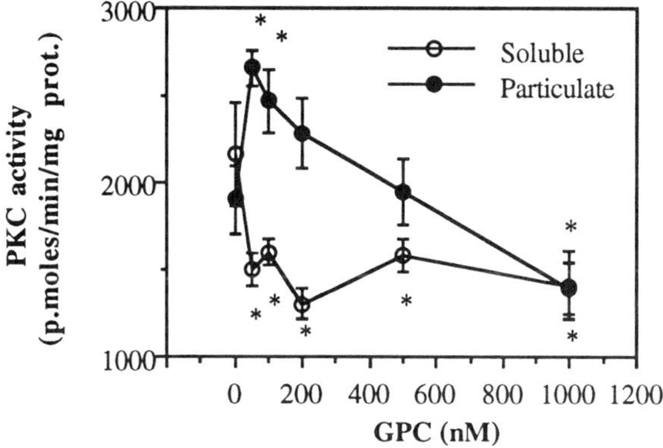

FIGURE 1. Effect of *in vitro* addition of GPC on PKC activity in rat brain cortex slices. Values are means ± SD of two experiments with triplicate samples (*$p<0.05$ vs. the activity in absence of added GPC, Dunnett's *t*-test).

ment with amphetamine, used in this case as a non-specific CNS stimulant, was unable to modify PKC activity either at 1 or at 5 hours. The effect of GPC at the dose and times investigated appeared to be limited to the cortex, no changes were in fact detected in hippocampus and striatum (data not shown).

The *in vitro* effect of GPC is shown in FIGURE 1. The drug at concentrations as low as 50 nM induced a 40% increase in the particulate PKC activity and a proportional decrease (31%) in the soluble fraction. The concentration-response curve was bell-shaped; the maximal effect was already obtained with the lowest dose assayed (50 nM). Increasing the dose to 100 and 200 nM produced less activation; with very high doses (1 micromolar) the activity of the enzyme was down-regulated both in the soluble and in the particulate fraction.

DISCUSSION

The results show that GPC induces *in vivo* and *in vitro* translocation of PKC activity in rat cerebral cortex followed by enzyme down-regulation. No effect is observed at the hippocampal level. The activation/down-regulation process of PKC seems to be a characteristic behavior of this enzymatic system following stimulation involving proteolysis of the enzyme. It is presently unknown whether the observed effect is exerted directly on the enzyme or takes place through an indirect mechanism linked to the cholinergic activation induced by the drug. A further point under investigation is the possibility of interaction of GPC with the various subset of receptors for excitatory amino acids. It is tempting to speculate that the area-specific interaction with PKC may be related to the facilitating action that GPC exert on electrocortico-graphic potentials.[7] The increase in PKC activity induced by GPC in rat brain cortex might be also related to the memory-facilitating activity of this compound; this notion is supported by the bell-shaped concentration-response curve, which is reminiscent of the one observed in passive avoidance experiments.[4,5] Within this context, it has been shown that passive avoidance training preferentially increases PKC-γ immunoreactivity in cortical structures while active avoidance training translocates PKC-γ in hippocampus.[8]

The observation that both normal and pathological aging are accompanied by changes in PKC activity and ability to translocate[2] underscores the importance of assessing the effect of pharmacological interventions aimed at modulate the activity of this transduction system.

REFERENCES

1. ALKON, D. L., et al. 1991. Learning and memory. Brain Res. Reviews. **16:** 193–220.
2. MAGNONI, S., S. GOVONI, F. BATTAINI & M. TRABUCCHI. 1992. Changes in neuronal function downstream from the receptor in the aging brain: Protein kinases and phosphoproteins. Rev. Neurosci. **3:**249–270.
3. HEISE, G. A. 1987. Facilitation of memory and cognition by drugs. TIPS **8:** 65–68.
4. LOPEZ, C. M., S. GOVONI, F. BATTAINI, S. BERGAMASCHI, A. LONGONI, C. GIARONI & M. TRABUCCHI. 1991. Effect of a new cognition enhancer, alpha-GPC, on scopolamine induced amnesia and brain acetylcholine. Pharmacol. Biochem. Behav. **39:**835–840.
5. GOVONI, S., C. M. LOPEZ, F. BATTAINI & M. TRABUCCHI. 1992. Chronic treatment with an acetylcholine synthesis precursor, α-GPC, alters brain parameters linked to cholinergic transmission and passive avoidance behavior. Drug Dev. Res. **26:**439–447.
6. GOVONI, S., L. LUCCHI, F. BATTAINI & M. TRABUCCHI. 1992. PKC increase in rat brain cortical membranes may be promoted by cognition enhancing drugs. Life Sci. **50:**125–128.
7. LACOMBA, C., R. CAGIANO, O. MACI, J. VALERIO & V. CUOMO. 1992. Effects of L-alpha-GPC on the EEG power spectrum in the rat. Drug Dev. Res. **26:** 101–107.
8. BELDHUIS, H. J. A., H. G. J. EVERZ, E. A. VAN DER ZEE, P. G. M. LUITEN & B. BOHUS. 1992. Amygdala kindling-induced seizures selectively impairs spatial memory: Behavioral characteristics and effects on hippocampal neuronal PKC isoforms. Hippocampus **2:**397–410.

Cholinergic Neurotransmission in the Hippocampus of Aged Rats: Influence of L-α-Glycerylphosphorylcholine Treatment

F. AMENTA,[a,d] F. FRANCH,[b] A. RICCI,[a] AND J. A. VEGA[c]

[a] Sezione di Anatomia Umana, Istituto di Farmacologia, Università di Camerino, 62032 Camerino, Italy

[b] Sandoz Prodotti Farmaceutici S.p.A, 20135 Milano, Italy

[c] Clinica Neurologica Università "Tor Vergata" and I.R.C.C.S. Clinica S. Lucia, Roma, Italy

ABSTRACT: The influence of aging and of L-α-glycerylphosphorylcholine (GFC) treatment on the acetylcholine synthesizing and degradating enzymes choline acetyltransferase (ChAT) and acetylcholinesterase (AChE) and on cholinergic muscarinic M-1 and M-2 receptors were assessed in the hippocampus using immunocytochemical, histochemical and radioligand binding techniques, respectively. The investigation was performed on male Wistar rats of 2 months (young), 12 months (adult), and 27 months (old). Oral GFC was given at the dose of 100 mg/Kg/day from the 21st to the 27th month of age. ChAT revealed the highest immunostaining in the hippocampus of adult rats followed by young and old animals. The highest expression of AChE reactivity was noticeable in the hippocampus of adult rats followed by old and young animals. Treatment with GFC restored in part ChAT immunoreactivity and AChE reactivity in the hippocampus of aged rats. Muscarinic M-1 and M-2 receptors were labeled with [3H]-pirenzepine and [3H]-AF-DX-116 respectively. The density of M-1 muscarinic receptors decreased with age, whereas M-2 muscarinic receptors did not change. GFC treatment countered in part the loss of M-1 receptors in old rats and was without effect on M-2 receptors.

Experimental and clinical evidence suggests that cholinergic neurotransmission is involved in learning and memory processes.[1] Moreover, an impairment in cholinergic neurotransmission markers has been found in physiological aging and in senile dementia of the Alzheimer's type.[2]

The hippocampus is a cerebral region which plays an important role in learning and memory process and is particularly sensitive to aging (see ref. 3). We have recently shown that long-term treatment with L-α-glycerylphos-

[d] Send correspondence to: Prof. F. Amenta, Via A. Borelli 50, 00161 Roma, Italy; TEL: 39-6-4958291; FAX: 39-6-4452349.

phorylcholine (choline alphoscerate, GFC) is able to counter the age-dependent microanatomical changes occurring in the hippocampus.[3] In the present study we have assessed whether GFC administration has any effect on cholinergic neurotransmission markers in the hippocampus of aged rats.

METHODS

Male Wistar rats of 2 months (young), 12 months (adult), and 27 months (old) were used. At 21 months of age rats were divided into two groups, one of which was left untreated (control group). Rats of the second group were treated for 6 months with a daily oral dose of 100 mg/Kg of GFC.

Fifty percent of the animals were perfused through the left ventricle with fixative constituted by 4% paraformaldehyde, 0.5% glutaraldehyde, 0.2% picric acid and 10% saccharose in 0.1M phosphate buffer. The brain was removed, washed and frozen. Serial sections obtained at a $-20°C$ microtome cryostat were processed for the immunohistochemical detection of ChAT (using monoclonal antibodies against the enzyme) and for the histochemical demonstration of AChE. The product of immunoreaction was quantified by calculating the area occupied in a $500\mu m^2$ surface of the CA-1 and CA-3 fields of the hippocampus by image analysis. The intensity of AChE staining within pyramidal neurons layer of CA-1 and CA-3 field was assessed microdensitometrically.

The remaining rats were sacrificed by decapitation. The hippocampus was removed, weighed and homogenized. Membranes of the hippocampus were used for M-1 and M-2 muscarinic receptor assay using [3H]-pirenzepine and [3H]-AF-DX-116, respectively, as ligands.

RESULTS AND DISCUSSION

Dark-brown ChAT-immunoreactive nerve fibers were observed in sections of the hippocampus. The highest immunoreactivity was noticeable in adult rats followed by young and old animals (TABLE 1). Microdensitometric analysis of AChE revealed the highest enzyme reactivity in adult rats followed by old and young animals (TABLE 1). Treatment with GFC restored in part the reduced expression of ChAT and AChE in the hippocampus of old rats (TABLE 1).

Muscarinic M-1 receptors were decreased with increasing age (TABLE 1). The age-related changes involved the density of binding sites (B_{max} value) (TABLE 1) but not the affinity of [3H]-pirenzepine for receptor sites (*e.g.*, the dissociation constant or K_d value) (data not shown). No age-dependent changes were noticeable in the K_d or B_{max} value of [3H]-AF-DX-116 binding

TABLE 1. Cholinergic Neurotransmission Markers in the Hippocampus of Rats of Different Ages

	ChAT (A)	AChE (B)	M-1 Receptors (C)
Young (n = 10)	4.2 ± 0.3	32.7 ± 1.4	1170 ± 61
Adult (n = 8)	5.2 ± 0.6^a	45.7 ± 1.9^a	1010 ± 31^c
Old (n = 9)	3.9 ± 0.7	38.4 ± 2.6	850 ± 26^d
Old + GFC (n = 10)	4.5 ± 0.4^b	42.3 ± 1.9^b	980 ± 39^b

Values are the mean $\pm$ SEM. (A) is expressed as the percentage of a $500\mu m^2$ area including the CA-1–CA-3 fields occupied by the product of immunoreactive reaction; (B) is expressed in arbitrary units and represents the intensity of staining within pyramidal neuron layers of the CA-1–CA-3 fields; (C) is expressed in μmol/mg protein. $a = p < 0.001$ vs. young or old; $b = p < 0.01$ vs. old; $c = p < 0.01$ vs. young; $d = p < 0.001$ vs. young or adult.

(data not shown). Treatment with GFC restored in part the density of M-1 receptor sites in aged rats (TABLE 1), but was without effect on M-2 sites (data not shown).

GFC is a precursor in the biosynthesis of several brain phospholipids which increases the bioavailability of choline and acetylcholine in the nervous system.[4] In our work we have seen that the compound is able to restore the impairment of two enzymatic activities with a key role in cholinergic neurotransmission occurring in aging. Moreover, it restored the expression of muscarinic M-1 receptors, the manipulation of which has been proposed for the treatment for senile dementia.[5] The functional and practical relevance of the above observation should be clarified in future studies.

REFERENCES

1. BARTUS, R. B., R. L. DEAN, B. BEER & A. S. LIPPA. 1982. The cholinergic hypothesis of geriatric memory dysfunction. Science **217**:408–417.
2. AMENTA, F., W. L. COLLIER & D. ZACCHEO. 1991. Neurotransmitters, neuroreceptors and aging. Mech. Ageing Dev. **6**:249–273.
3. BRONZETTI, E., W. L. COLLIER, L. FELICI, D. ZACCHEO & F. AMENTA. 1992. Long term choline alfoscerate treatment counteracts age-dependent structural changes in the rat hippocampus. Drug Dev. Res. **26**:449–459.
4. SIGALA, S., A. IMPERATO, P. RIZZONELLI, P. CASOLINI, C. MISSALE & P. F. SPANO. 1992. L-α-glycerylphosphorylcholine antagonizes scopolamine-induced amnesia and enhances hippocampal cholinergic transmission in the rat. Eur. J. Pharmacol. **211**:351–358.
5. McKINNEY, M. & J. T. COYLE. 1991. The potential for muscarinic receptor subtype-specific pharmacotherapy for Alzheimer disease. Mayo Clin. Proc. **66**:1225–1237.

Gangliosides and Neurotrophic Factors in Neurodegenerative Diseases: From Experimental Findings to Clinical Perspectives

M. FUSCO,[a] G. VANTINI, N. SCHIAVO, A. ZANOTTI, R. ZANONI, L. FACCI, AND S. D. SKAPER

Fidia Research Laboratories, 35031 Abano Terme (PD), Italy

ABSTRACT: A large body of experimental data suggests that neurotrophic molecules and/or substances that facilitate their action could be pharmaceutical agents for neurodegenerative pathologies. In particular, it has been demonstrated that nerve growth factor (NGF) exerts a physiological role for forebrain cholinergic neurons, while brain-derived neurotrophic factor (BDNF) seems to play a relevant role in rescuing dopaminergic neurons following damage. In addition, gangliosides are reported to potentiate neurotrophic factor effects *in vitro* as well as *in vivo*. In this study we examined the effects of the monosialoganglioside GM1 in different experimental models. The responsiveness of forebrain cholinergic neurons following NGF ± GM1 was evaluated by assessing choline acetyltransferase (ChAT) activity in hippocampus, septal area and striatum of behaviorally impaired 24-month-old rats. NGF was intracerebroventricularly (i.c.v.) infused for 2 weeks while GM1 was given systemically for 3 weeks, starting from the beginning of NGF infusion. Moreover, the possible protective effects of GM1 were assessed following exposure of cultured cerebellar granule cells and dopaminergic mesencephalic neurons to different doses of 6-OH-DOPA, a metabolite of the dopamine pathway which has excitotoxic properties and has been hypothesized to participate in the pathology of Parkinson's disease. GM1 treatment to aged rats was seen to potentiate the NGF-induced increase of ChAT activity in the striatum ipsilateral to the NGF infusion. Moreover, in the striatum contralateral to the NGF infusion, GM1 increased ChAT activity above the control values, whereas NGF treatment alone did not affect enzymatic activity. GM1 treatment of cerebellar granule cells and mesencephalic neurons counteracted the dose- and time-dependent neurotoxicity of 6-OH-DOPA. These data support the notion that GM1 might prove useful in treating those pathological conditions where trophic factor deficits and/or excitotoxin-related toxicity play an important role.

The selective and progressive loss of neurons which characterizes a number of neurodegenerative pathologies (*e.g.*, cholinergic neurons in Alzheimer's

[a] *Send correspondence to:* Dr. M. Fusco, Fidia Research Laboratories, Via Ponte della Fabbrica 3/A, 5031 Abano Terme (PD), Italy; TEL: 39 49 8232 111; FAX: 39 49 810 927.

disease and dopaminergic neurons in the substantia nigra in Parkinson's disease) has been proposed to reflect both a deficit of neurotrophic factors[1] and an underlying excitotoxic process.[2] A large number of studies suggest that NGF exerts a trophic, physiological role for forebrain cholinergic neurons. In particular, a long-lasting and dose-dependent increase of ChAT activity occurs in the cholinergic forebrain regions of both newborn and adult animals[3,4] following i.c.v. administration of NGF. As a corollary, administration of anti-NGF antibodies induces in these same cholinergic regions a significant reduction of ChAT activity.[5] Another member of the NGF family, BDNF, has been shown to rescue dopaminergic neurons following damage.[6–8] These data, in turn, propose that NGF and BDNF might have the potential to became pharmaceutical agents in Alzheimer's and Parkinson's diseases.[9]

Gangliosides, a class of sialoglycosphingolipids, have been reported to facilitate NGF effects *in vitro* as well as *in vivo*. GM1 can potentiate NGF activity in preventing vinblastine-induced sympathectomy in developing animals[10] and can facilitate NGF effects in promoting recovery of forebrain cholinergic neurons otherwise destined to degenerate following different lesions.[11,12] Furthermore, several studies have shown that, *in vitro*, GM1 reduces excitatory amino acid (EAA)-related death of cerebellar granule cells under different experimental conditions and EAA cytotoxicity to other neuronal cell types.[13,14] *In vivo*, systemically administered GM1 diminishes brain neuronal damage induced by exogenous excitotoxins.[15]

Since basal forebrain cholinergic neurons of aged rodents, as in Alzheimer's disease, undergo degenerative changes associated with memory impairments, we used behaviorally impaired 24-month-old rats to evaluate the responsiveness of this neuronal system to NGF $\pm$ GM1. ChAT activity was assessed in hippocampus, septal area and striatum of aged rats treated with NGF (continuous i.c.v. infusion via osmotic mini-pumps; 3.5 µg/day for 2 weeks) $\pm$ GM1 (30 mg/kg, i.p. daily for 21 days starting from the date of mini-pump implantation). Controls received the corresponding vehicle.

In a different series of experiments, the neurotoxic properties of 2,4,5-trihydroxyphenylalanine (6-OH-DOPA) were investigated in cultured cerebellar granule cells and dopaminergic mesencephalic neurons in the presence and absence of GM1 ganglioside. In previous studies, 6-OH-DOPA toxicity has been shown to rely on the formation, by oxidation in solution, of a new compound capable of interacting with glutamate receptors of the AMPA/kainate subtype.[16]

NGF administration to 24-month-old rats increased ChAT activity in the forebrain. This effect was significant in the septal area and, more markedly, in the striatum ipsilateral to the infusion side. Systemic administration of GM1 did not modify either the ChAT activity in any region analyzed or the NGF-induced increase of ChAT activity in the septum and hippocampus. However, chronic GM1 treatment potentiated the NGF-induced increase of

ChAT activity in the striatum ipsilateral to the NGF infusion side. Moreover, in the striatum contralateral to the NGF infusion side, GM1 increased ChAT activity above control values, whereas NGF treatment alone did not significantly affect enzymatic activity.

Application of 6-OH-DOPA to either cerebellar granule cells or mesencephalic neurons resulted in a concentration- and time-dependent loss of neurons. The neurotoxicity of 6-OH-DOPA was glutamatergic-like, being antagonized by AMPA/kainate receptor subtype antagonists. GM1 treatment of these neuronal cultures was effective in protecting against neurodegeneration induced by either acute or chronic 6-OH-DOPA exposure.

The data reported here indicate that the monosialoganglioside GM1 has the capability to potentiate the effect of trophic factors also in an experimental paradigm involving aged animals. In addition, the previously reported ability of this compound to reduce EAA-related neurotoxicity was confirmed using cell cultures exposed to 6-OH-DOPA, a compound which produces a kainate-like toxicity and which may be formed as a consequence of L-dopa dysmetabolism. The sum total of these observations supports the notion that GM1 might prove useful in treating those pathological conditions where trophic factor deficits and/or EAA-related toxicity play an important role.

REFERENCES

1. APPEL, S. H. 1981. A unifying hypothesis for the cause of amyotrophic lateral sclerosis, Parkinsonism and Alzheimer disease. Ann. Neurol. **10:**499–505.
2. MELDRUM, B. & J. GARTHWAITE. 1990. Excitatory amino acid neurotoxicity and neurodegenerative disease. Trends Pharmacol. Sci. **11:**379–387.
3. GNAHN, H., F. HEFTI, R. HEUMANN, M. E. SCHWAB & H. THOENEN. 1983. NGF-mediated increase of choline acetyltransferase (ChAT) in the neonatal rat forebrain: Evidence for a physiological role of NGF in the brain? Dev. Brain Res. **9:**45–52.
4. FUSCO, M., B. ODERFELD-NOWAK, G. VANTINI, N. SCHIAVO, M. GRADKOWSKA, M. ZAREMBA & A. LEON. 1989. Nerve growth factor affects uninjured adult rat septohippocampal cholinergic neurons. Neuroscience **33:**47–52.
5. VANTINI, G., N. SCHIAVO, A. DI MARTINO, P. POLATO, C. TRIBAN, L. CALLEGARO, G. TOFFANO & A. LEON. 1989. Evidence for a physiological role of nerve growth factor in the central nervous system of neonatal rats. Neuron **3:**267–273.
6. HYMAN, C., M. HOFER, Y.-A. BARDE, M. JUHASZ, G. D. YANCOPOULOS, S. P. SQUINTO & R. M. LINDSAY. 1991. BDNF is a neurotrophic factor for dopaminergic neurons of the substantia nigra. Nature **350:**230–232.
7. KNUSEL, B., J. W. WINSLOW, A. ROSENTHAL, L. E. BURTON, D. P. SEID, K. NIKOLICS & F. HEFTI. 1991. Promotion of central cholinergic and dopaminergic neuron differentiation by brain-derived neurotrophic factor but not neurotrophin-3. Proc. Natl. Acad. Sci. USA **88:**961–965.

8. SPINA, M. B., S. P. SQUINTO, J. MILLER, R. M. LINDSAY & C. HYMAN. 1992. Brain-derived neurotrophic factor protects dopamine neurons against 6-hydroxydopamine and N-methyl-4-phenylpyridinium ion toxicity: Involvement of the glutathione system. J. Neurochem. **59:**99–106.

9. VANTINI, G. & S. D. SKAPER. 1992. Neurotrophic factors: From physiology to pharmacology? Pharmacol. Res. **26:**1–15.

10. VANTINI, G., M. FUSCO, E. BIGON & A. LEON. 1988. GM1 ganglioside potentiates the effect of nerve growth factor in preventing vinblastine-induced sympathectomy in newborn rats. Brain Res. **448:**252–258.

11. CUELLO, A. C., L. GAROFALO, R. L. KENIGSBERG & D. MAYSINGER. 1989. Gangliosides potentiate in vivo and in vitro effects of nerve growth factor on central cholinergic neurons. Proc. Natl. Acad. Sci. USA **86:**2056–2060.

12. ODERFELD-NOWAK, B., M. SKUP, J. ULAS, M. JEZIERSKA, M. GRADKOWSKA & M. ZAREMBA. 1984. Effect of GM1 ganglioside treatment on postlesion responses of cholinergic enzymes in rat hippocampus after various partial deafferentations. J. Neurosci. Res. **12:**409–420.

13. FAVARON, M., H. MANEV, H. ALHO, M. BERTOLINO, B. FERRET, A. GUIDOTTI & E. COSTA. 1988. Gangliosides prevent glutamate and kainate neurotoxicity in primary cultures of neonatal rat cerebellum and cortex. Proc. Natl. Acad. Sci. USA **85:**7351–7355.

14. FACCI, L., A. LEON & S. D. SKAPER. 1990. Excitatory amino acid neurotoxicity in cultured retinal neurons: Involvement of N-methyl-D-aspartate (NMDA) and non-NMDA receptors and effect of ganglioside GM1. J. Neurosci. Res. **27:**202–210.

15. LOMBARDI, G., R. ZANONI & F. MORONI. 1989. Systemic treatments with GM1 ganglioside reduce quinolinic acid induced striatal lesions in the rat. Eur. J. Pharmacol. **174:**123–125.

16. ROSENBERG, P. A., R. LORING, Y. XIE, V. ZALESKAS & E. AIZENMAN. 1991. 2-4-5-Trihydroxyphenylalanine in solution forms a non-N-methyl-D-aspartate glutamatergic agonist and neurotoxin. Proc. Natl. Acad. Sci. USA **88:**4865–4869.

Oral Cytidine 5′-Diphosphate Choline Administration to Rats Increases Brain Phospholipid Levels

J. AGUT,[a] I. LOPEZ G.-COVIELLA,[b] J. A. ORTIZ,[a] AND R. J. WURTMAN[c,d]

[c] *Department of Brain & Cognitive Sciences, Massachusetts Institute of Technology, Cambridge, Massachusetts 02139 USA*

[a] *Centro de Investigacion Grupo Ferrer, Barcelona 08028, Spain*

[b] *Departmento de Fisiologia, Universidad de La Laguna, S/C de Tenerife, Spain*

ABSTRACT: Exogenous cytidine 5′diphosphocholine (CDP-choline) is completely metabolized to circulating cytidine and choline. Both compounds enter the brain and can be used in phosphatidylcholine (PC) synthesis via the Kennedy (CDP-choline) cycle. We administered oral CDP-choline to 12 month-old rats (500 mg/kg/day) for 21, 42, or 90 days to determine whether this treatment would alter brain levels of PC and the other structural phospholipids, phosphatidylserine (PS) and phosphatidylethanolamine (PE). After 42 days, brain PC levels increased significantly (p < 0.01) by 23.3%; after 90 days PC increased by 30% (p < 0.01), PS by 37.2% (p < 0.01), and PE by 13% (not significant). The ratios of each of the phospholipids to total membrane phospholipids were unchanged. These data demonstrate that repeated oral CDP-choline administration can increase the amounts of phospholipids in brain membranes, thus providing a rationale for using this compound in brain diseases that damage neurons.

INTRODUCTION

CDP-choline is a key intermediate in the most important pathway mediating the incorporation of free choline into PC, a major membrane phospholipid;[1] it is also used as a drug in several countries to treat brain diseases associated with neuronal damage (*e.g.*, trauma). Oral administration of CDP-choline to humans or rats increases blood levels of two metabolites needed for PC synthesis, cytidine and choline.[2] In previous studies, we found that oral administration of CDP-choline for 27 months to mice increased brain PC, PE, and PS levels.[3] In the present study, we examined the time-course of this effect in 12-month-old rats.

[d] *Send correspondence to:* Richard J. Wurtman, M.D., E25-604 M.I.T., Cambridge, MA 02139 USA; TEL: (617) 253-6731; FAX: (617) 253-6882.

MATERIAL AND METHODS

Six groups of male Sprague-Dawley rats were housed in specific pathogen-free conditions, and given free access to food (A04, U.A.R., France) and water. Starting at 12 months of age, one group received CDP-choline, 500 mg/kg/day orally (10 ml/kg in water solution by gavage), once a day for 21 days, and a control group received the same volume of vehicle. Two additional groups received the same dose of CDP-choline via the diet for 42 or 90 days, and the remaining two groups were used as paired controls for each treatment period. At the end of each treatment period (21, 42, and 90 days), the rats were sacrificed by decapitation, their heads dropped into liquid nitrogen and the fronto-parietal cortex dissected.

Brain phospholipids were extracted according to the method of Folch *et al.*,[4] and subsequently purified by thin-layer chromatography as we have previously described.[3] The total amounts of each of the phospholipids were determined by phosphate assay. Data were analyzed by two-way analysis of variance (ANOVA). Statistical significance was taken as $p<0.01$.

RESULTS AND DISCUSSION

Phospholipid levels in the frontoparietal cortex of CDP-choline treated animals were significantly higher than those in animals not receiving the drug (TABLE 1). In rats treated with CDP-choline for 90 days, PC levels increased by 30.0 ($p<0.01$) and PS levels by 37.2% ($p<0.01$); PE levels increased (by 13%) but not significantly ($p>0.01$). Administration of CDP-choline for 42 days increased brain PC significantly by 23.3% ($p<0.01$). No changes were observed with the 21-day treatment period. None of the treatments altered the ratios of any of the three phospholipids to total membrane phospholipid content.

TABLE 1. Effects of Oral Administration of CDP-Choline for 21, 42, or 90 Days on Brain Phospholipid Levels

nmol/mg Protein	21 Days of Treatment		42 Days of Treatment		90 Days of Treatment	
	Control (10)	CDP-Choline (12)	Control (11)	CDP-Choline (10)	Control (7)	CDP-Choline (9)
PC	221 ± 20	250 ± 21	161 ± 14	$210 \pm 5^*$	182 ± 8	$260 \pm 14^*$
PS	84 ± 4	95 ± 4	41 ± 3	36 ± 5	51 ± 4	$70 \pm 2^*$
PE	171 ± 11	187 ± 10	156 ± 6	168 ± 4	194 ± 25	223 ± 7

Groups of 12 month-old male Sprague-Dawley rats received 500 mg/kg/day of CDP-Choline (or placebo) by gavage for 21 days, and in the diet for 42 and 90 days. Numbers within parenthesis represent the number of animals in each group. Values are means $\pm$ SEM. $^* p < 0.01$.

These data show that repeated oral administration of CDP-choline to rats can increase the levels of phospholipids in cerebral cortex membranes. By providing choline, exogenous CDP-choline can enhance brain levels of phosphocholine,[5] which is a precursor in the synthesis of PC. CDP-choline is also metabolized to yield cytidine;[2] this can generate CTP, needed to convert the endogenous phosphocholine to CDP-choline, which then becomes PC after the addition of diacylglycerol.

We previously showed that chronic administration of CDP-choline to aged mice (between the 3rd and 30th months) increased brain PC, PE and PS contents.[3] We demonstrate that this effect can occur in rats after much shorter treatment periods and that overall membrane phospholipid composition is preserved.

REFERENCES

1. KENNEDY, E. P. & S. P. WEISS. 1956. The function of cytidine coenzymes in the biosynthesis of phospholipids. J. Biol. Chem. **222:**193–214.
2. LOPEZ G.-COVIELLA, I., J. AGUT & R. J. WURTMAN. 1987. Metabolism of cytidine (5′)-diphosphocholine (CDP-choline) following oral and intravenous administration to the human and the rat. Neurochem. Internat. **11:**293–297.
3. LOPEZ G.-COVIELLA, I., J. AGUT, J. A. ORTIZ & R. J. WURTMAN. 1992. Effects of orally administered cytidine 5′-diphosphate choline on brain phospholipid content. J. Nutr. Biochem. **3:**313–315.
4. FOLCH, J., M. LEES & G. H. SLOAN-STANLEY. 1957. A simple method for the isolation and purification of total lipids from animal tissues. J. Biol. Chem. **226:** 497–509.
5. MILLINGTON, W. R. & R. J. WURTMAN. 1982. Choline and physostigmine enhance haloperidol-induced HVA and DOPAC accumulation. Eur. J. Pharmacol. **80:**431–434.

Effect of CDP-Choline on Cognition and Immune Function in Alzheimer's Disease and Multi-Infarct Dementia[a]

R. CACABELOS,[b] X. A. ALVAREZ, A. FRANCO-MASIDE, L. FERNÁNDEZ-NOVOA, AND J. CAAMAÑO

Institute for CNS Disorders, Basic and Clinical Neurosciences Research Center, La Coruña, Spain

ABSTRACT: The cholinergic dysfunction present in Alzheimer's disease (AD) might be due to a specific vulnerability of cholinergic neurons linked to neurotrophic imbalance, neuroimmune impairment, and/or direct effects of β-amyloid deposition and NFT formation in ACh neurons. The presence of abnormal epitopes exposed on neuronal membranes may contribute to the activation of resting microglia initiating a neuroimmune cascade leading to cell destruction. According to this hypothesis, a multifactorial treatment in AD should produce: 1) inhibition of β-amyloid and NFT formation; 2) restoration of neuronal membrane integrity; and 3) control of neuroimmune auto-aggression. Since interleukin-1 (IL-1) is an APP gene promoter showing a progressive increase in body fluids in parallel with mental deterioration in AD patients, we have studied the effects of CDP-choline on cognition, several biological parameters, and IL-1β production in AD and multi-infarct dementia (MID) in order to elucidate whether this compound alone or in combination with other drugs is able to restore immune function and improve mental performance in senile dementia.

PATIENTS AND METHODS

CDP-choline (Somazina, Ferrer International, Spain) was given daily (1000 mg, p.o.) for 3 months to: a) control subjects (N = 8; age 66.37 ± 4.42 years), b) early-onset AD patients (EOAD; N = 11; age = 60.36 ± 5.75 years), c) late-onset AD patients (LOAD; N = 7; age = 75.28 ± 3.14 years), and d) MID patients (N = 10; age = 69.9 ± 7.24 years), following NINCDS-ADRDA and DSM-III-R criteria (GDS/FAST range: 3–5). Neuropsychological assessment was performed with MMSE, GDS, FAST,

[a] Research reported here was supported by the EUROSPES Foundation, FIS (91/0051), and the Ramón Areces Foundation.

[b] *Send correspondence to:* R. Cacabelos, Institute for CNS Disorders, Basic and Clinical Neurosciences Research Center, 15004 La Coruña, Spain; TEL: 34-81-226546; FAX: 34-81-228617.

BCRS, BEHAVE-AD, Hamilton-D, and Hachinski scales. Serum IL-1β was measured by RIA.

RESULTS

After 3 months of treatment, CDP-choline improved memtal performance in controls (MMS-1 = 33.87 ± 1.05; MMS-3 = 34.75 ± 0.43; FAST-1 = 1.75 ± 0.43; FAST-3 = 1.62 ± 0.48), EOAD (MMS-1 = 19.83 ± 5.65; MMS-3 = 23.83 ± 6.11; FAST-1 = 4.11 ± 0.56; FAST-3 = 4.00 ± 1.24), LOAD (MMS-1 = 18.9 ± 6.93; MMS-3 = 21.71 ± 8.14; FAST-1 = 4.57 ± 0.90; FAST-3 = 4.71 ± 1.03), and MID (MMS-1 = 23.05 ± 9.22; MMS-3 = 27.1 ± 9.3; FAST-1 = 4.1 ± 1.3; FAST-3 = 3.5 ± 1.28). Hamilton scoring was reduced in all groups from 4.42 ± 2.66 to 3.28 ± 2.11 in controls, from 14.0 ± 6.67 to 11.72 ± 4.74 in EOAD, from 10.57 ± 5.60 to 8.85 ± 4.91 in LOAD, and from 17.1 ± 8.71 to 12.0 ± 9.47 in MID. Blood pressure (SBP/DBP) tended to be reduced with treatment in controls (134.75 ± 18.68/75.67 ± 9.15 vs. 128.75 ± 18.21/74.75 ± 6.01), EOAD (132.90 ± 5.75/86.54 ± 12.22 vs. 130.18 ± 15.15/80.81 ± 8.93), LOAD (156.0 ± 10.02/85.42 ± 7.61 vs. 144.28 ± 8.74/83.0 ± 8.34), and MID (148.6 ± 12.88/94.4 ± 17.46 vs. 139.6 ± 13.34/84.7 ± 8.22) as well as heart rate.

Basal serum IL-1β levels were 171.17 ± 38.65, 213.63 ± 37.56, 184.35 ± 12.65, and 187.67 ± 48.01 pg/ml in controls, EOAD, LOAD, and MID, respectively. The significant increase ($p < 0.05$) in the concentration of serum IL-1β observed in EOAD patients was restored to normal values (177.32 ± 37.29, $p < 0.02$) after chronic treatment with CDP-choline.

DISCUSSION AND CONCLUSION

In our sample, more than 60% of patients with senile dementia showed a genetic pattern with more than two generations affected. Furthermore, about 90% of patients with LOAD had symptomatology of cerebrovascular impairment with an Hachinski score higher than 5. According to the present results, it seems that CDP-choline influences mental performance, cerebrovascular parameters and neuroimmune function, showing a mild antidepressant effect. Some reports indicate that high levels of IL-1 correlate in part with mental deterioration in AD. In this regard, IL-1β might be an indicator of brain damage in AD. Our results show a clear increase in the basal concentration of serum IL-1 in EOAD which is reverted to normal values after CDP-choline treatment. In conclusion, CDP-choline shows some benefit as a palliative-restorative treatment in senile dementia, improving mental performance in 60–80% of patients, reducing vascular risk factors, and stabilizing immune function in AD.

REFERENCES

1. WURTMAN, R. J., J. K. BLUSZTAJN, I. H. ULUS, *et al.* 1990. Choline metabolism in cholinergic neurons: Implications for the pathogenesis of neurodegenerative diseases. Adv. Neurol. **51:**117–125.

2. NITSCH, R. M., J. K. BLUSZTAJN, A. G. PITTAS, B. E. SLACK, J. H. GROWDON & R. J. WURTMAN. 1992. Evidence for a membrane defect in Alzheimer disease brain. Proc. Natl. Acad. Sci. USA **89:**1671–1675.

3. AGUT, J., I. L. G. COVIELLA, & R. J. WURTMAN. 1984. Cytidine 5′-diphosphocholine enhances the ability of haloperidol to increase dopamine metabolites in the striatum of the rat and to diminish stereotyped behavior induced by apomorphine. Neuropharmacology **23:**1403–1406.

4. AGNOLI, A., M. FIORAVANTI & H. LECHNER. 1985. Efficacy of CDP-choline in chronic cerebral vascular diseases (CCVD). *In* Novel Biochemical, Pharmacological and Clinical Aspects of Cytidinediphosphocholine. V. Zappia, E. P. Kennedy, B. I. Nilsson & P. Galletti, Eds. 305–315. Elsevier. New York.

5. LOZANO, R. 1989. Estudio de la evolución del deterioro piscoorgánico en el ancíano. Tratamiento con CDP colina. Rev. Esp. Geriat. Gerontol. **24**(Supl. 1):**65–72.

6. CACABELOS, R., M. BARQUERO, P. GARCÍA, X. A. ALVAREZ & E. VARELA DE SEIJAS. 1991. Cerebrospinal fluid interleukin 1 (IL-1β) in Alzheimer's disease and neurological disorders. Meth. Find. Exp. Clin. Pharmacol. **13:**455–458.

7. CACABELOS, R., A. FRANCO-MASIDE & A. ALVAREZ. 1991. Interleukin 1 in Alzheimer's disease and multi-infarct dementia: Neuropsychological correlations. Meth. Find. Exp. Clin. Pharmacol. **13:**703–708.

8. GRIFFIN, W. S. T., L. C. STANLEY, C. LING, *et al.* 1989. Brain interleukin 1 and S-100 immunoreactivity are elevated in Down's syndrome and Alzheimer's disease. Proc. Natl. Acad. Sci. USA **86:**7611–7615.

9. CACABELOS, R. 1991. Alzheimer's disease. JR Prous Publishers. Barcelona.

10. CACABELOS, R. 1991. Neuroimmune function in mental disorders. Ann Psiquiat. **2:** 135–154.

11. MCGEER, P. I., S. TAKAGI, H. AKIYAMA & E. G. MCGEER. 1988. Immune system response in Alzheimer's disease. *In* Current Communications in Molecular Biology. The molecular Biology of Alzheimer's Disease. C. E. Finch & P. Davis, Eds. 47–50. CSH. New York.

Acetyl-L-Carnitine and Alzheimer's Disease: Pharmacological Considerations beyond the Cholinergic Sphere[a]

A. CARTA,[b] M. CALVANI, D BRAVI, AND S. Ní BHUACHALLA

*Sigma-Tau Pharmaceuticals, Department of Scientific Affairs,
Gaithersburg, Maryland 20878 USA*

ABSTRACT: Since ALCAR and L-carnitine are "shuttles" of long chain fatty acids between the cytosol and the mitochondria to undergo β-oxidation, they play an essential role in energy production and in clearing toxic accumulations of fatty acids in the mitochondria. ALCAR has been considered of potential use in senile dementia of the Alzheimer type (SDAT) because of its ability to serve as a precursor for acetylcholine. However, pharmacological studies with ALCAR in animals have demonstrated its facility to maximize energy production and promote cellular membrane stability, particularly its ability to restore membranal changes that are age-related. Since recent investigations have implicated abnormal energy processing leading to cell death, and severity-dependent membrane disruption in the pathology of Alzheimer's disease, we speculate that the beneficial effects associated with ALCAR administration in Alzheimer patients are due not only to its cholinergic properties, but also to its ability to support physiological cellular functioning at the mitochondrial level. This hypothetical mechanism of action is discussed with respect to compelling supportive animal studies and recent observations of significant decrease of carnitine acetyltransferase (the catalyst of L-carnitine acylation to acetyl-L-carnitine) in autopsied Alzheimer brains.

Acetyl-L-carnitine (γ-trimethyl-β-acetylbutyrobetaine, ALCAR), the acetyl ester of L-carnitine, is currently under investigation for application in patients with Alzheimer's disease (AD). Although ALCAR's cholinergic effects are established[1,2] it is not known if this alone is responsible for its effects in AD. Recently published studies have pointed to altered energy metabolism as a salient destructive element in the neuropathological sequence leading to the clinical picture of AD.[4,5] There is a growing body of scientific evidence suggesting an effect of ALCAR at a sub-cellular level in the brain.

[a] Research reported here was supported by Sigma-Tau, U.S.
[b] *Send correspondence to:* Dr. Angelico Carta, Sigma-Tau Pharmaceuticals, Department of Scientific Affairs, 200 Orchard Ridge Drive, Gaithersburg, MD 20878 USA; TEL: (301) 948-1041; FAX: (301) 948-8627.

Animal pharmacological studies with ALCAR in the central nervous system have shown that it stimulates alternative utilization of lipid substrates and ketone bodies as it does in muscle tissue. ALCAR (75 and 500 mg/kg/i.p.) administered to aged albino Fisher rats caused a decrease in levels of lactic acid and sugar phosphates indicative of a reduction in brain glycolytic flow with a concomitant increase in phosphocreatine and adenosine triphosphate levels.[6] Additionally, ALCAR (150 mg/kg/day/i.p. for six months) reduces age-related increases of sphingomyelin thereby acting as a preventive measure against membrane fluidity changes.[7] ALCAR exerts a selective effect on certain enzymes crucial in the regulation of neuronal energy production.[7] In hippocampal mitochondria, ALCAR (100 mg/kg/i.p.) lowered citrate synthase and malate dehydrogenase activity.[8] The activity of the electron transport chain cytochrome oxidase activity was increased in striatum and hippocampus. These data agree with those from other studies indicating that ALCAR substantially increases the amount of a 16kDa mitochondrial inner protein (probably subunit IV of cytochrome oxidase) which decreases with age in the striatum.[9] Additionally, ALCAR erases the reduction of subunit I of cytochrome oxidase (Complex I)mRNA by acting on mitochondrial DNA transcription processes.[10]

Treatment with ALCAR restores levels of mitochondrial transcripts in aging rats; pre-treatment with ALCAR further boosts these levels.[11] Pre-treatment with ALCAR causes a 46% decrease in state 4 oxidation rate in senescent Fisher rats and doubles the respiratory control ratio in synaptic mitochondria of these rats compared with controls. This phenomenon is seen as an ALCAR-induced decrease in proton leakage. Age-related reductions in cholesterol and phospholipid content in synaptic mitochondria are also reversed by pre-treatment with ALCAR.[11]

Pathological damage at the membranal level in the Alzheimer's brain is well documented, and evidence of abnormal energy metabolism in AD brains is convincing.[4,5] Therefore, there is an attractive argument that the beneficial effects of ALCAR in AD patients[12,13] are a result of this drug's ability to stabilize membrane activity and provide a reservoir of energetic substrates that help maintain the cellular energy production process at a close-to-normal level, thereby preventing excessive loss of neurons. Perhaps the most compelling rationale for a comprehensive mechanism of action ALCAR in AD is provided by the post-mortem finding of significantly decreased carnitine acetyltransferase activity (25–40%) in discrete regions and isolated cerebral microvessels of 36 AD brains.[14] Although this is not the sole enzymatical defect observed in the AD brain, it is especially interesting since the oxidative metabolism of cerebral microvessels relies on fatty acids rather than glucose.

REFERENCES

1. IMPERATO, A., M. G. SCROCCO, O. GHIRARDI, M. T. RAMACCI & L. ANGELUCCI. 1991. In vivo probing of the brain cholinergic system in the aged

rat: Effects of long-term acetyl-L-carnitine. Ann. N.Y. Acad. Sci. **621:**90–97.

2. DOLEZAL, V. & S. TUCEK. 1981. Utilization of citrate, acetylcarnitine, acetate pyruvate and glucose for the synthesis of acetylcholine in rat brain slices. J. Neurochem. **36:**1323–1330.

3. FRITZ, I. B. 1963. Carnitine and its role in fatty acid metabolism. *In* Advances in Lipid Research. R. Paoletti & D. Kritchevsky, Eds. 285–292. Academic Press. New York.

4. PETTEGREW, J. W., K. PANCHALINGAM, W. E. KLUNK, R. J. MCCLURE & L. R. MUENZ. 1991. Alterations of membrane and energy metabolism in probable alzheimer's disease: A preliminary longitudinal in vivo ^{31}P NMR spectroscopy study. Am. Acad. Neurol. Abst., Boston, April, 1991.

5. WURTMAN, R. J., J. K. BLUSZTAJN, I. H. ULUS, I. LOPEZ G.-COVIELLA, R. L. BUYKUYSAL, J. H. GROWDON & B. E. SLACK. 1990. Choline metabolism in cholinergic neurons: Implications for the pathogenesis of neurodegenerative disease. *In* Alzheimer's Disease. Advances in Neurology. R. J. Wurtman, S. Corkin & J. H. Growdon, Eds. 117–126. Raven Press. New York.

6. AURELI T., A. MICCHELI, R. RICCIOLINI, M. E. DiCOCCO, M. T. RAMACCI, L. ANGELUCCI, O. GHIRARDI & F. CONTI. 1990. Aging brain: Effect of acetylcarnitine treatment on rat brain energy and phospholipid metabolism: A study by ^{31}P/^{1}H/NMR spectroscopy. Brain Res. **526:**108–112.

7. AURELI, T., G. CAPUANI, A. MICCHELI, O. GHIRARDI, M. T. RAMACCI & E. CONTI. 1991. Changes in brain membrane phospholipid composition during aging: Effect of acetylcarnitine. J. Neurochem. **57**(Suppl):S115.

8. VILLA, R. F. & A. GORINI. 1991. Action of acetyl-L-carnitine on different cerebral mitochondrial populations from hippocampus and striatum during aging. Neurochem. Res. **16**(10):1125–1132.

9. VILLA, R. F., L. TURPEENOJA, G. BENZI & A. M. GIUFFRIDA-STELLA. 1988. Action of L-acetylcarnitine on age-dependent modifications of mitochondrial membrane protein from rat cerebellum. Neurochem. Res. **13:**909–976.

10. GADALETA, M. N. 1990. Aging and mitochondrial DNA transcription process. It. Biochem. Soc. Trans. **1:**64.

11. GADALETA, M. N., V. PETRUZZELLA, M. RENIS, F. FRACASSO & P. CANATATORE. 1990. Reduced transcription of mitochondrial DNA in the senescent rat: Tissue dependence and effect of acetyl-L-carnitine. Eur. J. Biochem. **187:**501–506.

12. SANO, M., K. BELL, L. COTE, G. DOONEIEF, A. LAWTON, L. LEGLER, K. MARDER, A. NAINI, Y. STERN & R. MAYEUX. 1992. Double-blind parallel design pilot study of acetyl-L-carnitine in patients with Alzheimer's disease. Arch. Neurol. **49:**1137–1141.

13. SPAGNOLI, A. *et al.* 1991. Long-term acetyl-L-carnitine treatment in Alzheimer's disease. Neurology **41**(11):1726–1732.

14. KALARIA, R. N. & S. I. HARIK. 1992. Carnitine acetyltransferase activity in the human brain and its microvessels is decreased in Alzheimer's disease. Ann. Neurol. **32:**583–586.

Activation PET as an Instrument to Determine Therapeutic Efficacy in Alzheimer's Disease[a]

W. D. HEISS, J. KESSLER, I. SLANSKY, R. MIELKE, B. SZELIES, AND K. HERHOLZ

Max-Planck-Institut für Neurologische Forschung and Neurologische Universitätsklinik, Köln, Germany

ABSTRACT: Forty patients with probable Alzheimer's disease (AD) were selected from a pool of 80 patients and assigned to 4 groups. Each received either social support, cognitive training only, or cognitive training in combination with pyritinol or phosphatidylserine. Treatment duration was 6 months. Before and after treatment the patients underwent neuropsychological testing as well as measurement of the regional cerebral metabolic rate for glucose using positron emission tomography (PET) and 2[^{18}F]-fluoro-2-deoxy-D-glucose (FDG). Before treatment, the groups were comparable in respect to resting and activated glucose pattern achieved by a visual recognition task. They did not differ in scores of a neuropsychological test battery. After the treatment period the group with cognitive training + phosphatidylserine showed a significant glucose enhancement during the stimulation tasks in various brain regions, and an improvement in cognitive functioning compared to the other groups. The group with cognitive training + pyritinol had better stimulation effect as that of the social support group indicating that a combination of cognitive training + pharmacological intervention was superior than that of cognitive training alone.

INTRODUCTION

Various forms of therapeutic interventions have been used in the treatment of AD, the most common form of dementia. These treatments attempt to reverse or retard the course of the illness by improving the synaptic transmission, by enhancing glucose utilization of the neurons or by stabilizing membrane functioning.[1] The underlying histopathological changes cannot be influenced by therapeutic strategies available today. The clinical demonstration of such treatment effects in AD, however, is a tedious task necessitating large numbers of patients and long observation periods.[2,3] Cost-benefit calculations limit large-scale clinical trials to those drugs which have been shown to possess

[a] This work was supported by BMFT grant No. 070 1763 A/8.
[b] *Send correspondence to:* W. D. Heiss M.D., MPI für Neurologische Forschung, Gleueler Str. 50, 50937 Köln (Lindenthal), Germany; TEL: 49-221-4726-220; FAX: 49-221-4726-298.

some potential therapeutic efficacy. Based on the mode of action as demonstrated in animal experiments, the rationale of a drug's effect can be tested in selective clinical studies in which a quantifiable parameter related to the course and severity of the disease is used as the target variable. The impairment of memory and other cognitive disturbances is related to a decrease in glucose metabolism in brain regions predominantly affected by AD,[4,5] and this relationship became stronger during specific activation.[6] Therefore, increase of glucose utilization at rest and during activation might indicate improved synaptic function and cognitive performance.

METHODS

Eighty patients with probable AD according to current diagnostic criteria[7] were randomly assigned to four groups each receiving either social support, cognitive training only or in combination with pyritinol (2 × 600 mg/d) or phosphatidylserine (4 × 100 mg/d). All patients were mildly to moderately demented and scored between 14 and 25 on MMSE. Before and after a 6-month treatment period the patients underwent neuropsychological testing as well as measurement of regional cerebral metabolic rate for glucose (rCMRGl in μmol/100g/min) using PET and FDG at rest and during stimulation with a continuous visual recognition task. For statistical analysis of the changes in neuropsychological performance, regional metabolism at rest and during activation, 10 representative patients from each group were selected and matched with regards to age, sex, and severity of dementia.

RESULTS

Only the phosphatidylserine group showed a tendency for improvement in most of the neuropsychological tests, and no worsening was observed. The other groups showed no improvement, and in some cases a slight tendency of cognitive decline. The neuropsychological results are summarized in TABLE 1. In respect to resting global and regional CMRGl the four groups showed no differences in the first PET study before the treatment period began. The activation pattern achieved by the continuous visual recognition task, which consisted of graphic material, numbers, words, and letter of sequences adapted to the individual performance capacity, did not differ among the groups. During the observation period, resting metabolism decreased slightly in all groups except the one receiving cognitive training and phosphatidylserine where increases were found (most markedly in the temporo-parietal region, (FIG. 1a). During stimulation the group after cognitive training and phosphatidylserine was able to activate rCMRGl significantly (ANOVA,

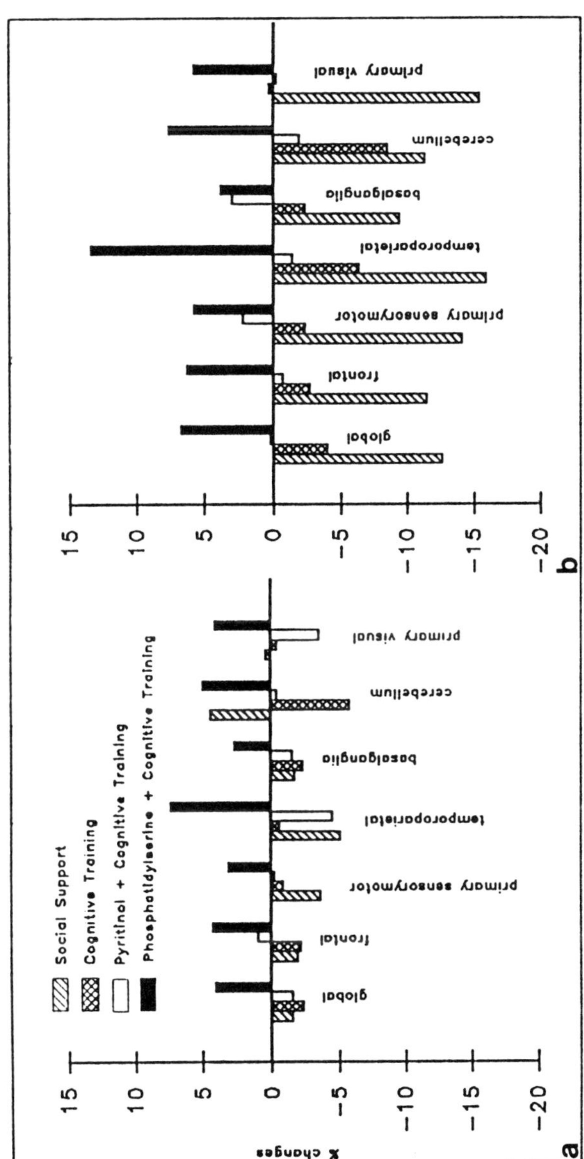

FIGURE 1. Δ Differences in glucose metabolism during the treatment period. **a:** Resting condition; **b:** Stimulation condition.

TABLE 1. Neuropsychological Test Battery

	Social Support		Cognitive Training		Cognitive Training + Pyritinol		Cognitive Training + Phosphatidylserine	
	a	b	a	b	a	b	a	b
MMST (30)[a]	19.6 ± 3.8	19.01 ± 6.0	22.1 ± 3.59	20.7 ± 6.49	22.8 ± 3.20	22.4 ± 5.93	21.7 ± 4.10	23.5 ± 5.81[c]
Verbal selective reminding task (max. 8)	3.74 ± 1.14	3.66 ± 1.82	3.88 ± 1.32	3.69 ± 2.22	4.41 ± 1.73	3.98 ± 1.88	4.31 ± 1.04	4.93 ± 0.86
Orientation (8)	5.50 ± 1.95	5.44 ± 2.50	5.1 ± 2.13	5.87 ± 1.80	5.90 ± 1.19	6.55 ± 1.01	5.50 ± 1.77	6.70 ± 1.33[c]
Praxia (max. 10)	6.10 ± 2.37	7 ± 2.90	8.3 ± 1.82	8.62 ± 1.84	8 ± 2.44	7 ± 2.66	7.8 ± 2.39	8.50 ± 2.01
Fragmented picture test[b] (50)	5.11 ± 4.88	3.11 ± 5.75	5.10 ± 3.10	3.25 ± 9.60	6.50 ± 5.80	5.22 ± 4.08	4.0 ± 2.53	4.1 ± 3.63
Reaction time	0.82 ± 0.19	0.85 ± 0.22	0.77 ± 0.24	0.80 ± 0.27	0.68 ± 0.13	0.77 ± 0.24	0.77 ± 0.17	0.69 ± 0.22
Block span test (7)	3.50 ± 1.54	3.65 ± 1.70	4.65 ± 0.91	4.37 ± 1.27	4.06 ± 1.87	4.10 ± 1.94	4.14 ± 1.51	4.80 ± 1.54[c]
"Supermarket"	10.30 ± 4.44	9.44 ± 5.72	11.20 ± 4.13	13.87 ± 5.51	14.7 ± 8.87	13.8 ± 8.03	13.40 ± 5.23	13.7 ± 5.10

a = before treatment; b = after treatment.

[a] Numbers in parentheses are maximum scores.

[b] Score of improvement from the first to the second presentation.

[c] 5–10% level of significance.

post hoc Wilcoxon tests) better than the other groups (comparison to social support $p < 0.01$ left temporo-parietal and $p < 0.05$ right sensomotoric region), but also the cognitive training plus pyritinol group did better than the social support group ($p < 0.02$ left temporo-parietal, $p < 0.05$ sensomotoric and right temporo-parietal regions). In the cognitive training plus phosphatidylserine group the extent of activation-induced CMRGl (% change from stimulated CMRG11 to stimulated CMRG12, FIG. 1b) increased significantly when compared to the other groups, with the largest differences to the social support group in global ($p < 0.02$), temporo-parietal ($p < 0.0008$), frontal ($p < 0.04$), sensomotoric and cerebellar CMRGl ($p < 0.03$), and to the cognitive training group in the temporo-parietal region ($p < 0.008$).

CONCLUSION

This longitudinal study demonstrates that synaptic and neuronal function might be improved, and progress of the AD might be mitigated by specific medical treatment in combination with cognitive training. The data suggest that the effect of symptomatic treatment can be best demonstrated by a test reflecting synaptic and neuronal activity, such as task-related metabolic activation, while the resting metabolism, which reflects mainly the basic demand of the tissue and corresponds to the number of preserved neurons, is only affected to a lesser extent.

REFERENCES

1. WURTMAN, R. J., S. CORKIN, J. H. GROWDON, E. RITTER-WALKER, Eds. 1990. Advances in Neurology, Vol. 51. Alzheimer's disease. Raven Press. New York.
2. WHALLEY, L. J. 1989. Drug treatments of dementia. Br. J. Psychiatry **155:** 595–611.
3. MAYEUX, R. 1990. Therapeutic strategies in Alzheimer's disease. Neurology **40:** 175–180.
4. HERHOLZ, K., R. ADAMS, J. KESSLER, B. SZELIES, M. GROND & W. D. HEISS. 1990. Criteria for the diagnosis of Alzheimer's disease with positron emission tomography. Dementia **1:**156–164.
5. RAPOPORT, S. I. 1991. Positron emission tomography in Alzheimer's disease in relation to disease pathogenesis—a critical review. Cerebrovasc. Brain Metab. Rev. **3:**297–335.
6. KESSLER J., K. HERHOLZ, M. GROND & W. D. HEISS. 1991. Impaired metabolic activation in Alzheimer's disease—a PET study during continuous visual recognition. Neuropsychologia **29**(3):229–243.
7. MCKHANN, G., D. DRACHMAN, M. F. FOLSTEIN, R. KATZMAN, D. PRICE & E. M. STADLAN. 1984. Clinical diagnosis of Alzheimer's disease. Neurology. **34:** 939–944.

The Use of the Computerized Neuropsychological Test Battery (CNTB) in an Efficacy and Safety Trial of BMY 21,502 in Alzheimer's Disease

NEAL R. CUTLER,[a,c] RAJESH C. SHROTRIYA,[b]
JOHN J. SRAMEK,[a] AMY E. VEROFF,[a] RANDALL D. SEIFERT,[a]
LINDA A. REICH,[b] AND DENISE YEE HIRONAKA[a]

[a] *California Clinical Trials, Beverly Hills, California 90211 USA*
[b] *CNS Clinical Research, Bristol-Myers Squibb Co., Wallingford, Connecticut 06492 USA*

ABSTRACT: BMY 21,502 is a nootropic which protects memory and enhances long-term potentiation according to preclinical findings. Alzheimer's disease (AD) patients who were diagnosed by DSM-III-R and NINCDS-ADRDA criteria were enrolled in a 12-week double-blind investigation of BMY 21,502 vs. placebo at 300 mg tid. The study design included a 1-week placebo lead-in and a 4-week placebo washout in addition to the 12-week double-blind treatment period. Efficacy was assessed with the Alzheimer's Disease Assessment Scale (ADAS) and the Computerized Neuropsychological Test Battery (CNTB) at weeks 4, 8, 12, and 16. Clinical Global Impression (CGI) assessments were also performed biweekly. Sixty-nine patients (28M, 41F; mean age 72 years, range 54 to 92 years) were enrolled in the study. Baseline Mini-Mental Status Examination (MMSE) scores ranged from 16 to 26 (mean 23.5) in patients on active drug (n = 34), and from 15 to 26 (mean 22.5) in placebo patients (n = 35). Baseline efficacy scores were comparable for drug and placebo patients ($p > 0.05$). Twelve (35%) patients who received BMY 21,502 withdrew from the study, 8 (24%) due to adverse events. Three (9%) patients who received placebo withdrew from the study, all due to adverse events. Patients on active drug who were valid for analysis of efficacy (n = 22) showed a mean decrease in ADAS of -1.5 at week 12, vs. a mean change of -0.5 in patients who received placebo (n = 32), although there was no significant difference between the two ($p > 0.05$). Correlations between the CNTB summary scores and ADAS cognitive subscores were, nevertheless, highly significant at baseline ($r = -0.83$, $p = 0.0001$) and week 12 ($r = -0.83$, $p = 0.0001$). Correlations between the word list learning, spatial, and naming subtests of the ADAS and CNTB were also highly significant ($p = 0.0001$). Although modest, the findings for active drug vs. placebo response in

[c] *Send correspondence to:* Neal R. Cutler, M.D., 8500 Wilshire Blvd. 7th Floor, Beverly Hills, CA 90211 USA; TEL: 310-854-4949; FAX: 310-854-5419 or -3965.

this study suggest that BMY 21,502 should be further investigated, with a larger study population, in order to fully determine the compound's potential efficacy.

Numerous studies have suggested a cholinergic genesis for the pathology of Alzheimer's disease (AD).[1–5] As part of the cholinergic hypothesis, the role of nootropics in AD has been investigated, with primarily preclinical evidence to date.[6–9] In order to explore the use of a metabolic enhancer in AD, BMY 21,502 is under development, with the hope that its ability to protect memory and its ability to enhance long-term potentiation which were found in preclinical studies will reduce cognitive deficits in AD patients.

In vivo preclinical studies found that BMY 21,502 improved visual discrimination acquisition in monkeys in doses ranging from 0.08 to 140 mg/day. Pretreatment with the compound also reduced scopolamine-induced amnesia in rats in a light-dark step-through apparatus, the most remarkable effect seen with 0.64 and 1.25 mg/kg. In a preclinical investigation in rats with lesions of the nucleus basalis, rats who were treated with BMY 21,502 made fewer errors in the food foraging task than those treated with vehicle, although there was no significant difference in time to completion between drug- and placebo-treated rats. There were additional positive findings using a T-maze relearning task and a water-escape task in rodents. However, BMY 21,502 demonstrated minimal effect in the electroshock model and the radial-arm task.

Preliminary pharmacokinetic studies in young and elderly volunteers revealed that peak plasma concentrations occurred at approximately 1 hour post-dose with oral administration, and that the half-life of the compound is approximately 1.5 hours. A single, escalating-dose study in young healthy males tested tolerability of BMY 21,502 in seven panels of six subjects. Four of each panel received active drug (25, 50, 100, 150, 200, 250, and 300 mg) and two received placebo. All seven doses appeared to be well tolerated, with only mild to moderate, transitory side effects noted. This study was replicated in the healthy elderly population, subjects ranging in age from 65 to 81 years. There were no observations of clinically significant laboratory values, vital signs, ECGs or EEGs and adverse events were predominantly mild to moderate, all transient. Two adverse events, one case of nausea and one of fatigue, were rated as severe. In a subsequent rising, multiple-dose study in healthy elderly subjects, 300 mg tid was found to be well tolerated. Adverse events did not appear to have any relationship to dose.

Based upon these early clinical findings, the present double-blind, multiple-dose, placebo-controlled study of 300 mg tid of BMY 21,502 in AD patients was designed. A one-week placebo washout preceded 12 weeks of double-blind treatment and a 4-week post-treatment placebo washout. Patients were screened to exclude any medical, neurologic, or psychiatric disorder or other abnormality which could interfere with efficacy or safety assessments. Efficacy assessments included the Clinical Global Impression (CGI) (assessed bi-weekly), and the Alzheimer's Disease Assessment Scale (ADAS) and Computerized Neuropsychological Test Battery, which were performed at weeks 4, 8, 12, and 16. The Mini-Mental Status Examination (MMSE), the Geriatric Evaluation by the Relatives' Rating Instrument (GERRI), and a Word Fluency Test were also performed at weeks 4, 8, 12, and 16. Safety assessments included continuous monitoring of vital signs, clinical laboratory evaluations at baseline and weeks 6 and 12, and ECG at week 12, liver function tests at weeks 2, 4, 8, 10, and two weeks post-treatment. A physical examination was performed at screening as well as the end of the study.

Sixty-nine patients (mean age 72 years, range 54 to 92 years; 28M, 41F) who met NINCDS-ADRDA and DSM-III-R criteria for AD, had a Reisberg Global Deterioration Scale score of 3 or 4, and who had an MMSE between 18 and 26 inclusive were enrolled in the study. Thirty-four patients were randomized to active drug, and thirty-five were randomized to placebo. Patients randomized to active drug had a mean baseline MMSE score of 23.5, and the placebo patients had a mean MMSE of 22.5 ($p > 0.05$). Baseline efficacy scores (ADAS, CGI, and CNTB) were also comparable for drug and placebo patients ($p > 0.05$).

Overall, the drug effect observed in this study was minimal. There were no significant differences between drug and placebo patients with respect to change in ADAS from baseline values at any of the four assessment times ($p > 0.05$). Fifty-four patients completed 12 weeks of study; 22 in the BMY 21,502 and 32 in the placebo group. Patients who received drug showed their greatest reduction in ADAS (-1.5) at week 12 compared to placebo (-0.5); whereas placebo patients had their greatest reduction (-0.7) at week 8. There were no significant week 12 differences between CGI improvement scores for the patients who received BMY 21,502 and patients who received placebo (BMY 21,502, 3.64; placebo 3.69) ($p > 0.05$). Of the 34 patients randomized to receive BMY 21,502, 8 were withdrawn due to adverse events, 1 withdrew due to lack of efficacy, 2 withdrew consent, and 1 was lost to follow-up. Of the placebo patients, three were withdrawn due to adverse events. The total percentages of discontinuations were 35% for patients on drug and 9% for patients on placebo.

Although the drug-related findings in this study were disappointing, the correlations we found between the ADAS and CNTB batteries were very promising, and contribute to the validation of the CNTB as an alternative standardization of neuropsychological assessment. The CNTB was developed as a comprehensive compilation of several standard cognitive function tests, such that it would determine language, word list learning, and spatial capabilities. The CNTB offers a wider range of sensitivity and practical utility than most noncomputerized batteries. Of particular importance is the CNTB's capacity as an "expert system" which standardizes the timing of the battery administration and tabulates the data (10).

Pearson correlations which were performed to analyze the relationship between patient performance on the ADAS and the CNTB revealed highly significant coefficients. The correlation between the ADAS cognitive sub-scores and the CNTB total scores was -0.83, both at baseline and at week 12. Correlations between the ADAS total score and CNTB summary score at baseline and week 12 were -0.83 and -0.79, respectively. The word list learning subtests (ADAS Word Recall vs. CNTB Word List Learning/Selective Reminding) had correlations of -0.70 and -0.64 at baseline and week 12. Correlations between Constructional Praxis and Visual Matching were -0.64 and -0.54, respectively, and correlations between the ADAS Naming subtest and the Boston Naming Test (short-form) were -0.68 and -0.71, respectively. This analysis found p-values of 0.0001 for all correlations.

These correlations comprise an additional installment in the validation process for this battery. The CNTB has been shown to have excellent test-retest reliability, as was demonstrated in a controlled study of ceranapril, an ACE inhibitor for the treatment of Alzheimer's disease. With these indications of inter-administration reliability, in addition to correlations observed between the CNTB and the ADAS, we can be confident that the CNTB is a viable alternative in neuropsychological testing for progress in AD.

Although efficacy findings were not significant for this population, it is possible that a trial in a larger population would prove more informative with respect to the mechanism of action and potential effects of BMY 21,502. The Pearson correlations between the ADAS and CNTB in this trial indicate that the CNTB may be useful in such a study in order to standardize cognitive assessment in a large, multicenter design.

REFERENCES

1. WHITEHOUSE, P. J., D. L. PRICE, R. G. STRUBLE, *et al.* 1986. Alzheimer's disease and senile dementia: Loss of neurons in the basal forebrain. Science **215:**1237.
2. WALLER, S. B., M. J. BALL, M. A. REYNOLDS & E. D. LONDON. 1986. Muscarinic and choline acetyltransferase in postmortem brains of demented patients. Can. J. Neurol. Sci. **13:**523–528.
3. SUNDERLAND, T., P. N. TARIOT, R. M. COHEN, *et al.* 1987. Anticholinergic sensitivity in patients with dementia of the Alzheimer type and age-matched controls. Arch. Gen. Psychiatry **44:**418–426.
4. DAVIS, B. M., R. C. MOHS, B. S. GREENWALD, *et al.* 1985. Clinical studies of the cholinergic deficit in Alzheimer's disease. I. Neurochemical and neuroendocrine studies. J. Am. Geriatr. Soc. **33:**741–748.

5. COYLE, J. T., D. L. PRICE & M. R. DELONG. 1983. Alzheimer's disease: A disorder of cortical cholinergic innervation. Science **219:**1184–1190.
6. GOTTFRIES, C. G. 1990. Pharmacological treatment strategies in Alzheimer type dementia. Eur. Neuropsychopharmacol. **1:**1–5.
7. PARNETTI, L., P. MECOCCI, A. PETRINI, *et al.* 1989. Neuropsychological results of long-term therapy with oxiracetam in patients with dementia of Alzheimer type and multi-infarct dementia in comparison with a control group. Neuropsychobiology **22:**97–100.
8. GAINOTTI, G., U. NOCENTI & E. SENA. 1989 Can the pattern of neuropsychological improvement obtained with cholinergic drugs be used to infer a cholinergic mechanism in other nootropic drugs? Prog. Neuropsychopharmacol. Biol. Psychiatry **13:**S47–59.
9. NICHOLSON, C. D. 1989. Nootropics and metabolically active compounds in Alzheimer's disease. Biochem. Soc. Trans. **17:**83–85.
10. VEROFF, A. E., N. R. CUTLER, J. J. SRAMEK, *et al.* 1991. A new assessment tool for neuropsychologic research: The computerized Neuropsychological test battery. J Ger. Psychiatr. Neurol. **4:**211–217.

Index of Contributors